CHEMOTHERAPY

Volume 5
Penicillins and Cephalosporins

CHEMOTHERAPY

Volume 1 **Clinical Aspects of Infections**
Prophylaxis; life-threatening infections; infection in leukaemia; surgical infection; anaerobic infection; respiratory and urinary tract infections; amikacin.

Volume 2 **Laboratory Aspects of Infections**
Sensitivity testing; assay methods; animal models of infection; sisomycin; tobramycin.

Volume 3 **Special Problems in Chemotherapy**
Tuberculosis; genital tract infections; antibiotic resistance and mode of action; topical chemotherapy and antisepsis.

Volume 4 **Pharmacology of Antibiotics**
Tissue concentrations; pharmacokinetics; untoward effects of antibiotics.

Volume 5 **Penicillins and Cephalosporins**
Penicillins and cephalosporins; betalactamases; new agents.

Volume 6 **Parasites, Fungi, and Viruses**
Parasitic infections; fungal infections; chemotherapy of viruses; co-trimoxazole.

Volume 7 **Cancer Chemotherapy I**
Symposia — new drugs and approaches; cell and pharmacokinetics; potentiators of radiotherapy; in vitro screening systems; immunological aspects.

Volume 8 **Cancer Chemotherapy II**
Free papers — new drugs and approaches; cell and pharmacokinetics; mechanisms of action; new analogues; cancer chemotherapy of specific organs.

CHEMOTHERAPY

Volume 5
Penicillins and Cephalosporins

Edited by
J.D. Williams
The London Hospital Medical College
London, U.K.

and
A.M. Geddes
East Birmingham Hospital
Birmingham, U.K.

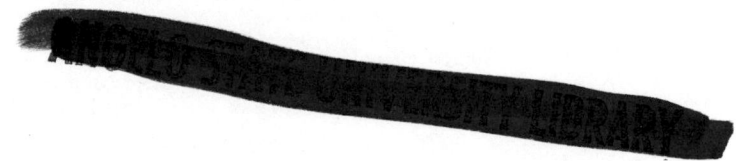

Plenum Press · New York and London

Library of Congress Cataloging in Publication Data

International Congress of Chemotherapy, 9th, London, 1975.
 Penicillins and cephalosporins.

 (Chemotherapy; v. 5)
 1. Penicillin—Congresses. 2. Cephalosporin—Congresses. I. Williams, John David, M.D. II. Geddes, Alexander McIntosh. III. Title. IV. Series.
 RM260.2.C45 vol. 5 [RM666.P35] 615'.58s [615'.329'23] 76-1943
 ISBN 0-306-38225-3

Proceedings of the Ninth International Congress of Chemotherapy
held in London, July, 1975 will be published in eight volumes,
of which this is volume five.

©1976 Plenum Press, New York
A Division of Plenum Publishing Corporation
227 West 17th Street, New York, N.Y. 10011

United Kingdom edition published by Plenum Press, London
A Division of Plenum Publishing Company, Ltd.
Davis House (4th Floor), 8 Scrubs Lane, Harlesden, London, MW10 6SE, England

All rights reserved

No part of this book may be reproduced, stored in a retrieval system, or transmitted,
in any form or by any means, electronic, mechanical, photocopying, microfilming,
recording, or otherwise, without written permission from the Publisher

Printed in the United States of America

CHEMOTHERAPY

Proceedings of the
9th International Congress of Chemotherapy
held in London, July, 1975

Editorial Committee

K. Hellmann, *Chairman* (Anticancer)
Imperial Cancer Research Fund, London.

A. M. Geddes (Antimicrobial)　　J. D. Williams (Antimicrobial)
East Birmingham Hospital.　　*The London Hospital Medical College.*

Congress Organising Committee

W. Brumfitt	I. Phillips	H.P. Lambert
K. Hellmann	M.R.W. Brown	P. Turner
K.D. Bagshawe	D.G. James	A.M. Geddes
H. Smith	C. Stuart-Harris	D. Armitage
E.J. Stokes	R.G. Jacomb	D. Crowther
F. Wrigley	D.T.D. Hughes	D.S. Reeves
J.D. Williams	T. Connors	R.E.O. Williams

International Society
of Chemotherapy Executive - to July 1975

P. Malek	H.P. Kuemmerle	H. Ericsson
C. Grassi	Z. Modr	G.M. Savage
G.H. Werner	K.H. Spitzy	H. Umezawa
	P. Rentchnick	

Preface

The International Society of Chemotherapy meets every two years to review progress in chemotherapy of infections and of malignant disease. Each meeting gets larger to encompass the extension of chemotherapy into new areas. In some instances, expansion has been rapid, for example in cephalosporins, penicillins and combination chemotherapy of cancer - in others slow, as in the field of parasitology. New problems of resistance and untoward effects arise; reduction of host toxicity without loss of antitumour activity by new substances occupies wide attention. The improved results with cancer chemotherapy, especially in leukaemias, are leading to a greater prevalence of severe infection in patients so treated, pharmacokinetics of drugs in normal and diseased subjects is receiving increasing attention along with related problems of bioavailability and interactions between drugs. Meanwhile the attack on some of the major bacterial infections, such as gonorrhoea and tuberculosis, which were among the first infections to feel the impact of chemotherapy, still continue to be major world problems and are now under attack with new agents and new methods.

From this wide field and the 1,000 papers read at the Congress we have produced Proceedings which reflect the variety and vigour of research in this important field of medicine. It was not possible to include all of the papers presented at the Congress but we have attempted to include most aspects of current progress in chemotherapy.

We thank the authors of these communications for their cooperation in enabling the Proceedings to be available at the earliest possible date. The method of preparation does not allow for uniformity of typefaces and presentation of the material and we hope that the blemishes of language and typographical errors do not detract from the understanding of the reader and the importance of the Proceedings.

        K. HELLMANN, Imperial Cancer Research Fund
        A. M. GEDDES, East Birmingham Hospital
        J. D. WILLIAMS, The London Hospital Medical College

Contents

The Beta Lactam Antibiotics - Penicillins and
    Cephalosporins 1
  G. T. Stewart

Clinical Relevance of Ampicillin/Cloxacillin for IV Use . . . 7
  C. Regamey, L. Barrelet, and F. A. Waldvogel

Experiences with Amoxicillin in Full-Term and Pre-Term
    Neonates 13
  L. Weingärtner, U. Sitka, and R. Patsch

Comparative Activity of Amoxycillin, Ampicillin, and
    Benzylpenicillin Against Streptococci Causing
    Bacterial Endocarditis 19
  M. J. Basker and C. E. Moon

A Multicentre Study of Talampicillin and Ampicillin
    in General Practice 25
  O. P. W. Robinson

Pharmacological and Clinical Studies with Talampicillin,
    an Ester of Ampicillin 31
  P. J. Wilkinson, A. L. Thomas, D. S. Reeves,
  and J. Symonds

Pharmacokinetic Studies of Serum Levels and Urinary
    Excretion of Ticarcillin after Intravenous and
    Intramuscular Administration to Patients with
    Normal and Abnormal Renal Function 37
  M. J. Parry and H. C. Neu

The Use of Ticarcillin in the Treatment of Acute
    Urinary Tract Infections 45
  H. D. Short and L. O. Gentry

Microbiology of Carfecillin, the α-Phenyl Ester
 of Carbenicillin   51
 M. J. Basker and R. Sutherland

Chemotherapeutic Activity of Carfecillin, the α-Phenyl
 Ester of Carbenicillin, in the Treatment of
 Experimental Mouse Infections   57
 K. R. Comber and G. Valler

Pharmacological and Clinical Studies with Carfecillin,
 an Orally Administered Ester of Carbenicillin   63
 P. J. Wilkinson, D. S. Reeves, and R. Wise

Determination of Indanyl Carbenicillin in Urine with
 Blood   71
 M. P. de Carvalho and A. M. Ferreira

In Vitro Activity and Clinical Use of Indanyl
 Carbenicillin   75
 G. Fontana and M. Laudi

Clinical Experience with Geopen (Carbenicillin)   83
 Ž. Ivić

Indanyl Carbenicillin and Urinary Infections   87
 R. Pedrotti and V. Forte

Oral Treatment with Carindacillin Patients Suffering
 from Urinary Tract Infections   93
 L. Cioni, N. Pilone, and L. Moriconi

Carindacillin in the Therapy of Urinary Tract Infections . .   99
 T. Germinale and C. Giglio

Urinary Levels of Carindacillin in the Pediatric Age 103
 A. Ferro, G. Ceccarelli, and G. R. Burgio

Clinical Pharmacological Studies with Bacampicillin 109
 L. Magni, B. Sjöberg, J. Sjövall, and J. Wessman

Clinical and Bacteriological Study on Bacampicillin
 in Skin and Soft Tissue Infections 115
 E. Skog, E. Sandström, and G. Wallmark

Bacampicillin in Respiratory Tract and Urinary
 Tract Infections 123
 B. Ursing, M. Lindroth, and C. Kamme

CONTENTS

Clinical Study of Bacampicillin in Urinary Tract
 Infections – A Comparison with Ampicillin 131
  W. J. Kaipainen, T. Timonen, and V. Raunio

Bacampicillin in Acute Tonsillitis 137
  P.-H. Jeppsson, O. Nylén, S. Jönsson, and
  P. Branefors-Helander

Clinical Study on Bacampicillin in Otitis Media
 Acuta and Sinusitis Acuta 145
  O. Olsson and C. Henning

Clinical, Bacteriological, and Pharmacological Study of
 Bacampicillin in Chronic Maxillary Sinusitis 151
  V. Raunio, K. Jokinen, and S. Karjalainen

Mecillinam and Pivmecillinam – New Beta-Lactam
 Antibiotics with High Activity Against
 Gram-Negative Bacilli 159
  F. Lund, K. Roholt, L. Tybring, and
  W. O. Godtfredsen

The Disposition of Mecillinam and Pivmecillinam in Man . . . 167
  J. Andrews, M. J. Kendall, and M. Mitchard

Plasma Profile and Urinary Excretion of Mecillinam
 After Pivmecillinam 173
  R. L. Parsons, G. M. Hossack, and G. M. Paddock

Mecillinam: Factors Affecting In Vitro Activity 183
  D. S. Reeves, R. Wise, M. J. Bywater, and S. R. Stern

The Activity of Mecillinam (FL1060), in Combination
 with Other Antibiotics, Against H. influenzae
 and Streptococcus faecalis 191
  R. Wise, G. A. J. Ayliffe, J. M. Andrews, and
  K. A. Bedford

Laboratory and Clinical Studies with Mecillinam 199
  D. McGhie, M. J. Robertson, A. M. Geddes, and
  K. C. L. Lim

A Clinical Investigation of Pivmecillinam, a Novel
 β-Lactam Antibiotic, in the Treatment of
 Urinary Tract Infections 205
  R. Wise, D. S. Reeves, J. M. Symonds, and
  P. J. Wilkinson

Antibacterial Activity of Eight Cephalosporins
  (Cefamandole Included) on Two Common
  Respiratory Pathogens (Haemophilus
  influenzae and Diplococcus pneumoniae) 211
 E. Yourassowsky, E. Schoutens, and
 M. P. Vanderlinden

Relationship between Lytic and Inhibitory
  Concentrations of Cephalosporins 219
 J. M. T. Hamilton-Miller

Cephacetrile: Plasma Concentrations During and
  After Constant Infusion 223
 K. G. Naber, H. G. Meyer-Brunot, and I. Reitz

Clinical Evaluation of Cefoxitin 229
 G. K. Daikos, H. Giamarellou, K. Kanellakopoulou,
 and G. Piperakis

Synergistic Interaction of Cephalosporins and Human
  Serum on Gram-Negative Bacteria 235
 P. Orsolini and M. R. Milani

A Comparative Study of Ceftezol (Demethyl-Cefazolin)
  and Cefazolin: Absorption, Distribution,
  and Metabolism 241
 S. Ishiyama, I. Nakayama, H. Iwamoto, S. Iwai,
 I. Sakata, I. Murata, and H. Mizuashi

In Vitro and In Vivo Evaluation of Two New Orally
  Active Cephalosporin Derivatives 247
 O. Zak, C. Schenk, and W. A. Vischer

A New Parenteral Cephalosporin. SK&F 59962: Serum
  Levels and Urinary Recovery in Man 253
 P. Actor, D. H. Pitkin, G. Lucyszyn,
 J. A. Weisbach, and J. L. Bran

Pharmacokinetics of Cephradine 259
 E. Bergogne, N. Lambert, and J. L. Rouvillois

Studies on the Diffusion of Cephradine and
  Cephalothin into Human Tissue 263
 D. Adam. A. G. Hofstetter, W. Jacoby, and B. Reichardt

Dosage Schedule of Antimicrobial Agents 271
 Y. Ban, Y. Shimizu, Y. Kawada, and T. Nishiura

Schedule of Intermittent Cephalothin Therapy 277
 K. Shimada and H. Kato

CONTENTS

Absorption and Excretion Studies of Cephalosporins
      in Human Subjects 283
  A. G. Paradelis

Ocular Penetration and Clinical Evaluation of
      Ceftezole for Ocular Infections 293
  M. Oishi

Preliminary Studies of the Penetration Cephacetrile
      (Celospor®) into Human Cerebrospinal Fluid 299
  H. G. Meyer-Brunot, C. Schenk, and A. V. Lomar

Tissue Concentrations of Cefazolin in Man 305
  E. Sinagowitz, K. Pelz, A. Burgert, W. Kaczkowski,
  H. Sommerkamp, and M. Westenfelder

Cephazolin Sodium - An In Vivo and In Vitro Evaluation
      of 100 Patients with Urinary Tract Infections
      in a District General Hospital 311
  D. M. D. Rimmer

Treatment of Bacterial Pneumonia with Cefazolin 315
  M. T. Foster, Jr.

Identification of Beta-Lactamases by Analytical
      Isoelectric Focusing 319
  M. Matthew and A. M. Harris

The Combined Effect of Protein-Binding and
      Beta-Lactamases on the Activity of
      Penicillins and Cephalosporins 325
  S. Selwyn and C. Lam

Bacterial Biotransformation of Ampicillin, Amoxicillin
      and Oxacillin In Vitro and in Urine of Patients
      with Bacteriuria 331
  M. Arr, H. Graber, T. Perenyi, and E. Ludwig

Substrate Profiles of β-Lactamases Against Newer
      β-Lactam Antibiotics 337
  B. Wiedemann, V. Krcmery, and H. Knothe

Beta-Lactamase Resistance of Cephazolin and Other
      Cephalosporins 341
  C. S. Goodwin and J. P. Hill

Interactions of New Cephalosporins with Some
      Cephalosporinases 347
  R. Labia

The Activity of Haemophilus influenzae β-Lactamase 355
    S. Kattan, P. Cavanagh, and J. D. Williams

Ampicillin Resistance and Beta-Lactamase Activity
        in Clinical Isolates of Shigella sonnei 361
    H. C. Neu and A. Prince

Inhibition of Bacterial Cell Wall Synthesis by
        Amphomycin 365
    S. Ōmura, H. Tanaka, M. Shinohara, R. Ōiwa,
    and T. Hata

Effect of Primycin on DNA 371
    A. Daróczy, T. M. Jovin, and F. Hernádi

Pipemidic Acid, a New Synthetic Antibacterial Agent 379
    P. Adamowicz, J. F. Delagneau, P. de Lajudie,
    M. Pesson, and M. Reynier

Clinical Studies of Pipemidic Acid in the Field of
        Pediatrics 385
    S. Nakasawa, E. Tanaka, and H. Sato

In Vitro and In Vivo Studies on Antibiotics from
        Skin Micrococcaceae 391
    S. Selwyn, P. D. Marsh, and T. N. Sethna

Antimicrobial Substances from the Larval Isolates
        of Greater Wax Moth, Galleria mellonella L. 397
    A. Paszewski and J. Jarosz

Advantages of New Tetracycline-Complexes in Human Therapy . . 403
    I. L. Kahán, F. Kulka, and E. Vigh

Nifurpipone in Urinary Tract Acute Infections 411
    M. Laudi, G. Fontana, U. Ferrando, C. Benvenuti,
    and G. Sesia

The Use of Cinoxacin in Urinary Tract Infections 417
    A. H. Bennett

List of Contributors 419

THE BETA LACTAM ANTIBIOTICS - PENICILLINS AND CEPHALOSPORINS

G.T. Stewart

Department of Community Medicine

University of Glasgow. U.K.

INTRODUCTION

There are five criteria by which maintenance and development of activity in this leading group of antibiotics can be assessed:

1) Width of antimicrobial spectrum
2) Action on penicillinase-forming bacteria
3) Pharmacological improvements
4) Non-toxicity
5) Diminution of allergic responses

1) Width of Spectrum

It has to be remembered that earlier natural penicillins like penicillin G and penicillin N (as Abraham reminds us) possess considerable intrinsic activity against certain gram-negative bacilli, especially of the coli-typhoid group. Ampicillin and its homologues have extended this activity to a wider range of organisms in the same group as well as to haemophilus, to Proteus mirabilis, and to various streptococci. There is evidence of increasing resistance in hospital and non-hospital strains of E.coli to ampicillin, less so to its derivatives and homologues, though precise comparisons are difficult in the face of differences in local patterns of use, abuse and recording of data. The work of our colleagues in the Scandinavian countries on Bacampicillin and Mecillinam is therefore of special interest. Carbenicillin, with relatively weak activity against Pseudomonas and Proteus spp. is still useful though also threatened by resistant organisms. Rodriguez suggests a novel use for it against ampicillin-resistant haemophilus. Mecillinam is active against Friedlander and

Aerobacter as are (sometimes) some of the cephalosporins including the newcomers cephacetrile, cephazolin, cefamandole and cephoxitin as well as cephalothin, cephaloridine and cephalexin. Cephaloglycine has, rightly, slipped into obscurity and one wonders if the same fate might or even should befall some of the newer derivatives.

2) Action on penicillinase-forming bacteria

Here there is less to report about the drugs though knowledge of the inactivating enzymes and their production grows impressively. Our Conference has given detailed attention to this problem, as the contributions of experts like Chabbert, Costerton, Richmond, Sabath, Voropaeva, Bobrowski and a number of others have shown in several of our sessions. Pride of place among the several useful penicillinase-stable anti-staphylococcal beta-lactams seems to belong still to cloxacillin though I am interested to note among the revivals that interesting derivative quinacillin, remarkable for its narrow selective action against staphylococci and resistance to hydrolysis by several forms of constitutive and inducible beta-lactamase.

3) Pharmacological improvements come from intensive attempts to produce and maintain better levels in blood, tissue-fluids and tissues by improved absorption or slower excretion. There is, commendably, more emphasis on oral medication. There is also, lamentably, a dearth of good information about the indications for parenteral therapy and about the conditions, technical and otherwise, under which the effects of such therapy are most beneficial. In this connection one welcomes the scrupulous pharmacological measurements of absorption, retention and excretion made by Meyer-Brunot and his colleagues in Germany. It is reassuring to note that some advantages can still be obtained by simple kitchen methods used by O.P.W. Robinson's expert chemical colleagues to produce talampicillin, the phthalyl ester of ampicillin. Quinn suggests an explanation for the high activity of cefazolin which attains levels in tissue and also in bile in excess of most other cephalosporins.

4) Reduced toxicity

The aim here must surely be to emulate or at least not to depart from the non-toxicity of penicillin G and ampicillin. This remarkable property is retained only when the side chain is kept simple as in these two substances. Differences and improvements nowadays come mainly from alterations or elaboration of the side chain. It is a fact of beta-lactam biochemistry that elaboration usually increases toxicity. So, without disrespect to most of the derivatives now available, one can say that almost any future alteration of the beta-lactam molecule is liable to be an exercise in toxigenesis. To date, there is no evidence that any of the derivatives are less toxic than the simpler penicillins and cephalosporins. It is important therefore to remember - and occasionally in bad microbial situations to employ - the fact that penicillin G can be given in high dosage and maintained in the blood and tissues at very high levels for weeks on end without toxicity. One does read of occasional nephropathies and cephalopathies but these are still and always were exceptional. When organic toxicity does arise with benyl penicillin or with cephalothin it is most likely to be due to the cation (Na^+ or K^+) which can produce electrolyte imbalance in high doses. Some of the encephalopathies and neuropathies which I have seen or read about were almost certainly due to the procaine in procaine penicillin.

5) <u>Allergy</u>

This is now a rare disorder in the Western World. Among the reasons for reduction may be mentioned the removal of polymers, protein residues and other macromolecular complexes formed during manufacture or in storage. Such complexes can induce or elicit allergy in trace amounts. It was not realised therefore for many years that they were undetectable by the conventional methods of chemical and microbiological assay required by the B.P., U.S.P., F.D.A. and other regulatory agencies. Methods of assay and manufacture have now improved, but it is still possible in some countries or under some conditions for allergenic residues to be present in therapeutic preparations particularly since most beta-lactams, natural and semi-synthetic, tend to polymerise in solution to give macromolecules which serve as carriers for antigenic haptens formed from degradation products like penicillenates. We know a lot about the behaviour of penicillin G in this respect but very little about the new beta-lactams which tend to form antigenic fractions of baffling complexity. Syndromes such as the eosinophilic oliguria of methicillin and the mononucleosis rash of ampicillin have never been satisfactorily explained. There is a need to include in monitoring schedules some provision for immediate investigation of any untoward reactions even if they are seemingly transient. All beta-lactams are potentially immunogenic because they or their degradation products or polymers can act as haptens. Fortunately, the laws of hapten inhibition usually operate favourably, so the monovalent fractions and possibly the monomolecular drugs themselves act as inhibitors. When natural inhibitory mechanisms fail, the formol-lysine inhibitors described by de Weck and his colleagues would appear to offer a promising and highly rational approach to prevention and control. Since cross-reactions between penicillins and cephalosporins appear to depend upon similarities in side chains rather than upon the common lactam structure, it will be logical to explore further the derivatives with non-benzyl and non thio-enyl side chains among the cepahlosporins.

Allergy is, as I have said, a rare difficulty nowadays. Its importance is that it is so often unpredictable and that it may still be severe or fatal. To guarantee safety, if beta-lactams must be used in hypersensitive subjects, it is wise to keep epinephrine and oxygen at hand and no advance has yet eliminated this necessity.

GENERAL ADVANCES

Most of the practical advances during the past 15 years have come from experimentation with derivatives of the 6-APA and 7-ACA molecular nuclei. There are, however, some backroom results which might well have a greater bearing upon future developments.

(a) Chemical improvements have led not only to the production of 6-APA by chemical methods from natural penicillin but also to the conversion of penicillins into cephalosporins.

(b) In the total synthesis of cephalosporins referred to by Abraham, the sulphur atom in the dihydrothiazine ring can be replaced by an oxygen atom to yield, for instance, an oxycephalosporin with activity comparable to cephalothin. This finding raises many interesting possibilities. We know, for instance, that the thio-enyl ring in cephalothin is equivalent in antimicrobial activity to an unsubstituted benzyl ring but it was not known that activity could be retained with loss of the reactive sulphur atom in the fused lactam ring. This could point to methods of stabilising the lactam structure as well as to losing the sulphur-linked degradation products which play a role in allergy and cross-reactions.

(c) The production from Streptomyces spp. of 7-methoxy analogues of cephalosporin C with a straight (d-alpha-amino-adipyl-) side chain points the way to interesting new structures, especially if benzyl or thio-enyl derivatives are used as side chains. Cefoxitin is one such which seems, according to Daikos and his colleagues in Greece, to have promising activity though it is not clear how well it compares in vitro and in vivo with its non-methoxy analogue.

It is impossible in a summary such as this to do justice to the many studies and advances which are being reported in world literature or even in that part which has been reported at this Conference. Ultimately, the struggle between host and germ depends upon natural processes of adaptation and resistance. In using antimicrobials medically, we intervene in a situation of growing epidemiological complexity. Often the most we know - if we even know that - is the immediate outcome. So for the sake of safety as well as decency toward the future, we need to look where we are going. In this respect, our Conference has been better than most in its attempts during several sessions to assess the implications as well as the immediate results of the use of antimicrobials. When this is done with regard to penicillins and cephalosporins, as by Crain, Kunin, Gale, Howard and others, it is evident in terms of existing knowledge that this family of beta-lactam antibiotics is still by far the most important in background, present use and potential.

CLINICAL RELEVANCE OF AMPICILLIN/CLOXACILLIN FOR IV USE

C. Regamey, L. Barrelet, and F.A. Waldvogel

Infectious Disease Division, Department of Medicine

Hôpital cantonal, 1211 Geneva 4, Switzerland

Most of the gram negative bacilli (especially enterobacteriaceae) which are highly resistant to ampicillin (A) produce penicillinases which inactivate the antibiotic by hydrolyzing the beta-lactam ring. It has been postulated that the adjunction of an inhibitor of beta-lactamases would block the enzymes and allow therefore undestroyed A to exert a more prolonged bactericidal effect on apparently A resistant strains. Cloxacillin (C) is one of these inhibitors of penicillinases produced by E. coli, Klebsiella, Proteus sp., E. cloacae and Ps. aeruginosa. It exerts its inhibitory effect by a marked affinity for the beta-lactamases and forms relatively stable enzyme substrate complexes (1-3).

The combination of A and C was shown to act synergistically against bacilli resistant to A in vitro, in animal experiments and in urinary tract infections. The concentrations of both antibiotics found to achieve synergism seemed at first too high to be used for the treatment of systemic diseases, although large doses of these penicillins can be given intravenously without serious side effects. This prospective study was undertaken in order to evaluate the prevalence of A resistant gram negative bacilli septicemia and to determine their in vitro susceptibility to the combination of A and C. Finally, the study tried to answer the question whether a certain combination of A/C could be used clinically by comparing these in vitro results with serum concentrations of A and C obtained after the intravenous infusion of 4 g A and 1 g C.

During a one year period 178 different strains of gram negative bacilli were isolated from blood cultures of patients hospitalized at the University Hospital of Geneva: half of the isolates were E. coli, followed by Klebsiella (21%), Ps. aeruginosa (11%), Enterobacter,

Proteus sp. and Serratia. The first disc diffusion antibiotic susceptibility testing was performed following the recommendations of the ICS report (4) and 63 strains (35%) were resistant to A (zone size ≤ 11 mm). Of these 63 strains, 50 isolates (all enterobacteriaceae and 6 Ps. aeruginosa) were then studied further as to their susceptibility to the combination A/C: a second antibiogram with 3 discs containing 25 mcg A, 10 mcg C, and a combination with 25 mcg A and 25 mcg C, respectively, was performed. Despite the fact, that all bacilli had zone sizes ≤ 11 mm around the A disc, 7 E. coli, 5 Klebsiella, 1 Enterobacter, 1 Serratia and 1 Ps. aeruginosa showed significantly larger zone sizes around the A/C disc (12-24 mm). Thus, the A/C combination increased the susceptibility of 15 strains or 30% of the A resistant bacilli.

To quantitate the synergism, all 15 strains showing increased susceptibility to the A/C combination were studied by the two dimensional broth dilution checkerboard method, using Muller-Hinton broth adjusted to pH 7.4 and an inoculum of 5×10^5 cells-ml. Concentrations of 4 to 512 mcg/ml A and 8 to 256 mcg/ml C alone and in all combinations were tested. MICs and MBCs (lowest concentrations in which less than 0.03% of the original inocula of organisms remained viable) were determined. MICs were in general equal to the MBCs. Table 1 gives the results of the checkerboards for the 7 strains of E. coli and shows at least an eightfold reduction of the MICs of A in combination with C. The MICs of the 5 Klebsiella strains fell twofold and the MBCs at least fourfold with final MIC and MBC concentrations of 64-128 mcg/ml A and 16 to 64 mcg/ml C. Single strains of Enterobacter, Serratia and Ps. aeruginosa were susceptible to the synergism with MICs of 4/32, 16/8, 32/32 mcg/ml, respectively.

Synergism was graphically appreciated by drawing isobolograms for all 15 strains. MICs and MBCs were plotted on an arythmetic scale, with the A and C concentrations represented on opposing axes.

Table 1

RESULTS OF THE TWO DIMENSIONAL BROTH DILUTION CHECKERBOARD METHOD FOR THE 7 SUSCEPTIBLE STRAINS OF E. COLI

	MIC Ampicillin (µg/ml)	MIC Ampicillin/Cloxacillin combination (µg/ml)	
1.	256	8/32	16/16
2.	256	32/32	64/16
3.	128	4/32	16/16
4.	256	8/32	16/16
5.	512	32/32	64/16
6.	128	<4/32	4/16
7.	>256	16/32	32/16

For each strain either the MIC or MBC isobol bowed significantly toward the coordinates.

Synergism was also studied by establishing killing curves to determine the time-course of the bactericidal effect of A and C alone and in combination. Serial colony counts from a starting inoculum of approximately 5.8×10^5 bacteria/ml were performed with Muller-Hinton broth cultures. Viable bacteria/ml were counted at 2,4,8 and 24 hours. All 7 E. coli strains and 2 of the 5 Klebsiella strains were tested. Antibiotic concentrations were chosen from MBCs obtained with the checkerboards (64/8, 64/16, 32/8, 16/16 and 64/32 mcg/ml A/C). For all E. coli, the number of viable bacteria/ml fell to less than 100/ml within 24 hr whereas the colony count in the medium containing A or C alone was similar to the growth curve of the control in broth. The synergism was less spectacular with the 2 strains of Klebsiella: the log drop was 1.3 and 2.8 with A/C concentrations of 64/32 mcg/ml.

The last part of this study concerns the serum concentrations and other pharmacologic data obtained after the parenteral administration of a large dose of A simultaneously with C, namely 4 g A and 1 g C (AMPICLOX, Beecham).

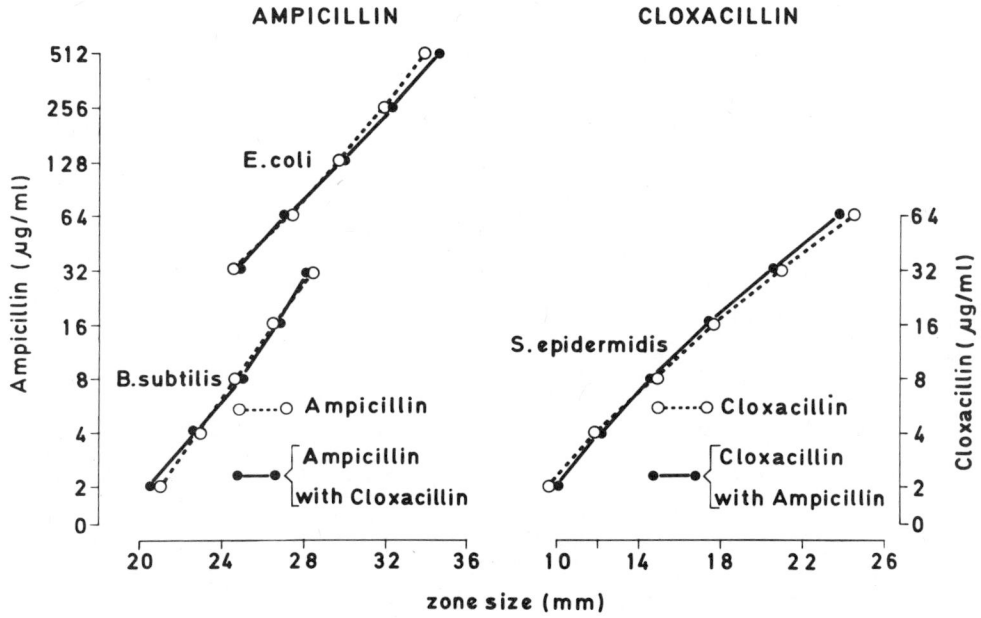

Fig. 1. Recovery of A and C. The combination of the two antibiotics did not interfere with the dosages of each separately.

Six healthy male volunteers received within 30 min intravenously 56 mg/kg A (approx. 4 g) and 14 mg/kg C (approx. 1 g) with a constant-infusion pump. Fourteen blood samples were drawn at short intervals for up to 5.5 hr. The serum concentrations of the two antibiotics were determined by an adapted agar-well diffusion method (5) using E. coli NCTC 8661 as an indicator organism for the determination of A concentrations between 32 and 512 mcg/ml (figure 1). Cloxacillin which was added in concentrations up to 128 mcg/ml to the A standards did not interfere with the dosage of A.B. subtilis ATCC 6633 was used as indicator organism for the dosage of concentrations of A from 2 to 32 mcg/ml and a S. epidermidis from Geneva for C.

Figure 2 shows the average serum concentrations measured simultaneously for A and C. The peak concentration of A was 235 mcg/ml with a standard error (SE) of 11 mcg/ml; at 1 hr the average concentration was 117 ($\pm$ 8) and at 2 hr 43 ($\pm$ 5) mcg/ml. The peak concentration of C was 85 ($\pm$ 7) mcg/ml; average concentrations were 32 ($\pm$ 3) and 8 ($\pm$ 1) mcg/ml after 1 and 2 hr, respectively.

The serum concentrations of A and C plotted for each volunteer declined exponentially. The $T\frac{1}{2}$ of A was calculated from 1 to 5.5 hr

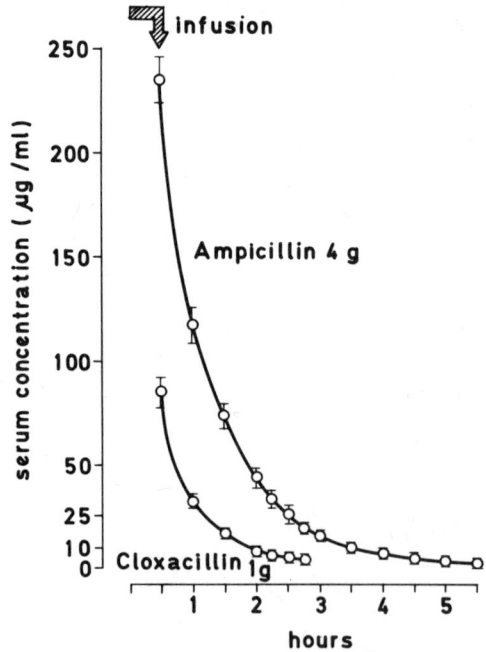

Average serum concentrations (with standard error) after an iv infusion of 56 mg/kg (4 g) A and 14 mg/kg (1 g) C in 6 volunteers.

(12 samples) and averaged 0.8 hr (47 ± 3 min). The $T_{\frac{1}{2}}$ of C calculated with 4 to 6 values from 1 to 2.75 hr was shorter, 0.5 hr (31 ± 3 min), it is responsible for a modification of the A/C serum concentration ratio; this ratio was 4/1 at 1 hr and 5/1 at 2 hr.

The agar diffusion antibiotic susceptibility testing using conventional discs defined in the ICS study (4) as well as one disc containing the combination of 25 mcg A and 25 mcg C was an excellent screening procedure to detect the gram negative bacilli susceptible to the synergism of A/C. Strains unsusceptible to the synergism had no inhibition zone around the A/C disc, whereas susceptible strains had zone sizes between 12 and 24 mm. Susceptible strains of E. coli, Enterobacter and Serratia were all cephalothin resistant, implying that their beta-actamase synthesis was chromosomal (6). The synergism was confirmed by other procedures including bactericidal studies such as two dimensional broth dilution checkerboards and killing curves. E. coli, Enterobacter and Serratia were most susceptible: they were inhibited by 32 mcg/ml A or less with 4 to 32 mcg/ml C when an inoculum of 5×10^2 cells/ml was tested. Moreover starting with an inoculum of 6×10^5 cells/ml, we recovered after 24 hr less than 100 E. coli/ml in the killing curve studies. These experiments showed that the synergistic action of A/C expressed itself not only as a one log decrease in the colony count at 4 hr as compared with the count obtained with A, but as an almost complete bactericidal action. Klebsiella were less susceptible. Hamilton-Miller (7) found that the inhibition of Klebsiella beta-lactamases by C was less active than by methicillin.

The question which arise from these results is whether this synergism is of clinical relevance in septicemias. Large doses of A and C can be administered without serious side effects. The serum concentrations reached after an intreavenous infusion of 4 g A and 1 g C reached peak levels of 285/85 mcg/ml A/C and for at least 1 hr the measured serum concentrations were above in in vitro determined MBCs of the susceptible strains. Our results show that when a synergistic effect is obtained against enterobacteriaceae, it involves mostly C concentrations of 16 or 32 mcg/ml. Our in vivo results demonstrated that this concentration of C was present for only approximately 1.5 hr. It seems therefore that the combination of 4 g A and 1 g C might not be ideal. A 3:2 or 2:2 combination of the two antibiotics would give more favorable serum concentration ratios for a prolonged period. The latter combination is prescribed currently in certain Swiss hospitals. It would bear the additional advantage of giving appropriate antistaphylococcal coverage with adequate doses of C in cases of septicemia of unknown origin.

Patients presenting with septicemia due to gram negative bacilli are often treated with A before microbiological results are available. However, as shown by this study, more than a quarter of all enterobacteriaceae isolated from blood cultures in Geneva are A resistant. Could the simultaneous addition of C to A diminish the risk of inadequate initial antibiotic coverage ? The A/C combination has been shown to give favorable results in urinary tract infections (1) because urinary concentrations of A and C are high. We feel that the addition of C to A enhances also the gram negative antibacterial spectrum of A in septicemia but that a larger dose of C in combination with A might come closer to the demonstrated in vitro synergism.

References

1. Sabath LD, et al. New Engl. J. Med. 277:232; 1967.
2. Sabath LD, Abraham EP. Nature 204: 1066; 1964.
3. Bach JA, et al. Antimicrob. Ag. Chemother. 1966: 328; 1967.
4. Ericsson HM, Sherris JC. Acta Pathol. Microbiol. Scand. Sect. B, Suppl. 127, 1971.
5. Bennett JV, et al. Appl. Microbiol. 14: 170; 1966.
6. Roupas A, Pitton JS. Antimicrob. Ag. Chemother. 5: 186; 1974.
7. Hamilton-Miller JMT. Biochem. J. 87: 209; 1963.

EXPERIENCES WITH AMOXICILLIN IN FULL-TERM

AND PRE-TERM NEONATES

L. Weingärtner, U. Sitka and R. Patsch.

Paediatric Clinic (Director: Prof. Dr. sc. med. L Weingärtner) and Institute for Medical Microbiology and Epidemiology (Director: Prof. Dr. sc. med. S. Ortel) of Martin-Luther-University, Halle-Wittenberg, G. D. R.

The fact that one often needs an effective and non-toxic broad spectrum antibiotic in the treatment of neonates instigated our trials with amoxicillin. For this purpose 12 full-term and 7 pre-term neonates were given 1 dose of 50mg/kg orally during the first 2 days of life. A second group of 7 full-term neonates of the same age were given 2 doses of amoxicillin 50mg/kg orally at 12 hour intervals. In every case we determined serum levels and calculated elimination constants and serum half lives.

The amoxicillin serum level determinations were made in agar diffusion tests (punched plate process). The assay organism used was Sarcina Lutea ATCC 9431. Laboratory reference standard material with a potency of 850mg was used. After 18 hours incubation time at $37°C$ the zones of inhibition were measured and the antibiotic concentration in the serum were determined in the semi-logarithmic system against the homologous standard.

The mean serum level of amoxicillin in the first group of full-term neonates was 23 mcg/ml at 2 hours. After 4 hours the mean level had risen to 52 mcg/ml. After absorption had been completed and the amoxicillin had been distributed the serum level dropped, and after 6 hours it was around 33 mcg/ml. After 10 hours nevertheless it was still around 15mcg/ml (figure 1). These values almost coincide with those found by Simon with the same quantity of amoxicillin, i.e. 50mg/kg serum concentration in full-term neonates. His values lie slightly lower than ours but were also at their peak after 4 hours.

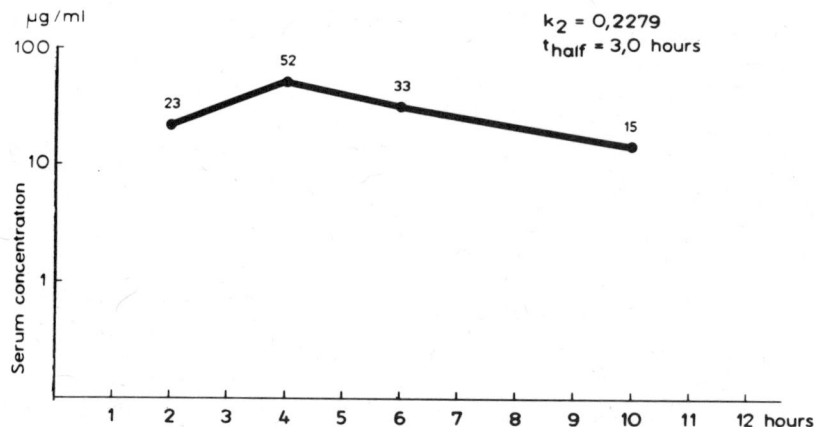

Fig. 1. Mean serum concentration of Amoxicillin in 8 newborns, 1 x 50 mg/kg oral administration.

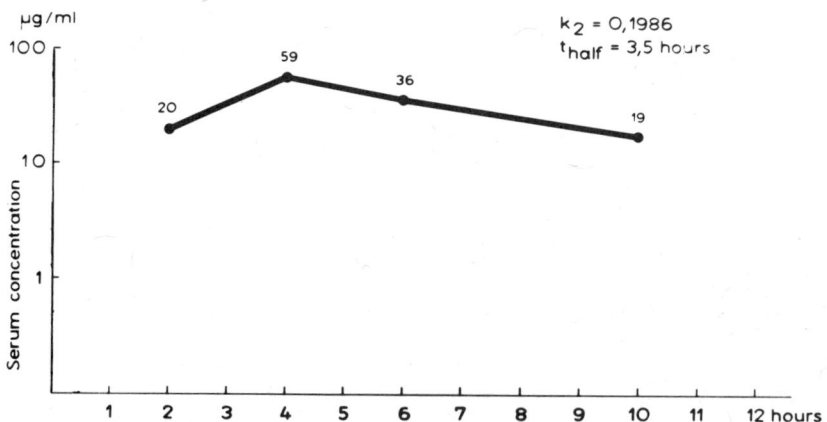

Fig. 2. Mean serum concentration of Amoxicillin in 7 prematures, 1 x 50 mg/kg oral administration.

The same trial with 7 pre-term babies showed in contrast to our experiences with ampicillin only little deviation from the curve shown in figure 1, Weingärtner, Sitka and Patsch. Mean value after 2 hours was 20mcg/ml. The climax of the curve was again reached after 4 hours, with 59mcg/ml. The drop in concentration resembles the curve of full-term neonates. Only the 10 hour value at 19 mcg/ml was a little higher, figure 2.

As conversion and excretion of drugs in pre-term babies is usually slower than in full-term babies, one must assume that the absorption of amoxicillin was good although it was less favourable in pre-term than in full-term neonates.

In the 2nd group of full-term neonates of 1 or 2 days old who were given 2 doses of 50 mg/kg amoxicillin at 12 hourly intervals, the 4 hour value was not determined. However, the mean 6 hour value of 30 mcg/ml was about the same as in the first group of full-term neonates. The decline after 10 hours to 15mcg/ml did not differ significantly either. Then, in order not to put the children under too great a strain, we took another value after the 2nd dosing with amoxicillin, after 24 hours, figure 3.

The average values of about 5 mcg/ml found, showed a higher concentration than we could expect after having given one dose to the first 2 groups of full-term neonates and pre-term neonates. If one interpolates the course of the serum levels in figures 1 and 2 from the 4th to the 10th hour further, one gets values for the full-term neonates which lie slightly under 1 mcg/ml and for pre-term babies values which lie slightly above 1 mcg/ml. In order to examine this question we again took serum levels from 4 full-term babies of 1 or 2 days age after having given them 50mcg/kg amoxicillin and found mean levels of 26.4 mcg/ml after 6 hours and 1.6 mcg/ml after 24 hours.

On comparison of the 24 hour values the concentrations were 2 to 3 times higher after 2 doses of 50 mg/kg amoxicillin in 12 hourly intervals. Therefore there was a type of cumulative effect under these circumstances after 2 applications of amoxicillin within 24 hours. In contrast to us, Cohen et al. who gave patients 30mg/kg amoxicillin in 6 hourly intervals over 7 days did not find this cumulative effect. However, the conditions of both trials cannot easilly be compared as we were working with healthy babies and dosages of amoxicillin differed.

The elimination constant k_2 was 0.2279, or 0.1986. The serum half lives t_2 were assessed as 3 hours in full-term neonates and 3.5 hours in pre-term neonates. They are therefore in contrast to the results of Cohen et al. who calculated serum half lives of under 2 hours.

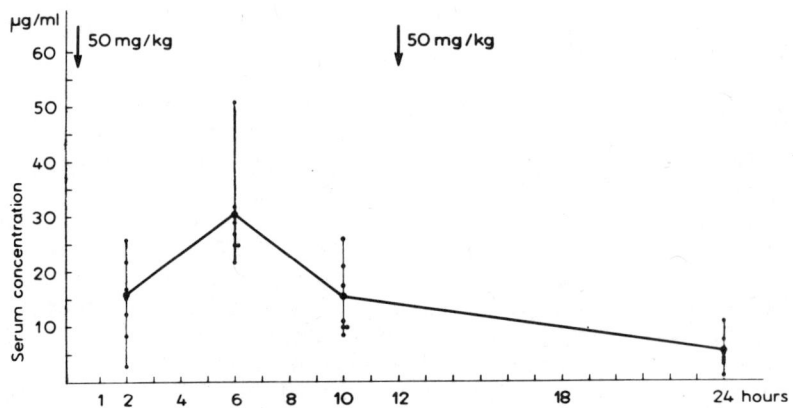

Fig. 3. Mean serum concentration of Amoxicillin in 7 newborns, 50 mg/kg oral administration two times a day.

Table 1. Mean serum concentrations and standard deviations of Amoxicillin, µg/ml, in 7 prematures and 8 newborns, 1 x 50 mg/kg oral administration

Hours	2	4	6	10
Prematures (n = 7)	20 ± 7	59 ± 13	36 ± 10	19 ± 5
Newborns (n = 8)	23 ± 10	52 ± 13	33 ± 11	15 ± 5

The serum levels of amoxicillin found by us in full-term and pre-term neonates showed small variations as you can see from the mean values and standard deviations in table 1.

One can conclude from these results that one oral dose of amoxicillin given every 24 hours to full-term and pre-term babies can be enough when sensitive strains are involved. If one wants to be sure and also combat moderately sensitive strains, amoxicillin should be given in 12 hourly intervals. In this way even a considerable proportion of coli, which are as you know inhibited with 5 mcg/ml, are reached. It can also be shown that absorbtion, which has its own laws in full-term and pre-term babies is from good to very good.

The drug is without doubt suitable for the treatment of various illnesses in neonates. Among other indications it would also be very useful for neonatal listeriosis, for which we were the first to recommend ampicillin, Weingärtner et al. The growth of listeriae is already inhibited at a serum level of 1.1 mcg/ml. One can therefore assume a bactericidal effect. If there is a serious illness in the neonatal period we would recommend dosing 3 times with amoxicillin to be on the safe side.

Summary

Trials were done with amoxicillin in full-term and pre-term neonates of 1 or 2 days age. The children were given 50mg/kg amoxicillin orally. Serum levels were determined in the agar diffusion test and the elimination constant and serum half lives were calculated.

With a dosage of 50mg/kg amoxicillin the full-term neonates have peak serum values after 4 hours of 52 mcg/ml and the pre-term neonates 59 mcg/ml. The 10 hour values were 15 mcg/ml for the first group and 19 mcg/ml for the second.

With a single dose of amoxicillin serum levels of between 1 and 1.6 mcg/ml were determined after 24 hours. If the children were given 50mg/kg twice a day serum levels of about 5 mcg/ml were reached after 24 hours.

Amoxicillin can be recommended as an effective and suitable antibiotic for pre-term and full-term neonates. The drug should generally be given in 12 hourly and only in a serious illness should this be raised to an 8 hourly dose.

Bibliography

Cohen; J. A. Raeburn; J. Devine; J. Kirkwood; B. Elliott;
F. Cockburn a. J. O. Forfar:
Pharmacology of some oral penicillins in the newborn infant
Arch. Dis. Childh. 50 (1975) 230 - 234.

Simon C.:
Antibiotics in Newborns and young Babies.
Mschr. Kinderheilk. 123 (1975) 38 - 40.

Weingärtner, L.; R. Patsch; W. Weigel a. R. Müller:
Ampicillin - a semi-synthetic penicillin - in Pregnancy and
Pre-Term and Full-Term Neonates.
Mschr. Kinderheilk. 116 (1968) 63 - 68.

Weingärtner, L.; U. Sitka; R. Patsch a. D. Herrmann:
Pharmacokinetic studies of Carbenicillin (Pyopen) in Newborns
and Prematures.
VII. Internat. Congress of Chemotherapy, Prague 1971.
Advan. antimicrob. antineoplastic. chemother. 1 (1972) 99 - 102.

COMPARATIVE ACTIVITY OF AMOXYCILLIN, AMPICILLIN AND BENZYLPENICILLIN AGAINST STREPTOCOCCI CAUSING BACTERIAL ENDOCARDITIS

M. J. Basker and C. E. Moon

Beecham Pharmaceuticals Research Division

Brockham Park, Betchworth, Surrey, England

About 70% of cases of bacterial endocarditis are caused by α-haemolytic or non-haemolytic streptococci collectively known as Streptococcus viridans which are identical to those commonly found in the mouth. Other streptococci frequently implicated in the disease are Group D streptococci, mainly enterococci, but also S. bovis, which may be of increasing importance (Wilkowske et al, 1971; Gross et al, 1975).

The traditional treatment of streptococcal endocarditis is with a penicillin, used either alone or in combination with an aminoglycoside. Preliminary work has shown that amoxycillin is a penicillin with good activity against Gram-positive cocci and with outstanding oral absorption characteristics (Sutherland et al, 1972), properties that make it a suitable agent for use in the treatment of endocarditis. Results are reported here which compare the activities of amoxycillin, ampicillin and benzylpenicillin against streptococci associated with bacterial endocarditis.

RESULTS

The activity of amoxycillin against streptococci is shown in Fig. 1 in comparison with ampicillin and benzylpenicillin and it can be seen that the penicillins inhibited the growth of all three groups of organisms at low concentrations. The viridans streptococci were the most sensitive, and the enterococci were the least sensitive of the streptococci tested, with the strains of S. bovis showing intermediate sensitivity. Amoxycillin was as active as benzylpenicillin against viridans streptococci and

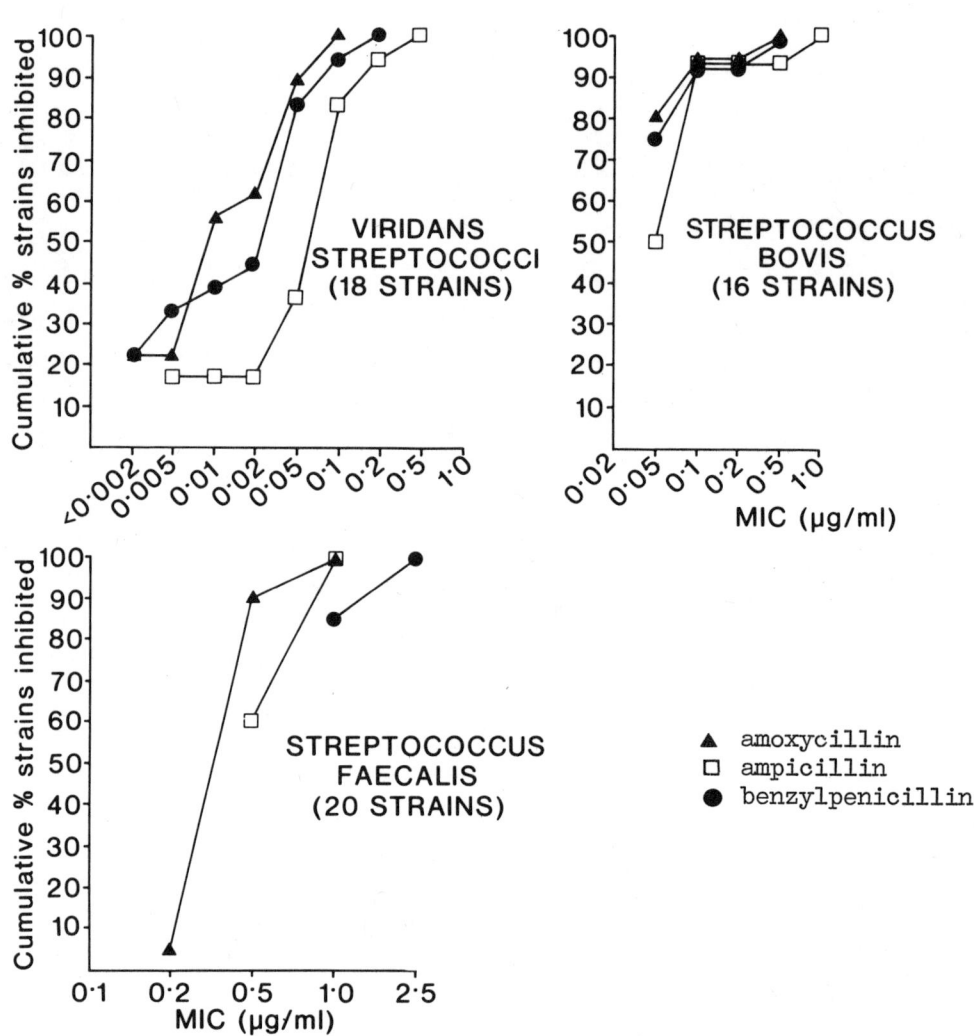

FIG. 1. Cumulative percent inhibition of Streptococcus viridans, Streptococcus bovis and Streptococcus faecalis by amoxycillin, ampicillin and benzylpenicillin.

inhibited 50% of the strains at concentrations of 0.01µg/ml or less. A number of strains were rather less sensitive and required concentrations of 0.05-0.1µg amoxycillin/ml for inhibition. These strains were also more resistant to ampicillin and to benzylpenicillin. Ampicillin was less active than the other two penicillins against the viridans streptococci and MIC values ranged from 0.005-0.5µg/ml. The strains of S. bovis were rather less sensitive than the viridans streptococci to the penicillins and the range of Minimum Inhibitory Concentrations varied from 0.05-1.0µg/ml. Again amoxycillin was as active as benzylpenicillin, and both compounds were rather more active than ampicillin. Amoxycillin was the most active of the penicillins against the test strains of enterococci, being twice as effective as benzylpenicillin, and inhibited most strains at 0.5µg/ml. Ampicillin was slightly less active than amoxycillin against S. faecalis but was more active than benzylpenicillin against these organisms.

The Minimum Bactericidal Concentrations of the compounds against the three groups of streptococci are illustrated in Table 1. In these tests, the penicillins showed pronounced activity against viridans streptococci and S. bovis but appeared to demonstrate poor bactericidal activity against S. faecalis. Thus, the MBC values of the penicillins were only slightly higher than the MIC values against viridans streptococci and S. bovis but were considerably higher (>100µg/ml) for the enterococci.

TABLE 1. Minimum Bactericidal Concentrations of amoxycillin, ampicillin and benzylpenicillin

Organism	Amoxycillin		Ampicillin		Benzylpenicillin	
	MIC*	MBC	MIC	MBC	MIC	MBC
S. viridans	0.02	0.05	0.05	0.1	0.02	0.05
S. bovis	0.1	0.5	0.2	0.5	0.1	0.5
S. faecalis	0.5	>100	0.8	>100	1.0	>100

* Minimum Inhibitory Concentrations were determined by serial dilution in Todd-Hewitt Broth (5ml) inoculated with 10^6 cells/ml. After 18hours incubation at 37°C the tubes were examined for inhibition and the MIC value was taken as the lowest concentration preventing visible growth. MBC values were considered to be the lowest concentrations of antibiotic that caused a 99.99% kill of the culture and were determined by streaking onto agar 0.03ml aliquots (4mm loop subculture) taken from tubes not showing visible growth after 18 hours incubation at 37°C.

However, results in Fig. 2 show the marked bactericidal activity of amoxycillin in a viable count experiment against S. faecalis. Amoxycillin caused a 99.0% fall in the viable count by 6 hours but thereafter, the rate of kill declined and at 24 hours, 10^2–10^3 bacteria/ml were still viable. The addition of gentamicin, however, resulted in a considerable increase in the bactericidal

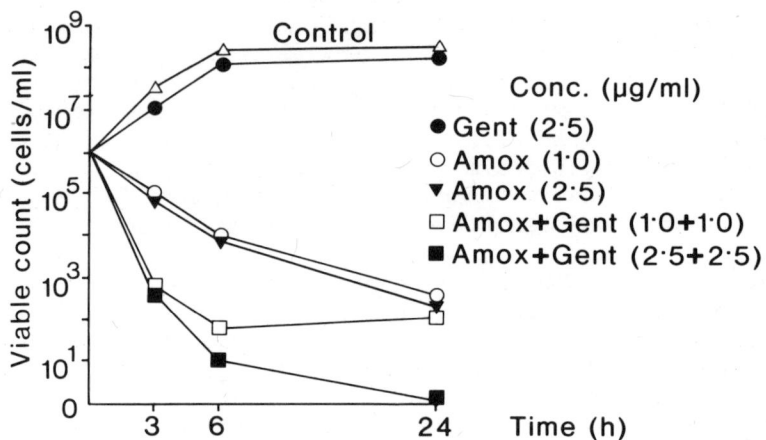

FIG. 2. Bactericidal activity of amoxycillin, gentamicin and combinations against Streptococcus faecalis F1.

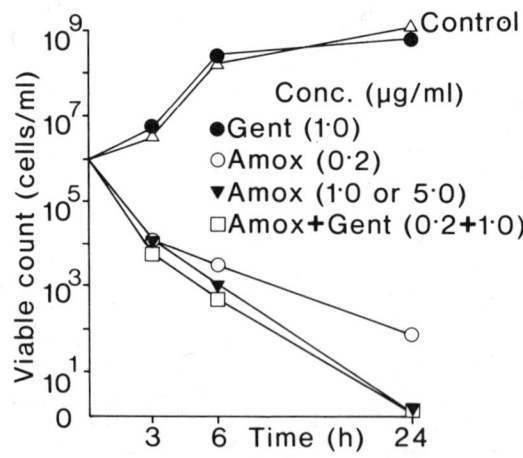

FIG. 3. Bactericidal activity of amoxycillin, gentamicin and a combination against Streptococcus salivarius V1.

activity and a combination of 2.5µg amoxycillin/ml and 2.5µg gentamicin/ml brought about a total kill of the culture within 24 hours.

Amoxycillin also reduced the viable count of a viridans streptococcus (S. salivarius) by 99.0-99.9% at low concentrations (0.2 and 0.5 µg/ml) by 6 hours and reduced the 24 hour count to zero at a concentration of 0.5µg/ml. The bactericidal activity of amoxycillin was however, enhanced by the addition of an ineffective concentration of gentamicin and a combination of 0.2µg amoxycillin/ml + 1.0µg gentamicin/ml was slightly more effective than 1.0µg amoxycillin/ml alone (Fig. 3). Similarly, amoxycillin produced marked reductions in the viable counts of S. bovis S1, reducing the numbers 90.0-95.0% within 6 hours and sterilising the culture at a concentration of 2.5µg/ml at 24 hours. Again gentamicin increased the bactericidal effects of amoxycillin.

DISCUSSION

Before the advent of antibiotics, bacterial endocarditis was invariably fatal as the bacteria invaded and severely damaged heart valves, resulting in heart failure. Problems in treatment are still encountered as the organisms are deeply embedded in heart valves and vegetations but nowadays, mortality tends to be highest in the elderly, or in people infected with organisms other than viridans streptococci. Endocarditis caused by viridans streptococci or S. bovis may be treated with a penicillin alone, although aminoglycosides such as streptomycin, kanamycin or gentamicin may be added to enhance bactericidal activity. Enterococci are less susceptible to the penicillins and enterococcal endocarditis is almost always treated with a combination of a penicillin and an aminoglycoside.

Oral ampicillin has been used successfully in the treatment of bacterial endocarditis caused by a variety of streptococci (Beaty et al, 1966; Toivanen et al, 1969) and the results reported here show that amoxycillin is more active than ampicillin and as active as benzylpenicillin against viridans streptococci and against S. bovis, and is more active than both these penicillins against enterococci. Thus, on the basis of in vitro activity and good oral absorption characteristics following administration to human subjects it would seem that amoxycillin would also make a suitable candidate for the treatment of the disease.

During the course of clinical trials, amoxycillin has been shown to be effective in the treatment of a limited number of cases of streptococcal endocarditis either alone, for the treatment of viridans streptococci, or in combination with gentamicin against endocarditis caused by enterococci (Mashimo, 1973; Seligman, 1974).

REFERENCES

Beaty, H. N., Turck, M., and Petersdorf, R. G. 1966. Annals of Internal Medicine, $\underline{65}$, 701.

Mashimo, K. 1973. Amoxycillin International Symposium, London, Sept. 1973. 123 (Excerpta Medica, Amsterdam, 1974).

Seligman, S. J. 1974. The Journal of Infectious Diseases, $\underline{129}$, (Supplement), S213.

Sutherland, R., Croydon, E. A. P., and Rolinson, G. N. 1972. British Medical Journal, $\underline{3}$, 13.

Toivanen, A., Toivanen, P., and Gronroos, J. A. 1969. Current Therapeutic Research, $\underline{11}$, 150.

Wilkowske, C. J., Facklam, R. R., Washington II, J. A., and Geraci, J. E. 1971. Antimicrobial Agents and Chemotherapy. 1970. 195.

A MULTICENTRE STUDY OF TALAMPICILLIN AND AMPICILLIN IN GENERAL PRACTICE

O.P.W. ROBINSON

BEECHAM PHARMACEUTICALS, U.K.

BEECHAM HOUSE, GREAT WEST ROAD, BRENTFORD, MIDDX.

Talampicillin (Talpen), the phthalidyl ester of ampicillin (fig. 1), like other thiazoldine esters of penicillins (Hamilton-Miller, 1967) is considered to be devoid of antibacterial activity. It is particularly well absorbed following oral administration and liberates free ampicillin into the circulation. Blood ampicillin levels obtained following oral doses of talampicillin are twice those achieved following equivalent oral doses of ampicillin (Clayton J.P. et al, 1974). Metabolic studies have indicated that ampicillin is liberated from the ester during talampicillin's passage through the gut mucosa by the action of tissue esterases and that no intact talampicillin is present in the peripheral blood (Jeffrey D.J. et al, 1975).

These properties suggested that talampicillin might have certain advantages over ampicillin in that therapeutic effects equivalent to ampicillin should be obtained with a smaller dose. Also, the incidence of gastrointestinal side effects associated with ampicillin might be reduced after talampicillin since the ester is devoid of any antibacterial activity and is virtually completely absorbed.

In view of these properties the clinical and bacteriological effectiveness of ampicillin and talampicillin was compared in patients suffering from presumed bacterial infections occurring in general practice.

607 patients suffering from infections of the respiratory tract, urinary tract or skin and soft tissue were treated for six days with either ampicillin or talampicillin. 44 General Practitioners took part in the study, each treating 10-20 patients who were allocated to ampicillin or talampicillin treatment on an alternate basis.

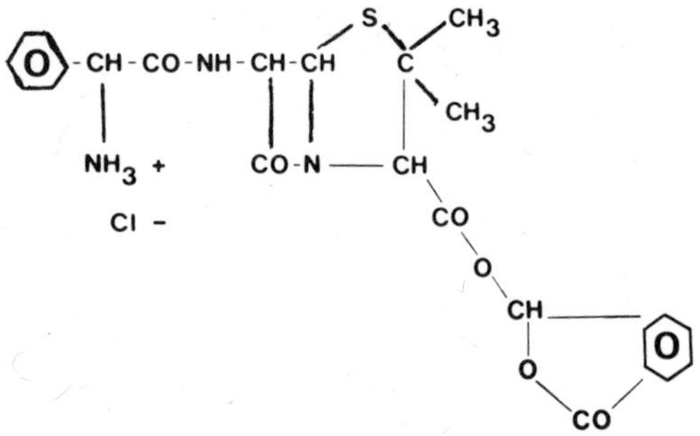

Fig. 1. Talampicillin HCl (Talpen) BRL 8988.

Table 1

	RESP. TRACT		URINARY TRACT		SKIN & SOFT TISSUE		TOTAL	
DRUG	A	T	A	T	A	T	A	T
PATIENTS	157*	149	73	82	64*	65	294*	296
SUCCESS (cure + improved)	96.8%	95.3%	91.8%	86.6%	87.5%	92.3%	93.5%	92.2%

* 1 Ampicillin treated patient had both respiratory and skin infection

The dosage of ampicillin given was 250 mg. q.i.d. and that of talampicillin was 185 mg. (containing the equivalent of 125 mg. ampicillin) q.i.d. Both substances were given as capsules half an hour before meals.

Swabs or cultures were taken from all patients before, and 24 hours after completing their treatment course, when they were also assessed clinically as "cured", "improved" or "failed". Side effects were sought in response to the question "how did you find the treatment?" Reported side effects were graded as mild, moderate or severe.

A bacteriological assessment was made subsequently and classified as :-

1. Successful   - if an initially sensitive organism was eradicated, the second culture being sterile or growing a resistant organism.

2. Partially   - if an initially sensitive organism was eradicated but
   successful   replaced by a different sensitive organism on the second culture.

3. Failure   - if an originally sensitive organism failed to be eradicated.

Patients in whom initial cultures showed no growth, resistant organisms or commensals were considered unassessable bacteriologically.

Results

299 patients (130 males and 169 females) aged 9-98 years (median 36 years) were treated with ampicillin and 308 patients (132 males and 176 females) aged 4-95 years (median 38 years) with talampicillin.

Clinical response within the three infection categories is shown in table 1. Six patients receiving ampicillin and 12 receiving talampicillin were not assessed owing to failure to record the diagnosis, thus 294 patients were assessed clinically after ampicillin and 296 after talampicillin. There was no significant difference between treatments, 93.5% patients being successfully treated (cured or improved) after ampicillin and 92.2% after talampicillin. There was also no significant difference when the three infection categories were considered separately.

Bacterial infection was confirmed by swab or culture in 190 patients (63.3%) receiving ampicillin and 183 patients (59.4%) receiving talampicillin. 33 of these receiving ampicillin and 39 receiving talampicillin were unassessable bacteriologically. The bacterial response of assessable infections is shown in table 2. Successful results were achieved in 83.4%

Table 2

	RESP. TRACT		URINARY TRACT		SKIN & SOFT TISSUE		ALL INFECTIONS	
TREATMENT	A	T	A	T	A	T	A	T
NO. INFECTIONS	74	71	48	46	35	27	157	144
SUCCESS	85.1%	91.5%	89.6%	93.5%	71.4%	74.1%	83.4%	88.9%
PARTIAL SUCCESS	-	4.2%	-	-	-	3.7%	-	2.8%
FAILURE	14.9%	4.3%	10.4%	6.5%	28.6%	22.2%	16.6%	8.3%

Bacterial response in three infection categories

Table 3

ORGANISM	CULTURES	SENSITIVE	RESISTANT
STAPH. PYOGENES	81	47	34 (42%)
ESCH. COLI	66	56	10 (15.2%)
COLIFORMS	33	28	5 (15.2%)
PROTEUS	15	14	1 (6.7%)
OTHER	180	167	13 (7.2%)
TOTAL	375	312	63 (16.8%)

Sensitivity results to ampicillin

Table 4

	AMPICILLIN (299)				TALAMPICILLIN (308)			
	+	++	+++	Total	+	++	+++	Total
DIARRHOEA	29	9	3	41 (13.7%)*	20	3	-	23 (7.5%)*
GASTRIC	5	1	-	6 (2%)	7	3	2	12 (3.9%)
RASH	3	1	1	5 (1.7%)	6	1	1	8 (2.6%)
MONILIA	1	5	-	6 (2%)	1	1	-	2 (0.6%)
OTHER	2	2	1	5 (1.7%)	8	2	3	13 (4.2%)

* ($p < 0.02$ $x^2 = 6.27$)

Incidence of side effects

patients in the ampicillin group and in 88.9% in the talampicillin group. Partial success occurred in 4 patients on talampicillin. 26 patients (16.6%) on ampicillin and 12 patients (8.3%) on talampicillin were classified as failures.

The sensitivity to ampicillin of organisms isolated from patients, as reported by the various pathological laboratories, is shown in table 3. 42% of Staph. pyogenes and 15.2% E.Coli were reported resistant to ampicillin.

The incidence and severity of side effects is shown in table 4. There was no significant difference in the incidence of side effects, 56 patients (18.7%) and 51 patients (16.6%) having side effects in the ampicillin and talampicillin groups respectively (7 patients in each group had 2 side effects). There was, however, a significant difference in incidence of diarrhoea which occurred in 41 patients (13.7%) on ampicillin and in 23 patients (7.5%) on talampicillin. ($p < 0.02$, $x^2 = 6.27$). The severity of diarrhoea was also greater after ampicillin.

Discussion and Conclusion

Talampicillin containing the equivalent of 125 mg. ampicillin has proved to be equally effective both clinically and bacteriologically to 250 mg. ampicillin when both preparations were given 4 times daily for 6 days in this study under general practice conditions. Although the total side effect incidence following both preparations was similar, there was a significantly reduced incidence of diarrhoea in the talampicillin group and it was less severe. This may be due to several factors - the smaller daily dose of talampicillin given, a possible reduced intrinsic irritant effect of talampicillin on the gut mucosa, or a reduced effect of talampicillin on the gut flora since the ester has no antibacterial activity until ampicillin is liberated from it into the circulation during absorption.

The results in this study agree closely with those reported by other authors (Knudsen E.T. and Harding J.H., 1975) who compared the same total daily dose of talampicillin given as 250 mg. (equivalent to 169 mg. ampicillin) three times daily to general practice patients with ampicillin 250 mg. given four times daily for 7 days. They also reported a significantly reduced incidence of diarrhoea after talampicillin.

The incidence of ampicillin resistant staphylococci (42%) in the present study confirms the prevalence of penicillinase producing staphylococci in general practice reported by other writers (Shaw E.J., 1974, Price D.J.E. et al, 1968).

It was encouraging to find that after fifteen years of extensive use, ampicillin resistance was found in only 15.2% of E.Coli isolates.

Acknowledgements

I should like to thank those General Practitioners from Clinical Research International and the Wessex Clinical Trials Organisation for co-operating in this study and Miss Jacky Urwin of Beecham Research Division for providing the stastical analysis.

References

Clayton J.P., Cole M., Elson S.W., Ferres H., 1974. Antimicrobial Agents and Chemotherapy 5 No. 6 p. 670-671.

Hamilton-Miller, 1967, Chemotherapia 12 p. 73.

Jeffery D.J., Jones K.H., Langley P.F., 1975, 9th International Congress of Chemotherapy.

Knudsen E.T. and Harding J.H., 1975, to be published.

Price D.J.E., O'Grady F.W., Shooter R.A. and Weaver P.C., 1968, Brit. Med. J. 3 p. 407.

Shaw, Elizabeth J., 1974, Practitioner 213 p. 484.

PHARMACOLOGICAL AND CLINICAL STUDIES WITH TALAMPICILLIN, AN ESTER OF AMPICILLIN

P.J. WILKINSON, A.L. THOMAS, D.S. REEVES AND J. SYMONDS*

DEPARTMENT OF MEDICAL MICROBIOLOGY

SOUTHMEAD HOSPITAL, BRISTOL, BS10 5NB, ENGLAND

Talampicillin (Talpen, Beecham Research Laboratories) is the thiazolidine carboxylic ester of ampicillin. After oral administration the ester is rapidly hydrolysed in the intestinal wall to release free ampicillin into the body (Jeffery et al, 1975). We initially did some studies in human volunteers to confirm the findings of Clayton et al (1974) that talampicillin gives higher blood levels than the same oral doses of ampicillin. A study was then undertaken in patients with infections from ampicillin-sensitive organisms to assess the pharmacology and clinical effectiveness of talampicillin.

METHODS

Volunteer Study

4 fasting healthy male volunteers took part, all of whom were known to have normal renal and hepatic function tests. 2 took 500 mg of a commercial preparation of ampicillin containing in 2 capsules at 0900 hours. Blood samples were taken at 0, 1, 2, 4, 6, 8 hours after the dose. All urine was collected for two 6-hour and one 12-hour consecutive periods following the dose. 4 days later these two volunteers took two 250 mg capsules of talampicillin containing a total of 338 mg equivalent of ampicillin, and the pattern of sampling repeated. The other two volunteers followed a similar protocol but reversed the order of the drugs. All urine and serum samples were assayed for ampicillin.

Clinical Protocol

43 established infections in 42 hospital patients were treated with talampicillin (500 mg ampicillin equivalent) at 12 hourly intervals for 7 days. The capsules were given before meals whenever possible, and a satisfactory regime was found to be twice daily administration at 0600 and 1700 hours. There were 38 urinary infections, 4 chest infections and one infection of a post-operative abdominal wound. All infections were judged to be clinically significant and would have normally been treated with ampicillin, and all were confirmed sensitive to ampicillin on disc testing as a criterion for inclusion in the trial. Many of the patients with urinary infections had indwelling catheters, or urinary tract pathology, or underwent urinary tract surgery.

The outcome of treatment was judged on clinical grounds and by bacteriological culture. In urinary infections follow-up specimens were cultured at 14 and 42 days after beginning treatment.

Serum and urine samples were collected when possible. Both were assayed for ampicillin. A range of haematological and biochemical parameters were measured before and after treatment to detect any toxic effects.

<u>Laboratory methods</u>. Standard bacteriological methods for isolation, identification and disc sensitivity testing were used. <u>Esch. coli</u> was typed where possible by O-antigen serotyping and <u>Proteus mirabilis</u> by Dienne's method. The minimal inhibitory concentration (m.i.c.) of ampicillin for all isolates was determined by an agar dilution method. Ampicillin in samples from volunteers and patients was assayed by a large-plate agar diffusion method using <u>Bacillus subtilis</u> (N.C.T.C.6633) as indicator organism. Doses were applied to the plates randomised in triplicate using 6 mm diameter antibiotic assay paper discs.

RESULTS

Volunteer Studies

The mean peak serum level in the 4 volunteers was 5.3 mg/l after 500 mg talampicillin (338 mg ampicillin) and 2.8 mg/l after 500 mg ampicillin (fig.1). Furthermore, the peak serum concentration occurred sooner with the talampicillin indicating more rapid absorption. The mean 24-hour urinary recovery of ampicillin was 51.8% after talampicillin and 26.3% after ampicillin (fig.2). Apart from mild eructations of a petrol-like taste no volunteers complained of any side-effect.

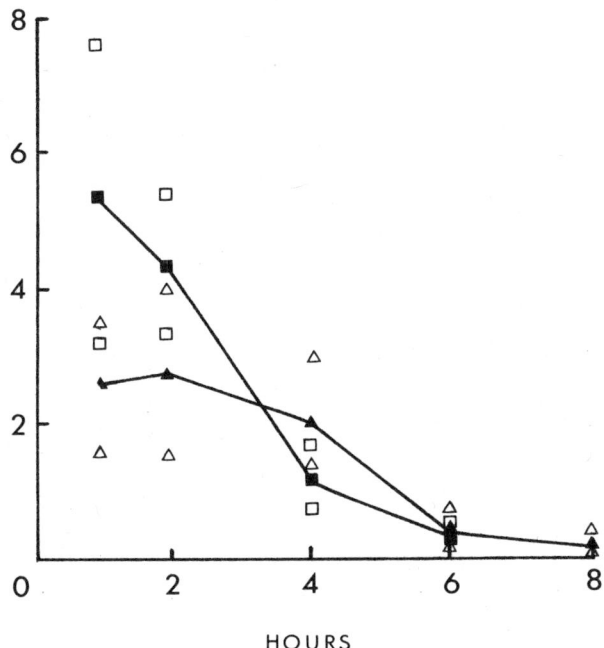

Fig.1: Serum levels (means and ranges) of ampicillin in 4 volunteers. Doses given as in figure.

Outcome of Infections Treated

28 of 38 urinary pathogens were absent from both follow-up specimens, including one case known retrospectively to be complicated by septicaemia. The four chest infections were cured on clinical and bacteriological criteria, but the single wound infection persisted and the organism (Esch. coli) became resistant to ampicillin. Neither the pre- nor the post-treatment strains from this wound infection were typeable, so it was not possible to exclude re-infection. All the bacteria isolated had m.i.c.'s of ampicillin of 8 mg/l or less with a single exception (see Table 1). The infecting organisms in the chest infections were 2 Haemophilus influenzae, 1 H. parainfluenzae, and 1 Strep. pneumoniae.

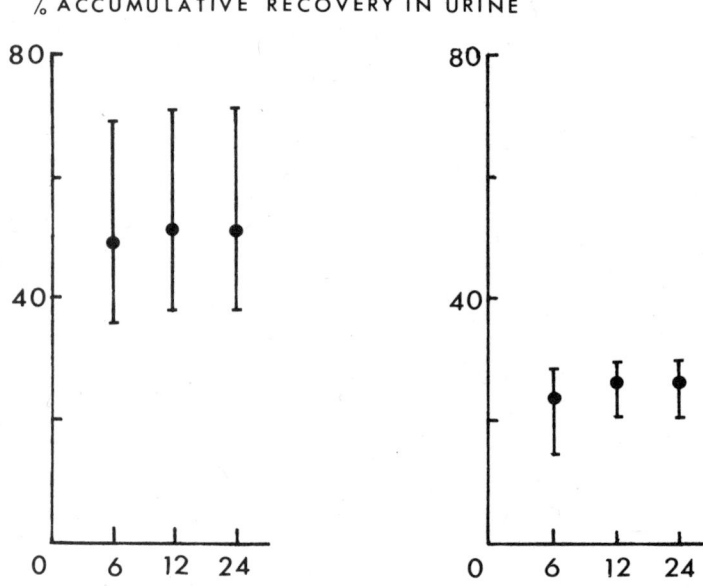

Fig.2: 24-hour cumulative urinary excretion of ampicillin in 4 volunteers.

Serum Levels

After the first dose of talampicillin, ampicillin levels were measured in 14 patients at 1, 2, 3, 4, and 6 hours afterwards, although not all samples were collected in every case. The mean peak serum concentration was 13 mg/l (S.D. 8.82; range 3.8-38.4 mg/l) (Fig. 3). The mean time to reach the peak level was 1.8 hours (range 1-5 hours).

Outcome of treatment	Esch. coli	Strep. faecalis	Proteus mirabilis	Other	Total
Cure	10	9	3	7	29
Failure	6*	1	2	–	9

* one strain resistant to ampicillin – m.i.c. 32 mg/l.

Table 1: Urinary infections: infecting organisms related to outcome.

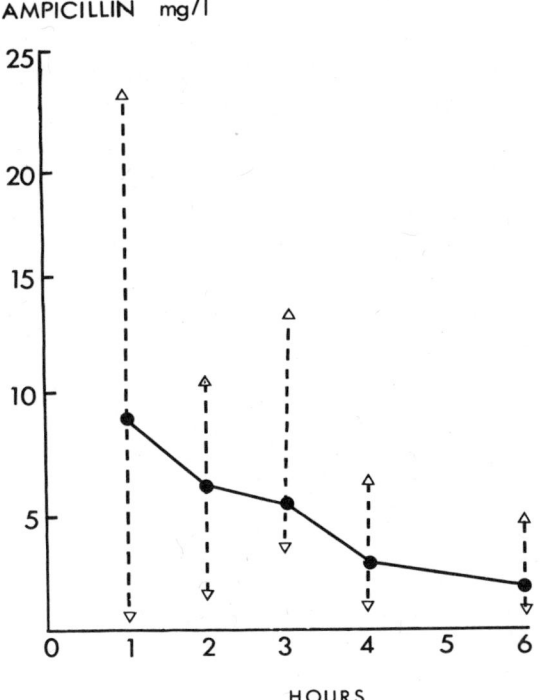

Fig.3: Serum levels (means and ranges) of ampicillin in 14 patients.

Urinary Levels

Urinary levels of ampicillin varied over a wide range (67 – 1026 mg/l) with a mean of 286 mg/l. The urinary recovery of the ingested dose in the first 48 hours of treatment was also variable (9% – 79%) with a mean of 42.3% (S.D. 16.74).

Tolerability and Side-Effects

Tolerability was good. Side-effects were few. 4 patients complained of a petrol-like after-taste, and the formulation has since been modified to eliminate this flavour One patient had vomiting relieved by anti-emetics. No patient had diarrhoea. Two patients, one of whom had received twice the dose in the protocol, developed a maculo-papular rash.

Toxicology

There were no changes in haematological or biochemical parameters which could be attributed to talampicillin.

DISCUSSION

Our results show that in both volunteers and patients talampicillin produces higher serum levels of ampicillin with a greater recovery of the ingested dose in the urine than is usually found from equivalent doses of ampicillin. Gastro-intestinal side-effects were virtually absent although they might have been expected from doses of conventional ampicillin sufficient to give equivalent serum levels on a multidose basis. Although diarrhoea is a well-quoted side effect of ampicillin treatment only a small number of studies actually report its incidence. In a large comparative study between talampicillin and ampicillin (Knudsen and Harding, 1975) the incidence of diarrhoea was 4.3 and 8.6% respectively, a statistically significant difference. Upper gastro-intestinal side-effects were more common with talampicillin and the unpleasant after taste was noted, as in the patients in our series. The cure rates of infections were virtually identical. Diarrhoea is an important side-effect since some infections in outpatients are relatively minor and this side-effect can be worse than the symptoms themselves. Furthermore, it may persist when the latter have subsided.

The cure-rate of urinary infections in this study we consider to be satisfactory at 76% considering the serious underlying urinary tract pathology in many patients, and that over 30% of the patients cured had an indwelling urethral catheter for some or all of the treatment period. What is needed is a comparative study against ampicillin to judge the clinical effectiveness of the two compounds against their respective incidences of side-effects.

REFERENCES

Clayton, J.P., Cole, M., Elson, S.W., Ferres, H. (1974). Antimicrobial Agents and Chemotherapy, $\underline{5}$, 670.

Jeffery, D.J., Jones, K.H., Langley, P.F. (1975). IXth International Congress of Chemotherapy.

Knudsen, E.T., Harding, J.H. (1975). IXth International Congress of Chemotherapy.

PHARMACOKINETIC STUDIES OF SERUM LEVELS AND URINARY EXCRETION
OF TICARCILLIN AFTER INTRAVENOUS AND INTRAMUSCULAR ADMINISTRATION
TO PATIENTS WITH NORMAL AND ABNORMAL RENAL FUNCTION

M.J. Parry and H.C. Neu
Division of Infectious Diseases
Departments of Medicine and Pharmacology
College of Physicians and Surgeons, Columbia University
New York, New York 10032 U.S.A.

SUMMARY

The pharmacokinetics of ticarcillin after intravenous and intramuscular administration were determined. In individuals with $C_{Cr} > 60$ ml/min, the $T_{1/2}$ was 71 ± 6 minutes after intravenous administration. Patients with C_{Cr} 30-60 ml/min had a $T_{1/2}$ of 3.0 ± 0.6 hours. The $T_{1/2}$ in patients with C_{Cr} 10-30 ml/min was 8.5 ± 2.1 hours, and in those with $C_{Cr} < 10$ ml/min, 14.8 ± 3.7 hours. Combined hepatic and renal failure increased the $T_{1/2}$ to 27.8 hours. Intramuscular administration of ticarcillin produced adequate urine levels in patients with normal renal function and therapeutic serum levels in those with renal failure. Urinary concentrations of ticarcillin during intravenous therapy were adequate at all levels of renal function. Ticarcillin was well cleared by hemodialysis with a $T_{1/2}$ of 3.4 ± 0.8 hours; peritoneal dialysis was minimally effective. A program for the use of ticarcillin in renal failure is presented.

The introduction of carbenicillin in 1967 (Acred et al, 1967) proved to be an important advance in the therapy of serious infections due to certain members of the Enterobacteriaceae and Ps. aeruginosa. In vitro studies of a thienyl penicillin derivative, ticarcillin (Neu and Winshell, 1970), showed this compound was twice as active as carbenicillin against Pseudomonas. Preliminary studies by several investigators (Rodriguez et al, 1973; Wise and Reeves, 1974) and by our own group (Parry and Neu, in preparation) have shown this agent to be effective in the treatment of serious gram negative infections. Since ticarcillin will be used to treat infections occurring in individuals with impaired renal function, we investigated the pharmacokinetics of ticarcillin in normal volunteers and in patients with varying degrees of renal insufficiency as well as in patients undergoing hemodialysis and peritoneal dialysis.

MATERIALS AND METHODS

Subjects for study included normal volunteers and patients admitted to the Columbia-Presbyterian Medical Center. Creatinine clearance (C_{Cr})/1.73m^2 was computed for each subject. Ticarcillin was administered in a dose of three grams intravenously or one gram intramuscularly to normal volunteers. Patients received 50 mg/kg intravenously or one gram intramuscularly. Venous blood samples were obtained at 0, 1/2, 2, 4 and 6 hours in most instances. In patients with markedly depressed renal function, 12 and 24 hour specimens were also obtained.

Peritoneal dialysis was performed using 1.5% Inpersol$^{(R)}$ solution perfused via a midline, lower abdominal catheter. Each pass was carried out over 45-60 minutes with a 10-15 minute dwell time. Venous blood and dialysate were assayed during dialysis. Dialysis clearance was computed for each of several passes and averaged for each patient.

Hemodialysis was carried out using a Travenol Ultraflow II$^{(R)}$ coil dialyzer. Fifty mg ticarcillin per kg body weight was given at the beginning of dialysis and arterial and venous blood was drawn at 1, 2, 3, 4 and 6 hours into dialysis. Coefficients of extraction and clearances were calculated for each patient sample.

Serum and urine levels of ticarcillin were determined using the agar plate technique and Ps.aeruginosa NCTC 10701 as the assay organism as previously described (Neu and Swarz, 1970). Patient urines and sera were diluted prior to assay with potassium phosphate buffer, 0.05M, pH 7.0, and standards were prepared in buffer or pooled human serum.

RESULTS

In subjects with normal renal function (C_{Cr} > 60ml/min), the half-life of ticarcillin was 71 $\pm$ 6 minutes (Table 1). Peak serum levels after a single dose of three grams administered intravenously over 5 minutes were 256.8 $\pm$ 81 ug/ml. Therapeutic blood levels were maintained for 1.5 hours following peak levels. Twenty patients with normal renal function given 50 mg ticarcillin per kg administered over 90-120 minutes every four hours achieved serum levels at the end of infusion (peak) of 203 ug/ml (range 144 - 335 ug/ml), and serum levels immediately prior to the next dose (trough) of 42 ug/ml (range 13 - 90 ug/ml) after repeated doses. No drug accumulation was noted with this dosing regimen.

TABLE 1

TICARCILLIN IN RENAL INSUFFICIENCY

Adjusted CrCl	Patient Number	Average Half-Life
> 60	5	71 ± 6 min
30 - 60	4	3.0 ± 0.6 hr
10 - 30	4	8.5 ± 2.1 hr
< 10	4	14.8 ± 3.7 hr

In mild renal insufficiency (C_{Cr} 30-60 ml/min), ticarcillin half-life was slightly prolonged to 3.0 ± 0.6 hours, and minimal drug accumulation was noted at normal dosing intervals. Moderately severe renal impairment, (C_{Cr} 10-30 ml/min), produced further prolongation of the half-life to 8.5 ± 2.1 hours, necessitating modification of the normal dosing interval. Drug accumulation was minimised and therapeutic levels maintained by administering two grams of ticarcillin every eight hours to these patients. Peak serum levels in patients receiving ticarcillin every eight hours averaged 267 ug/ml (range 190 - 390 ug/ml) and trough levels averaged 140 ug/ml (range 110 - 190 ug/ml).

Patients with severe renal insufficiency (C_{Cr} <10 ml/min), demonstrated further impairment of ticarcillin excretion, with a half-life of 14.8 ± 3.7 hours. Peak serum levels of 396 ug/ml (range 290-560 ug/ml) and trough levels of 222 ug/ml (range 220-225 ug/ml) were obtained using ticarcillin in a dosage regimen of two to three grams every twelve hours. No toxicity was noted in any patient achieving these serum levels. One patient with combined hepatic and renal failure had a ticarcillin half-life of 27.8 hours, necessitating doses every 24 hours.

Urinary concentrations of ticarcillin were adequate even in patients with renal insufficiency (Table 2). With normal C_{Cr}, peak concentrations of ticarcillin ranged from 650-2,475 ug/ml after a single three gram dose, and 3,200-18,000 ug/ml after multiple doses given every four hours. Urinary recovery of ticarcillin in individuals with normal renal function was 60-70% of the administered dose. Urinary concentrations in mild to moderate renal insufficiency (C_{Cr} 30-60 ml/min) were not noticeable different from those with normal renal function and ranged from 4,700-15,200 ug/ml after multiple doses. Seventy percent of the administered dose was recovered in the urine over twelve hours in one patient with a creatinine clearance of 40 ml/min. Except in the presence of anuria, urinary concentrations of ticarcillin were

TABLE 2

TICARCILLIN URINARY EXCRETION

CrCl (ml/min)	Peak Conc. (ug/ml)	12 hr recovery (%)
> 60	3200 - 18000	77
30-60	4700 - 15200	68
10-30	1100 - 6800	-
< 10	450 - 3900	-

well maintained and therapeutic even in severe renal insufficiency with peak levels of 1,100 - 6,800 ug/ml in patients with creatinine clearances from 10-30 ml/min, and 450 - 3,900 ug/ml in patients with creatinine clearances less than 10 ml/min.

Intramuscular administration of ticarcillin produced urinary levels in patients with normal renal function. Seventy-one percent of the administered dose was recovered in the urine over six hours with an average concentration of 2461 ug/ml (range 800 - 3,700 ug/ml). In three patients with normal renal function receiving one gram ticarcillin intramuscularly every eight hours, urinary concentrations averaged 2,056 ug/ml (range 1,075 - 2,650 ug/ml). Serum levels on this dosage regimen in patients with normal renal function were inadequate to treat systemic Pseudomonas or Enterobacter infections (< 30 ug/ml). However, in the presence of moderate to severe renal insufficiency, intramuscular administration of ticarcillin produced therapeutic serum levels. One patient with a creatinine clearance less than 5 ml/min given one gram of ticarcillin intramuscularly every six hours, maintained relatively constant serum levels of 395 - 405 ug/ml.

Ticarcillin was well cleared by hemodialysis (Table 3). Dialysis clearance averaged 33 $\pm$ 10 ml/min and extraction ratios were 0.16 and 0.23 for blood flow rates greater than and less than 200 ml/min respectively. The ticarcillin half-life in three patients undergoing dialysis was 3.4 $\pm$ 0.8 hours, representing an average 77% reduction in predialysis half-life.

Peritoneal dialysis was effective in removing only small amounts of ticarcillin from the blood and reduced the predialysis half-life by approximately one third to 10.6 $\pm$ 0.8 hours (Table 3). Preitoneal clearances were 7.2 $\pm$ 1.8 ml/min. Dialysis levels ranged from 10-30% of simultaneous serum levels.

TABLE 3

TICARCILLIN IN DIALYSIS

		Ticar.	Carb.*
Hemodialysis			
Extraction ratio BFR	200 ml/min	0.16	0.14
BFR	200 ml/min	0.23	0.21
Clearance (ml/min)		33	
Half-life (hours)		3.4	5.5
Peritoneal dialysis			
Clearance (ml/min)		7.2	
Half-life (hours)		10.6	

* data of Bullock, Cestero and Hoffman
Ann.Int.Med. 78 : 173, 1970

COMMENTS

Carbenicillin has been used in the therapy of gram negative infections at doses which require the monitoring of renal function with appropriate adjustments in dosage. Further adjustments must be made in the presence of combined hepatic and renal failure (Hoffman et al, 1970).

The pharmacokinetics of ticarcillin in renal insufficiency are similar to those of carbenicillin. The half-life of ticarcillin in subjects with normal renal function is 71 ± 6 minutes. This figure is in agreement with other investigators and is similar to that of carbenicillin. With decreasing renal function, ticarcillin clearance falls but the half-life excedes four hours (normal dosing interval) only after the creatinine clearance is less than 30 ml/min, necessitating little modification in dosage before this degree of renal impairment is reached. In patients with severe renal insufficiency the half-life of ticarcillin rose to 14.8 ± 3.7 hours. This is similar to the half-life of carbenicillin in renal failure (15.7 hours) (Hoffman et al, 1970) and the data of Davies et al (1974) who found the ticarcillin half-life to be 13.5 hours in nine patients with severe renal failure.

Hemodialysis is effective in reducing the half-life of both carbenicillin and ticarcillin. Extraction ratios for ticarcillin of 0.23 and 0.16 for blood flow rates less than and greater than 200 ml/min, respectively compare with those reported for carbenicillin of 0.21 and 0.14 (Hoffman et al, 1970) (Table 3). Other investigators have recently found ticarcillin to be well dialyzed with a half-life of 4.7 hours (Davies et al, 1974). Peritoneal dialysis is minimally effective in removing ticarcillin from the blood.

Despite the progressively increasing half-life of ticarcillin with renal insufficiency, we found that urinary concentrations of ticarcillin were therapeutic at all levels of renal function (Table 2). Only in the presence of anuria did inadequate concentrations of drug reach the lower urinary tract.

Intramuscular administration of ticarcillin produces therapeutic urinary levels, and has been successfully used in the treatment of urinary tract infections. In the presence of moderate to severe renal insufficiency, serum levels adequate to treat systemic Pseudomonas infection can be achieved using intramuscular therapy.

Guidelines have been constructed for ticarcillin dosage in renal failure (Table 4). Non-renal clearance is unimportant except in the presence of severe renal failure where adjustments must be made if there is concommittant hepatic failure. Drug accumulation has not been significant in patients treated with multiple doses of ticarcillin according to these guidelines and adequate therapeutic levels have been maintained.

TABLE 4

SUGGESTED TICARCILLIN DOSAGE FOR SYSTEMIC INFECTIONS
IN PATIENTS WITH ABNORMAL RENAL FUNCTION

Initial Loading Dose of 3 gm followed by

CrCl > 60	3 gm IV every 4 hours
30–60	2 gm IV every 4 hours
10–30	2 gm IV every 8 hours
<10	2 gm IV every 12 hours or
	1 gm IM every 6 hours
<10 + hepatic dysfunction	2 gm IV every 24 hours or
	1 gm IM every 12 hours
Peritoneal dialysis	2 gm IV every 12 hours
Hemodialysis	3 gm IV after each dialysis

REFERENCES

Acred, P., Brown, O.M., Knudsen, E.T., Rolinson, G.N. and Sutherland, R. (1967) Nature, 215, 25-30.

Davies, M., Morgan, J.R. and Anand, C. (1974) Chemotherapy, 20, 339-341.

Hoffman, T.A., Cestero, R. and Bullock, W.E. (1970) Annals of Internal Medicine, 73, 173-178.

Neu, H.C. and Swarz, H. (1970) Journal of General Microbiology, 58, 301-305.

Neu, H.C. and Winshell, E.B. (1970) Antimicrobial Agents and Chemotherapy, 385-389.

Rodriguez, V., Bodey, G.P., Horikoshi, N., Inagaki, J. and McCredie, K.B. (1973) Antimicrobial Agents and Chemotherapy 4, 427-431.

Wise, R. and Reeves, D.S. (1974) Chemotherapy, 20, 45-51.

THE USE OF TICARCILLIN IN THE TREATMENT OF ACUTE URINARY TRACT INFECTIONS

H. David Short and Layne O. Gentry

Baylor College of Medicine

Houston, Texas, U.S.A.

Infections caused by gram negative bacteria have become an increasing cause of morbidity and mortality in hospitalised patients. The urinary tract is a common site from which serious infections can arise and disseminate to cause systemic infections. Infections of the urinary tract under these circumstances are commonly caused by hospital-acquired gram negative bacteria, many of which are resistant to frequently used antibiotics. Agents commonly used to treat these resistant organisms have potentially serious side effects, such as nephrotoxicity, ototoxicity, excessive salt loads and platelet abnormalities. In an effort to decrease these risks of side effects and to increase the effectiveness of such agents, research of newer antibiotics continues.

Ticarcillin is a new, braod spectrium, semi-synthetic penicillin. It has an antibacterial spectrum similar to that of carbenicillin, including Proteus, Escherichia, Enterobacter and Pseudomonas species. One distinct advantage of this compound over existing antibiotics is that it is more potent against many of these bacterial species (1). This report describes our studies of the efficacy and safety of this compound in serious urinary tract infections, including urinary tract infections in the pregnant patient.

MATERIALS AND METHODS

Patients in this study were referred from the Emergency Center or Obstetric Inpatient Service, Harris County Hospital District, Houston, Texas. Informed consent was obtained from all patients according to the guidelines of the Human Experimentation Committee, Baylor College of Medicine.

Urinary tract infection was confirmed by bacterial culture of bladder urine ($>10^5$ colonies/ml urine). A diagnosis of cystitis was made if there was dysuria, frequency and urgency present, and if a catheterised bladder urine sediment contained significant pyuria (>10 WBC/HPF). Pyelonephritis was the diagnosis if dysuria, frequency, urgency and flank pain were present, the urine culture was positive and if at least three of the following five findings were present: flank or abdominal tenderness; elevated temperature ($>101°F$); elevation of a peripheral WBC count ($>12,000$ WBC/mm^3); pyuria (>10 WBC/HPF); the presence of WBC or granular casts.

The dose of ticarcillin was determined according to the investigator's assessment of the clinical illness and ranged from 3 to 12 grams intramuscularly (IM) or intravenously (IV) per day in divided doses. All patients with suspected bacteremia were given IV medication.

The following laboratory data were obtained before, during and after ticarcillin: WBC count and differential, haemoglobin, haematocrit, BUN, creatinine, electrolytes, urinalysis, alkaline phosphatase, SGOT and bilirubin. Initially, platelet count and bleeding time were done routinely, however these were discontinued after no abnormalities were found. Urine cultures were done before, during and after completion of therapy.

Ticarcillin concentrations in serum and uring were measured using a bioassay system with Pseudomonas aeruginosa as the test organism.

Intravenous pyelography was performed when underlying abnormalities were suspected; none of the pregnant patients had pyelography.

RESULTS

A total of 25 patients, mean age 28 years (range 16-60) were treated in this study. The classification and aetiology of urinary tract infection in the 25 patients are illustrated in Figure 1. Sixteen patients had pyelonephritis, nine had cystitis. Escherichia coli was the isolate in 11 patients with pyelonephritis, two of whom had concurrent bacteremia, and in six patients with cystitis. Enterobacter aerogenes and Pseudomonas aeruginosa were responsible for pyelonephritis in two and three respective patients. Cystitis was caused by Pseudonomas aeruginosa in two patients and by Staphylococcus aureus in one patient. The staphylococcal infection occurred in a patient who had been known to use IV drugs and had been treated with an indwelling catheter.

Figure 1. TYPE OF URINARY INFECTION

Etiology	Type	
	Pyelonephritis	Cystitis
Escherichia coli	11	6
Enterobacter aerogenes	2	
Pseudomonas aeruginosa	3	2
Staphylococcus aureus		1
Total	16	9

*Concurrent bacteremia in 2 patients

The results of ticarcillin therapy in nine pregnant patients is tabulated in Figure 2. Four pregnant patients with pyelonephritis were successfully treated and had no relapse during their pregnancy. One pregnant patient with cystitis was also successfully treated. Relapse or re-infection with a similar organisms occurred in two pregnant patients with pyelonephritis, but both were successfully treated with a second course of ticarcillin. In two pregnant patients with pyelonephritis, therapy failed to eradicate infection caused by susceptible bacteria, and repeat sensitivity studies on day three revealed these organisms to be resistant to ticarcillin. Both patients were successfully treated with another antibiotic to which the organisms were susceptible. It was impossible to tell if these organisms were actually resistant to ticarcillin with erroneous sensitivity studies, or if a dual infection with one sensitive and one resistant strain was present. Another alternative mechanism is the emergence of antibiotic resistance during therapy, however without specific species identification this mechanism remains unproven.

Figure 2. TICARCILLIN THERAPY IN PREGNANCY

Number Patients	Type of Infection	Results
4	Pyelonephritis	Treated, no relapse*
1	Cystitis	Treated, no relapse*
1	Pyelonephritis	Relapse, same organism
1	Pyelonephritis	Re-infection, new organism
2	Pyelonephritis	Infection persisted, emergence of resistant strain
9		

* During this pregnancy

Figure 3. TICARCILLIN THERAPY IN NON-PREGNANT PATIENTS

Number Patients	Type of Infection	Complications	Results
3	Pyelonephritis	None	Treated, no relapse
7	Cystitis	None	Treated, no relapse
4	Pyelonephritis	Obstruction	Infection persisted, emergence of resistant strain
2	Cystitis	None	Relapse, same organism
16			

The results of ticarcillin therapy in non-pregnant patients is summarised in Figure 3. Three patients with pyelonephritis and no underlying complicating factors were successfully treated. Seven patients with cystitis also responded to ticarcillin therapy.

In four patients with pyelonephritis and urinary tract obstruction infection was never eradicated, and organisms sensitive to ticarcillin were replaced by resistant strains. Two patients had multiple relapses of cystitis caused by a similar strain of bacteria. Both patients had been recently married.

The side effects encountered in this study were minimal. The most common side effect was pain at IM injection site, however in none of these patients was the discomfort so severe that the midication had to be discontinued. One patient developed an elevated alkaline phosphatase and SGOT during therapy on a dose of 12 grams per day. These values returned to normal within seven days following discontinuation of ticarcillin.

Of the pregnant patients treated, five have delivered normal term infants. One patient delivered a low birth infant but he has subsequently done well. Three patients have not delivered to date.

DISCUSSION

Infections of the urinary tract are common, especially in young women of child bearing age. There is evidence of incidence of infection in working women as compared to nuns, thus suggesting that sexual intercourse is one contributing factor (2). Our study population was predominantly women of the child bearing age, but the true incidence of infection is unknown. Recurrent cystitis was associated with recent marriage in two of our patients also suggesting that sexual intercourse is a contributing factor. Anatomic abnormalities of the urinary tract have also been shown to predispose to urinary tract infections, and are frequently caused by the more uncommon gram negative bacteria. Upper urinary tract abnormalities in pregnant women occur after the first trimester, including vesicoureteral reflux (3).

We found pyelonephritis to be common during pregnancy as was relapsing infection following therapy suggesting that pyelonephritis during pregnancy is similar to infection encountered in patients with abnormal urinary tract anatomy.

The infrequent side effects noted in this study are consistent with other studies of carbenicillin. The one patient with abnormal liver function tests during ticarcillin therapy was also a frequent user of IV drugs, suggesting another possible etiology.

SUMMARY

Twenty-five patients including nine pregnant women were treated with parenteral ticarcillin for acute urinary tract infection caused by susceptible bacteria. Ten of these patients had either a persistence of infection, relapse or re-infection and four of these were pregnant. Of the remaining six non-pregnant patients in this group, four had underlying abnormalities of the urinary tract and pyelonephritis, the other two had recurrent cystitis. Pregnant patients had the highest recurrence rate. Of the pregnant patients six have delivered healthy babies althoug one was premature. Abnormal liver function tests were the only side effects noted in one patient, however this patient had a past history of drug abuse. No evidence of platelet abnormality caused by high dose ticarcillin therapy was noted. Ticarcillin appears to be an effective, safe antibiotic for treatment of acute urinary tract infections even during pregnancy.

REFERENCES

1. Bodey, G.P. and Deerhake, Beverly. (1971). Appl. Microbiol., 21, 61-65.
2. Stamey, T.A. Urinary Infections. The Williams and Wilkins Co., Baltimore, Maryland, 1972.
3. Heidrick, W.P., Mattingly, R.F. and Amberg, J.R. Obstet. Gynecol. (1967) 29, 571.

MICROBIOLOGY OF CARFECILLIN, THE α-PHENYL ESTER OF CARBENICILLIN

M. J. Basker and R. Sutherland

Beecham Pharmaceuticals Research Division

Brockham Park, Betchworth, Surrey, England

Carbenicillin (α-carboxybenzylpenicillin) is a broad spectrum penicillin active against a wide range of bacteria including _Pseudomonas aeruginosa_ and is widely used in the treatment of serious infections caused by pseudomonas or other Gram-negative bacilli. Carbenicillin is poorly absorbed by the oral route and is effective only after parenteral administration, but certain α-esters of the compound are absorbed after oral administration and undergo hydrolysis in the body to liberate carbenicillin (English et al, 1972; Clayton et al, 1975). This report describes the _in vitro_ activity of one such ester, carfecillin.

Carfecillin (Sodium α-phenoxycarbonylbenzylpenicillin) is the α-phenyl ester of carbenicillin (Fig. 1) and since the ester group is in the side chain, the compound possesses a free carboxyl group in the C_3 position of the thiazolidine ring and can be expected to demonstrate antibacterial activity _per se_ unlike those penicillin esters where the ester group is in the thiazolidine ring. In aqueous solutions the rate of hydrolysis of carfecillin to carbenicillin is dependent on the pH value of the solution. Thus at pH 8.0, the $\frac{1}{2}$ life of carfecillin at 37°C at a concentration of 100μg/ml was 90 minutes, increasing to 150 minutes at pH 7.4, and to greater than 10 hours at pH 6.5. In nutrient broth, pH 7.4, the rate of hydrolysis was similar to that in buffer, pH 7.4. In contrast, the rate of hydrolysis of carfecillin to carbenicillin in human serum was much more rapid ($\frac{1}{2}$ life about 10 minutes) under the same experimental conditions. As a result of the activity of non-specific esterases present in serum and tissues carfecillin is hydrolised very readily to carbenicillin and so the activity of carfecillin in the clinical situation is entirely that of carbenicillin.

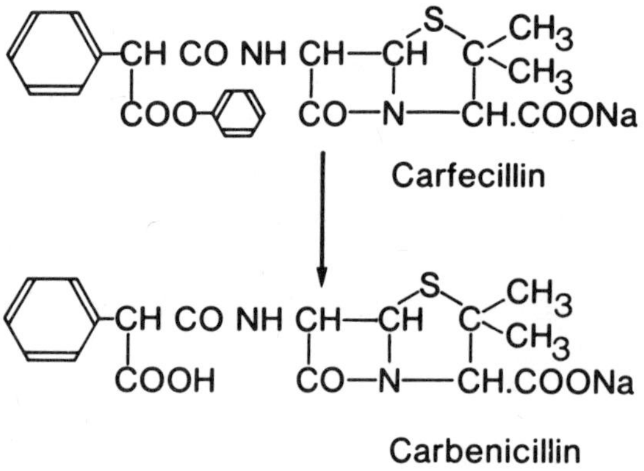

FIG. 1. Structure of carfecillin
(Sodium α-phenoxycarbonylbenzylpenicillin)

In tests *in vitro* for the measurement of antibacterial activity, the activity shown by carfecillin will depend, therefore, upon the extent to which hydrolysis to carbenicillin takes place. In general, conditions are more favourable for hydrolysis to carbenicillin in agar-dilution tests to measure Minimum Inhibitory Concentrations than in tests in liquid media. Against Gram-negative bacilli the Minimum Inhibitory Concentrations of carfecillin were generally about the same as, or slightly higher than, those of carbenicillin, but Klebsiella aerogenes was slightly more sensitive to carfecillin (Table 1). Against Gram-positive cocci, on the other hand, carfecillin was generally rather more active than carbenicillin. For example, carfecillin was twice as active as carbenicillin against penicillin-sensitive staphylococci and β-haemolytic streptococci, and 5 times more active against pneumococci and enterococci. However, results against the penicillin-resistant strain of Staphylococcus aureus suggest that carfecillin is less stable to staphylococcal penicillinase than is carbenicillin.

In the presence of serum the activity of carfecillin becomes that of carbenicillin as might be expected from the rapid rate of hydrolysis of carfecillin to carbenicillin in serum. This is illustrated by the results shown in Table 2 where it can be seen that in nutrient broth carfecillin was less active than carbenicillin against Ps. aeruginosa and more active than the latter against Staph. aureus, but in human serum the activities shown by the two compounds were the same.

Differences in activities of carfecillin and carbenicillin may be demonstrated more clearly in agar diffusion tests used for

TABLE 1. Minimum Inhibitory Concentrations of carfecillin and carbenicillin

MIC (µg/ml)

Organism	Carfecillin	Carbenicillin
E. coli	5.0	2.5
P. mirabilis	2.5	1.25
P. morganii	5.0	5.0
Ps. aeruginosa	50	25
K. aerogenes	125	250
Enterobacter sp.	12.5	5.0
Ser. marcescens	12.5	5.0
S. aureus	0.25	0.5
S. aureus+	125	25
Str. pyogenes	0.05	0.1
Str. pneumoniae	0.05	0.25
Str. faecalis	5.0	2.5

+ β-lactamase producing strain

TABLE 2. Minimum Inhibitory Concentrations of carfecillin and carbenicillin in the presence of serum

Organism	Medium	Carfecillin	Carbenicillin
Staph. aureus	nut. broth	0.25	1.0
	serum*	1.0	1.0
Pseudomonas aeruginosa	nut. broth	125	50
	serum	50	50

* 95% human serum

microbiological assays. Against <u>Ps. aeruginosa</u> NCTC 10701, a strain used for the assay of carbenicillin, an aqueous solution (pH 6.0) of carfecillin was about one fifth as potent as carbenicillin (Fig. 2), but in human serum the carfecillin standard line was the same as that of the carbenicillin standard line as a result of the rapid rate of hydrolysis to carbenicillin. In contrast, against <u>Sarcina lutea</u> NCTC 8340, a penicillin assay organism, carfecillin was from 10 to 20 times more potent than carbenicillin.

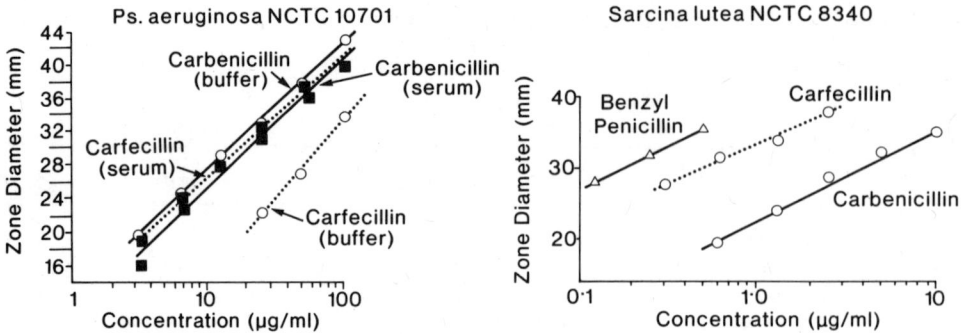

FIG. 2. Relative potencies of carfecillin and carbenicillin in microbiological assays against Ps. aeruginosa NCTC 10701 and Sarcina lutea NCTC 8340.

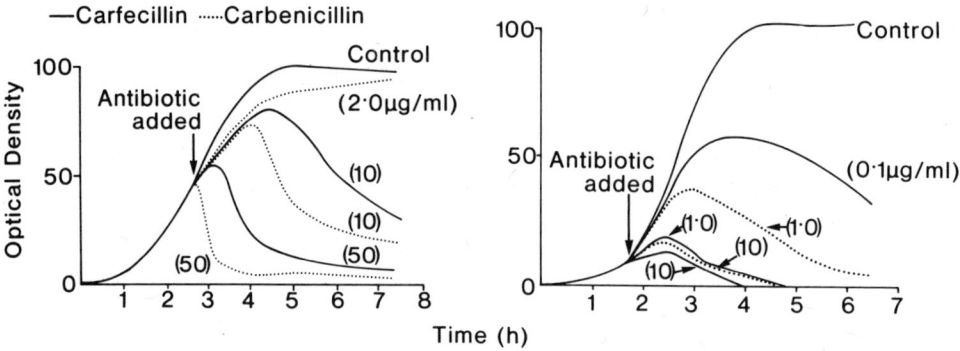

FIG. 3. Bacteriolytic activities of carfecillin and carbenicillin against E. coli (JT1) and S. aureus (Oxford)

A similar pattern emerged when the relative activities of carfecillin and carbenicillin were compared using a Bonet Maury Biophotometer continuous growth recorder. For instance, against a strain of E. coli (JT1) carbenicillin was more active than carfecillin as shown by the more rapid kill of carbenicillin compared with that of carfecillin (Fig. 3). However, against S. aureus (Oxford) the results were reversed and carfecillin produced a more rapid bacteriolytic effect than did carbenicillin (Fig. 3).

In conclusion, it is evident that carfecillin demonstrates an intrinsic antibacterial activity *in vitro* and is more active than carbenicillin against most Gram-positive cocci, but less active than the latter against Gram-negative bacilli. However, as carfecillin hydrolyses quite readily to carbenicillin in tests for antibacterial activity, the activity shown by carfecillin *in vitro* will be that of a mixture of carbenicillin and unhydrolysed ester, depending upon the extent to which hydrolysis takes place under the conditions of the test system. In the presence of serum or other body tissues, however, carfecillin is hydrolysed rapidly by non-specific esterases to carbenicillin and the activity shown in serum is entirely that of carbenicillin as is the case in the clinical condition (Wilkinson et al., 1975).

REFERENCES

Clayton, J. P., Cole, M., Elson, S. W., Hardy, K. D., Mizen, L. W., and Sutherland, R. 1975. J. Med. Chem., *18*, 172.

English, A. R., Retsema, J. A., Ray, V. A., and Lynch, J. G. 1972. Antimicrob. Ag. Chemother., *1*, 185.

Wilkinson, P. J., Reeves, D. S., Wise, R., and Allen, J. T. 1975. Brit. Med. J., *2*, 250.

We thank Dr. M. Cole for providing hydrolysis data.

CHEMOTHERAPEUTIC ACTIVITY OF CARFECILLIN, THE α-PHENYL ESTER OF CARBENICILLIN, IN THE TREATMENT OF EXPERIMENTAL MOUSE INFECTIONS.

K. R. Comber and G. Valler

Beecham Pharmaceuticals Research Division

Brockham Park, Betchworth, Surrey, England

SUMMARY

Carfecillin, the α-phenyl ester of carbenicillin was well absorbed after oral administration to infected and uninfected mice producing significant blood concentrations of carbenicillin whereas carbenicillin generally failed to produce detectable levels in mice by the oral route. Carfecillin showed activity of the same order as parenteral carbenicillin in the treatment of various intraperitoneal infections in mice including infections caused by certain ampicillin-resistant bacteria. Carfecillin was also effective in the treatment of experimental pyelonephritis in mice and was as active as parenteral carbenicillin in the treatment of renal infections caused by Pseudomonas aeruginosa and Escherichia coli.

Carbenicillin is widely used in the treatment of infections due to Gram-negative bacilli including Pseudomonas aeruginosa and other antibiotic-resistant bacteria (indole-positive Proteus, Serratia marcescens, Providencia) but the compound is poorly absorbed by the oral route and must be administered by injection. However, certain α-esters of carbenicillin have been shown to be absorbed after oral administration to animals or man, and to be hydrolysed rapidly in vivo to liberate carbenicillin (English et al, 1972, Clayton et al, 1975). This report describes the activity of one such ester, carfecillin, the α-phenyl ester of carbenicillin, in the treatment of experimental mouse infections.

METHODS

Intraperitoneal mouse infections. Albino mice (18-22g) were infected intraperitoneally with 0.5ml of a suspension of the test organism diluted in hog gastric mucin to give an infective inoculum of between 100 to 1000 Median Lethal Doses. In most tests the penicillins were administered as a single dose (0.2ml/20g) to groups of 5 or 10 mice immediately after infection, but in tests with Ps. aeruginosa the compounds were administered as divided doses at 0,2,4 and 6 hours after infection. The number of animals surviving 4 days after infection were recorded.

Experimental Pyelonephritis. Mice were infected intravenously with 0.2ml of a suitable dilution of the test organism in veal infusion broth, and the renal virulence of the bacteria was enhanced by intramuscular administration of 30mg/kg iron sorbitol citrate (Jectofer, Astra Chemicals Ltd) once a day for 4 days starting 18 hours after infection. Treatment with the penicillins started 24 hours after infection and continued 4 times a day at 2 hourly intervals for 4 days starting 18 hours after infection. Groups of 5 mice were killed at intervals after infection, the kidneys were removed and examined macroscopically and viable counts made of homogenates of the kidneys.

Oral absorption studies. Uninfected mice, and mice infected intraperitoneally with E. coli were dosed by the oral route with 0.2ml volumes of the penicillins. Groups of 5 mice were killed by cervical dislocation at intervals after dosing, blood was collected from the axillary region and the heparinised specimens were assayed microbiologically by large plate agar diffusion with Ps. aeruginosa NCTC 10701 as assay organism.

RESULTS AND DISCUSSION

Absorption studies. Results in Fig. 1 show the blood levels obtained in infected and uninfected mice with single oral doses of carfecillin, and for comparison values obtained with a single oral dose of ampicillin in uninfected mice are also presented. In general, carfecillin was well absorbed and mean peak carbenicillin blood concentrations of 17µg/ml were measured 5 minutes after an oral dose of 100mg carfecillin/kg and 22µg/ml at 20 minutes after a dose of 400mg carfecillin/kg to uninfected mice. Carfecillin was well absorbed in comparison with ampicillin and the antibiotic blood concentrations produced by the dose of 100mg carfecillin/kg were markedly higher than the levels obtained with 200mg ampicillin/kg. It is of interest that the absorption of carfecillin appeared to be delayed in mice infected intraperitoneally with Escherichia coli but the peak blood levels were notably higher in the infected animals (36µg/ml) than in uninfected animals (22µg/ml). A single oral dose of carbenicillin (400mg/kg) generally failed to produce detectable levels in the blood of infected mice, but at a dose of 1000mg carbenicillin/kg variable levels were measured in about 50% of the animals.

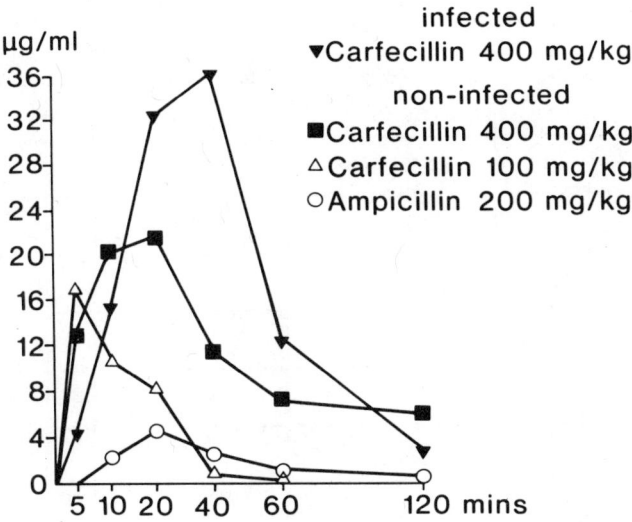

FIG. 1. Concentrations of Carbenicillin and Ampicillin in blood after oral administration in mice
▲——▲ Carfecillin 100mg/kg non-infected mice
■——■ Carfecillin 400mg/kg non-infected mice
▼——▼ Carfecillin 400mg/kg infected mice
●——● Ampicillin 200mg/kg non-infected mice

Intraperitoneal infections. The results of the mouse protection tests are shown in Table 1 where the activity of a single oral dose of carfecillin is compared with that of a single dose of carbenicillin given orally or by subcutaneous injection. In general, carfecillin showed activity of about the same order as subcutaneous carbenicillin and was distinctly more active than oral carbenicillin against Gram-negative bacilli. Against the Gram-positive cocci orally-administered carbenicillin showed activity about the same as that of carfecillin and this might have been due to the presence of benzylpenicillin in the carbenicillin, as the staphylococcus and streptococcus used were very sensitive to benzylpenicillin. Similarly, there was no significant difference in the activity of oral carfecillin or parenteral carbenicillin against infections due to Pseudomonas aeruginosa (Table 1). Oral carbenicillin was ineffective (CD/50 >1000mg/kg) against these pseudomonas infections. Carfecillin was also as active as parenteral carbenicillin in the treatment of infections

TABLE 1. Relative activities of carfecillin and carbenicillin against intraperitoneal mouse infections

Organism	Carbenicillin MIC (μg/ml)	CD/50 mg/kg		
		Carfecillin	Carbenicillin	
		Oral	Oral	Subcut.
E. coli (8)	25	374	>1000	125
E. coli (9)	5.0	110	>400	230
Salm. typhimurium (10)	2.5	187	490	130
P. mirabilis (13)	2.5	56	200	80
K. edwardsii (18)	12.5	97	300	115
Ser. marcescens (US1)	12.5	53	210	100
S. aureus (Smith)	1.25	13	19	4
S. pyogenes (CN10)	0.25	100	120	88
Ps. aeruginosa (11)	50	580 600	>4000	400 208
Ps. aeruginosa (30)	50	155 194	>4000	30 155

TABLE 2. Relative activities of carfecillin, carbenicillin and ampicillin against intraperitoneal infections due to certain ampicillin resistant organisms

Organism	Median Curative Dose (CD/50) mg/kg		
	Carfecillin (Oral)	Carbenicillin (Subcut.)	Ampicillin (Oral)
E. coli (415)	75	70	>1000
E. coli (487)	240	100	>1000
Prot. morganii (14)	31	33	>1000

* Carbenicillin was ineffective by the oral route (CD/50 >1000mg/kg)

caused by two ampicillin-resistant strains of E. coli and by a strain of Proteus morganii (Table 2). Ampicillin and oral carbenicillin were ineffective against these infections.

Experimental pyelonephritis. Carfecillin was as effective by the oral route as subcutaneous carbenicillin in the treatment of experimental pyelonephritis in mice caused by Ps. aeruginosa and an ampicillin-resistant strain of E. coli (Figs. 2 and 3) as judged by reduction in the numbers of macroscopic abscesses observed in the kidney and in the viable counts of the bacteria recovered from kidney homogenates. In these tests carbenicillin was relatively ineffective by the oral route against the pseudomonas and E. coli infections and ampicillin showed poor efficacy in the treatment of the infection due to E. coli.

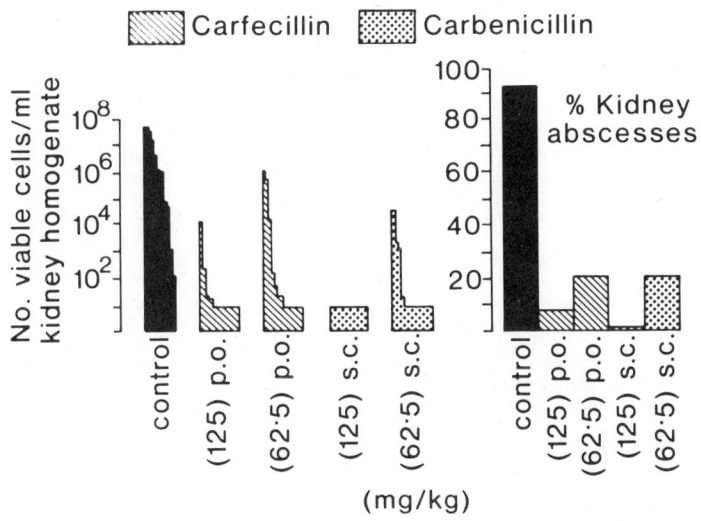

FIG. 2. Activity of carfecillin and carbenicillin against Pseudomonas aeruginosa in an experimental pyelonephritis model.

The results of these chemotherapeutic tests reported here show that carfecillin is well absorbed after oral administration to infected mice and confirm that the levels of carbenicillin liberated in the animal are adequate for the treatment of infection. These findings are in keeping with the results of clinical trials in man which showed that carfecillin was effective in the treatment of clinical infection (Wilkinson et al, 1975; Lees and Harding, 1974).

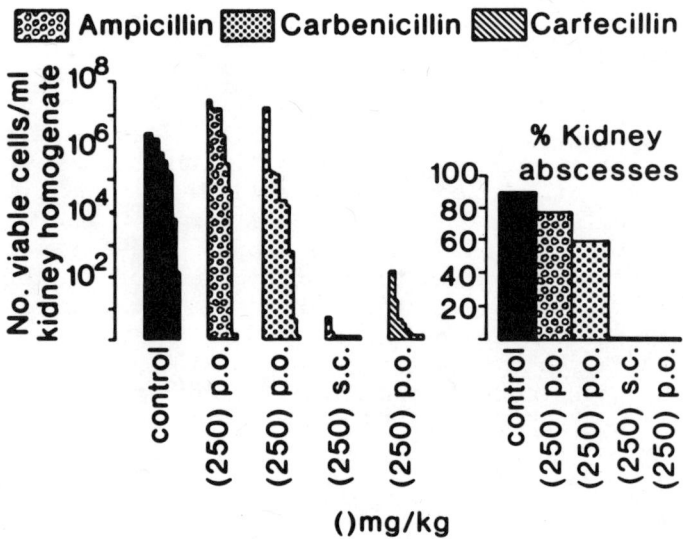

Fig. 3. Activity of carfecillin, carbenicillin and ampicillin against *Escherichia coli* JT415 in an experimental pyelonephritis model.

REFERENCES

Clayton, J. P., Cole, M., Elson, S. W., Hardy, K. D., Mizen, L. W. and Sutherland, R. (1975). J.Med.Chem., 18, 172.

English, A. R., Retsema, J. A., Ray, V. A. and Lynch, J. E. (1972). Antimicrob.Ag.Chemother., 1, 185.

Wilkinson, P. J., Reeves, D. S., Wise, R. and Allen, J. T. (1975). Brit.Med.J., 2, 250.

Lees, L. J. and Harding, J. M. (1974). Brit.J.Clin.Pract., 28, 349.

PHARMACOLOGICAL AND CLINICAL STUDIES WITH CARFECILLIN, AN ORALLY ADMINISTERED ESTER OF CARBENICILLIN

P.J. WILKINSON,* D.S. REEVES AND R. WISE

DEPARTMENT OF MEDICAL MICROBIOLOGY

SOUTHMEAD HOSPITAL, BRISTOL, BS10 5NB, ENGLAND

Carfecillin (Uticillin, Beecham Pharmaceuticals) is the phenyl ester of carbenicillin. The substitution of a phenyl group on the active side-chain enhances oral absorption, after which hydrolysis in the intestinal mucosa releases free carbenicillin into the circulation. The tablets of carfecillin now available commercially have been shown by Jones K.H. (1974) in healthy volunteers to give mean peak serum levels which are 37% better and 15 minutes earlier than those obtained from the formulation in gelatin capsules which was used throughout this series of studies. Details of method will not be given here, but are described elsewhere (Wilkinson P.J. et al., 1975).

VOLUNTEER STUDY

We first measured serum levels (Fig.1) in ten healthy volunteers after a single oral dose of carfecillin. The dose was 500 mg in four cases, equivalent to 397 mg of carbenicillin free acid, and 1000 mg in six cases, equivalent to 794 mg of free acid. Considerable individual variation was found but the larger dose gave the higher mean peak serum level of 5.5 µg/ml at 105 minutes, compared with 3.4 µg/ml at 90 minutes with the smaller dose. Four of these subjects continued to take carfecillin at 8-hourly intervals over the next four days and a higher mean peak up to 10 µg/ml was found on the larger dose regimen on day 2, but no further increase was apparent on day 4 (Fig.2). It was obvious that doses of this order would be inadequate for the treatment of systemic infections with Pseudomonas spp., or any but the most sensitive organisms.

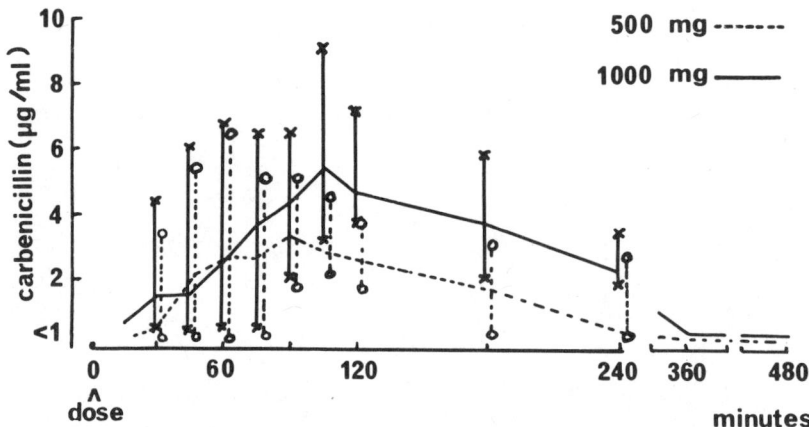

Fig.1 Mean serum levels (and ranges) of carbenicillin after single oral doses of carfecillin in ten healthy volunteers.

Four patients in severe renal failure (creatinine clearance ≤2.2 ml/min) were then given three doses of carfecillin 1000 mg at 4-hourly intervals to see if higher serum levels could be achieved in this situation (Fig.3). Considerably higher levels of up to 50 µg/ml were obtained by twelve hours, but a plateau seemed to be reached by this time and these levels still appeared inadequate for systemic antipseudomonal therapy.

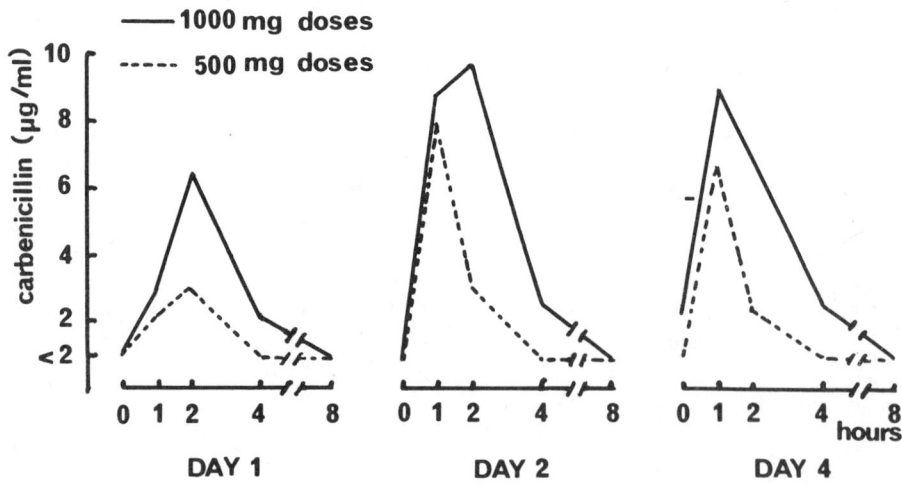

Fig.2 Mean serum levels of carbenicillin after 8-hourly oral doses of carfecillin in 4 healthy volunteers. Samples after dose at 0800 hours.

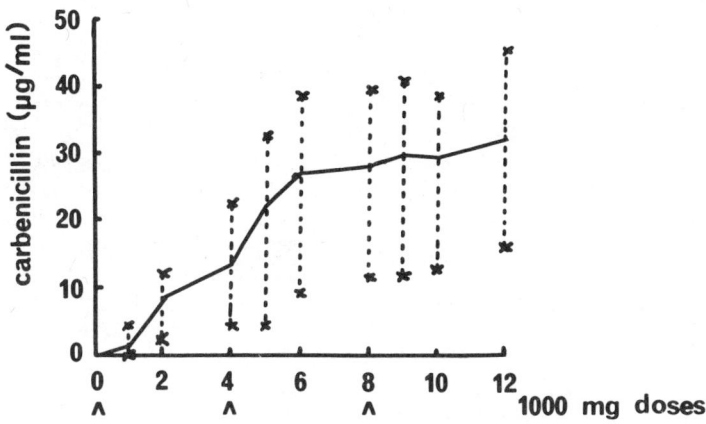

Fig.3 Mean serum levels (and ranges) of carbenicillin after oral doses of carfecillin in four volunteers in renal failure.

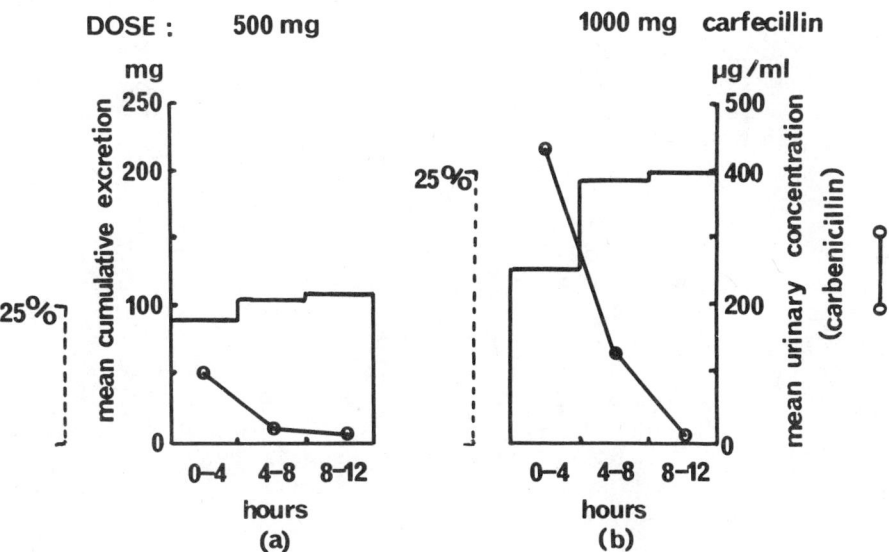

Fig.4 Urinary carbenicillin after single oral doses of carfecillin in ten healthy volunteers.

Urinary concentrations after a single dose of 500 mg of carfecillin (Fig.4a) were considered too low (mean peak 112 µg/ml in the first four hours) for treatment of urinary tract infections with <u>Pseudomonas</u>, but adequate after 1000 mg (Fig.4b) where a mean peak of 434 µg/ml was obtained in the same period. In all cases, about 25% of the administered drug was recovered in the urine. The urinary recovery in subjects receiving multiple doses was of the same order. Of the patients in renal failure, two were anuric, 1 had no detectable antibiotic in his urine, and 1 had a mean level of 49 µg/ml in a 12-hour collection. These results suggested that carfecillin in the larger dose might be expected to be an effective treatment of urinary infection with <u>Pseudomonas</u> spp., except in severe renal failure.

CLINICAL TRIAL

It was decided therefore to embark on a clinical trial of carfecillin at a dosage of 1000 mg 8-hourly for 7 days, treating urinary infections in hospital patients. 35 patients were treated in this way, having a mean age of 68.7 years (range 24-85) and a male:female ratio of 24:11. The criteria for inclusion in the trial were
1. Informed consent.
2. Two consecutive isolates of the same organism in pure growth and significant numbers ($>10^5$/ml) from mid-stream urinary specimens, or a single specimen taken from a catheter.
3. Sensitivity of isolate to carbenicillin by disc test.
4. Patient aged 16 or more and not pregnant.
5. No history of penicillin allergy.

The criteria of cure were bacteriological, namely failure to culture the initial isolate from the urine at 14 and 42 days after beginning treatment, whether or not infection with a different organism had occurred. The cure rate for all infections was 60% (21 cases out of 35), but was slightly higher for infections with <u>Pseudomonas</u> at 67% (8 out of 12). This was considered satisfactory in a relatively elderly and difficult group of hospital patients with a high incidence of urinary tract disease, and was particularly satisfactory in the difficult infections with <u>Pseudomonas spp</u>. The results of treatment are summarised in the Table, which gives details of the failures of treatment.

Serum levels were measured at 1 and 2 hours after the first dose of carfecillin in 18 of the patients (Fig.5), and were more variable than those of the volunteers, but of the same order of magnitude. The differences between the patients with moderate renal impairment (creatinine clearance less than 40 ml/min) and the remainder was not statistically significant.

Table: Details of Failures of Treatment

Infecting Organism	No.	Failed treatment	MIC (µg/ml) of carbenicillin for infecting organism	Primary and contributory pathologies in failures (if present)
Ps. aeruginosa	12	4	16.0 16.0 64.0 128.0	a) carcinoma of bladder b) benign prostatic hypertrophy c) chronic functional bladder hypotonia with persistent residual urine d) urethral stricture, peri-urethral abscess.
Esch. coli	9	6	10.0 0.25 1.0 8.0 4.0 1.0	a) carcinoma of colon (operated on last day of course of carfecillin) b) megaloblastic anaemia; female patient aged 82 c) prostatic hypertrophy d) prostatic hypertrophy e) prostatic hypertrophy f) ischaemic heart disease, female patient aged 75 yrs.
Proteus mirabilis	4	3	0.25 16.0 0.125	a) prostatic hypertrophy b) prostatic hypertrophy c) carcinoma of bladder
Staph. aureus	2	1	8.0	prostatic hypertrophy
Other	8	0	-	-

Satisfactory urinary concentrations were found in patients of both groups (Fig. 6), though no patient in our series had a creatinine clearance of less than 10 ml/minute and it is at such low levels that urinary excretion of carbenicillin is unlikely to be adequate for therapy of urinary tract infection.

TOXICOLOGY AND TOLERABILITY

The drug was remarkably well tolerated by patients and volunteers alike and in no case had its administration to be stopped. One healthy volunteer and two patients had mild diarrhoea but no

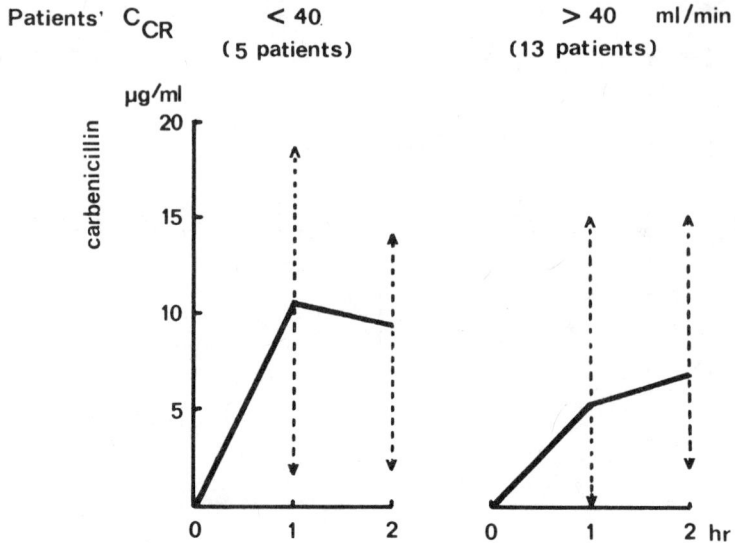

Fig.5 Serum carbenicillin levels in the two hours following the first dose of 1000 mg of carfecillin in 18 patients in relation to creatinine clearance (C_{CR}).

rashes, nausea or other side-effects were found. A comprehensive range of haematological and biochemical parameters were monitored before and after carfecillin and in no cases could any changes in these parameters be attributed to the drug. No free phenol was detected in the blood of any volunteer.

In a difficult group of patients, therefore, with a high incidence of severe urinary tract pathology, the cure rate obtained with carfecillin is considered to be satisfactory. Higher rates have been claimed in patients treated in general practice (Lees and Harding, 1974). For infections with Pseudomonas aeruginosa, it offers an oral treatment allowing domiciliary management of such patients with a saving in both cost and morbidity. Indeed, one paraplegic patient in our trial (Reeves, 1974) with multiple myeloma, vertebral collapse, a neurogenic bladder and staghorn renal calculi was successfully treated at home over a period of 1 year for successive recurrences of Pseudomonas urinary infection accompanied by pyrexia and rigors. The quality of his life was greatly improved in that he was spared the frequent hospital admissions to which he had grown accustomed and was able to remain at work for most of this period.

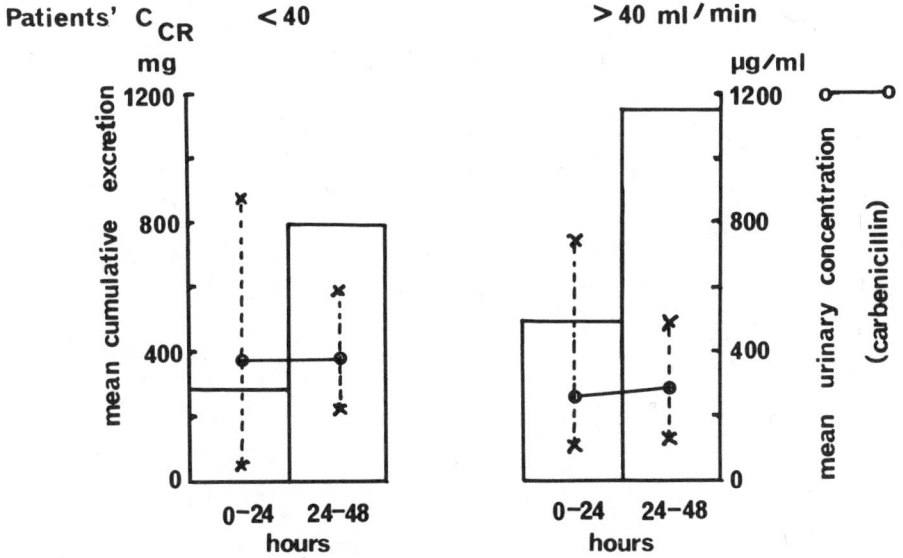

Fig.6 Urinary carbenicillin during the first 48 hours of treatment with oral carfecillin (1g. 8-hourly) in patients, in relation to creatinine clearance (C_{CR})

REFERENCES

1. Jones, K.H. (1974). Personal communication.
2. Wilkinson, P.J., D.S. Reeves, R. Wise and J.T. Allen (1975). Brit. med. J. 2, 250-252.
3. Lees, L.J. and Harding, J.W. (1974). Brit. J. clin. Pract. 28, 349-352.
4. Reeves, D.S. (1974). Brit. med. J. 4, 718-719.

DETERMINATION OF INDANYL CARBENICILLIN IN URINE WITH BLOOD

M. PINA DE CARVALHO   A. MATOS FERREIRA

Dept. Clinical Pathology   Urology Unit

Government Hospitals of Lisbon - Hospital do Rego

In a previous study the Authors[1] evaluated the efficacy of indanyl carbenicillin in patients with urinary tract infections which had been divided into two groups - one with acidification and the other with alkalinization of the urine.

The concentration of indanyl carbenicillin in some of the urine samples (determined by the plate diffusion technique) was practically nil and, as hematuria was found in two thirds of those samples, it was suspected that the presence of blood might interfere with the assessment of the urinary concentration of the drug.

MATERIALS AND METHODS

The study was performed with seven healthy, adult volunteers. The dose of 1 gr of indanyl carbenicillin was administered to the fasting volunteers and the urine was collected 0-4 and 4-8 hours after the oral intake of the drug.

Urinalysis was performed on all the samples collected. The pH values varied from 5.0 to 7.0 and glucose, ketone, protein or hemoglobin tests were negative in all of them.

Heparinized blood was added to the urine samples in amounts of 0.5 ml, 0.2 ml and 0.1 ml of blood per 100 ml of urine.

The technique used was the plate diffusion test (Wellcotest medium sensitivity test agar) and the standard strain was Pseudomonas aeruginosa - Elsworth NCTC-10701.

The inoculation of the plates was done with a swab following the Felmingham and Stokes[2] technique.

The samples were let to dry at the temperature of 37º during one hour and then four cylinders were placed in each plate; one cylinder filled with pure urine and the other three with samples of urine containing blood in the referred proportions.

The inhibition zones were compared with those obtained with successive dilutions of indanyl carbenicillin, using the same method and the same standard strain, in order to measure the urinary concentrations of the drug.

Furthermore, the inhibition zones were compared among themselves in order to evaluate the influence that the blood might have in the urine samples.

RESULTS

The urinary concentrations of indanyl carbenicillin varied between 150 µg and 1,200 µg per ml, the results agreeing with the values obtained by other authors (Butler et al[3]; Turck[4].

The differences in the inhibition zone sizes obtained with the pure urine and with the samples to which blood was added in the concentrations of 0.5 ml, 0.2 ml and 0.1 ml per 100 ml of urine were not significant.

DISCUSSION

In a study on urologic patients with urinary tract infections under treatment with indanyl carbenicillin, some of the samples had concentrations less than 2.5 µg/ml. About two thirds of these samples were hematuric, so it was thought that the presence of blood would inhibit the drug.

The addition of blood to the urine of volunteers to whom indanyl carbenicillin was administered did not influence the M.I.C. of the drug.

As all the urine in the first study[1] was heavily infected, production of carbenicillinase by the infecting strain could be responsible for the nil results.

CONCLUSIONS

In the present study, the addition of blood in different concentrations to the urine of subjects to whom indanyl carbenicillin was administered, did not change the inhibition zones obtained by the plate diffusion method.

BIBLIOGRAPHY

(1) MATOS FERREIRA, A.; CALAIS DA SILVA, F.E.; ROCHA MENDES, J. and PINA DE CARVALHO, M.: Indanyl Carbenicillin in Urinary Tract Infections. Influence of Urine pH. Acta Therapeutica 1(1):49-58, 1975.

(2) FELMINGHAM, D. and STOKES, E.J. (1972), Med. Lab. Technol. 29-198.

(3) BUTLER, K.; ENGLISH, A.R.; KNIRSCH, A.K.; KORST, J.J.: Metabolism and Laboratory Studies with Indanyl Carbenicillin; Delaware Medical J. 43:366, 1971.

(4) TURCK, M.: The Treatment of Urinary Tract Infections with an Oral Carbenicillin; J. Inf. Dis. 127 (Suppl.) 133, 1973.

IN VITRO ACTIVITY AND CLINICAL USE OF INDANYL CARBENICILLIN

G. Fontana and M. Laudi

Urological Department

Ospedale Maggiore di Torino, Italy

During the sixties, Staphylococcus undoubtedly held the rôle of "captain of men of death", as it was defined in a 1956 New England Journal of Medicine editorial. Examining the worldwide medical literature of the seventies, it can be considered that at present its place has been taken by Schizomycetes having low potential virulence, with the front line occupied by Gram-negative germs, among them the microorganisms of the normal intestinal flora or of other regions (respiratory, urogenital, etc.)

We know that these Schizomycetes are sufficiently "supervised" by the normal cellular and humoral factors of organic defense as also by the biological equilibrium of their natural habitat. Nonetheless, when the organic defenses do not appear very valid (newborns, prematures) or are impaired (severe burns, subjects wasted by cancer, patients undergoing immunodepressant treatment), and also when the biological equilibrium is altered by the uncontrolled and indiscriminate use of chemoantibiotics, these microorganisms take on a pathogenic guise and rank, so that it is correct to define them "opportunistic pathogens".

Numerous other eventualities can lead to an infection sustained by this type of microorganisms; in the urological field, it is enough to mention the endoscopic maneuvers which are effected with increasing frequency in diagnostic and therapeutic practice. In this case, obviously, the infection can also be exogenous but always with germs that owing to their great environmental diffusion, abundantly contaminate the instruments used.

Precisely in urology, Pseudomonas aeruginosa and numerous Enterobacteriaceae (coliforms, Proteus) are the "opportunistic pathogens" most frequently encountered.

Their common inheritance is the resistance to the chemoantibiotics, so that the introduction into clinical medicine of a new compound active on these Schizomycetes is always extremely interesting. In this sense, carbenicillin (alpha-carboxybenzylpenicillin) is certainly not a recent acquisition; as a matter of fact, its very low toxicity, the high blood and especially urine levels obtainable with it, and its activity against Pseudomonas aeruginosa, all the Proteus species and Escherichia coli have been known since 1967 (Acred et al 1967, Rolinson and Sutherland 1967, Robinson 1967, Brumfitt et al 1967, Knudsen et al 1967).

Nevertheless, this is a chemically unstable substance which is rapidly modified by acids, and therefore by the gastric juice (Renzini and Ferri 1974), and consequently poorly absorbed from the intestinal tract (Butler et al 1970).

The indanyl ester in position 5 of carbenicillin, chosen from among many analogues obtained in the Pfizer laboratories, constitutes an acid-stable carbenicillin derivative which is rapidly absorbed after oral administration (Butler et al 1973, Butler 1973). This compound is hydrolyzed, after absorption from the gastrointestinal tract, to metabolites of 5-indanol and carbenicillin which therefore constitutes the active principle.

The flourishing literature on this new antibiotic demonstrates the interest it has aroused in those who daily find themselves faced with the not easy problem of the therapy of infections from opportunistic pathogens of the above-mentioned strains (English et al 1972, Kayser et al 1973, Mioli and Tarchini 1973, Bastian and Bruhl 1973, Garcia Rodriguez et al 1974). Following this study line, our group of the Ospedale Maggiore di Torino Urological Department wished to put forward its experience on the use of indanyl carbenicillin, in the conviction that every antibiotic substance must be evaluated not only from the data already assumed but also and above all from the results obtained personally on the bacterial flora in one's hospital.

MATERIALS AND METHODS

The experimentation was conducted in vitro and in vivo. In vitro, with the collaboration of Dr. Savoia Dianella at the Istituto di Microbiologia dell'Università di Torino, indanyl carbenicillin's action was tested on 44 Gram-negative Schizomycetes strains some of which were isolated and some of which kept at the Institute.

The method used was that of determining the MIC in liquid culture medium (Grove and Randall 1955). In vivo, the antibiotic was administered to 40 patients from our Urological Department, in whom the clinical and laboratory data revealed the existence of an infectious process sustained by the bacterial strains already mentioned.

RESULTS

In tables 1, 2 and 3 are given the results of the in vitro susceptibility trials that were carried out with the serial dilutions method in a liquid medium on: 18 Pseudomonas aeruginosa strains, 16 indole-positive Proteus strains and 10 Proteus mirabilis strains (of which 2 penicillinase-producing strains).

Table 1
Susceptibility to indanyl carbenicillin of:

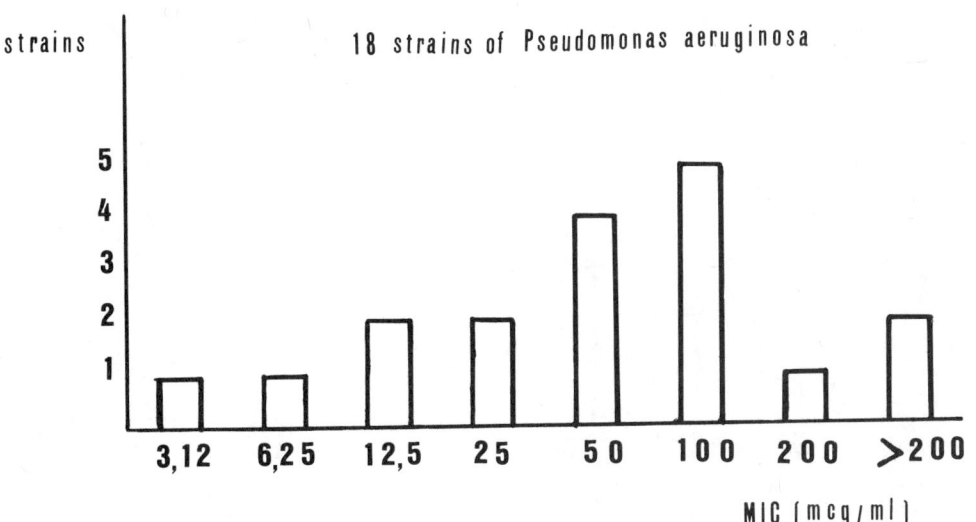

Table 2
Susceptibility to indanyl carbenicillin of:

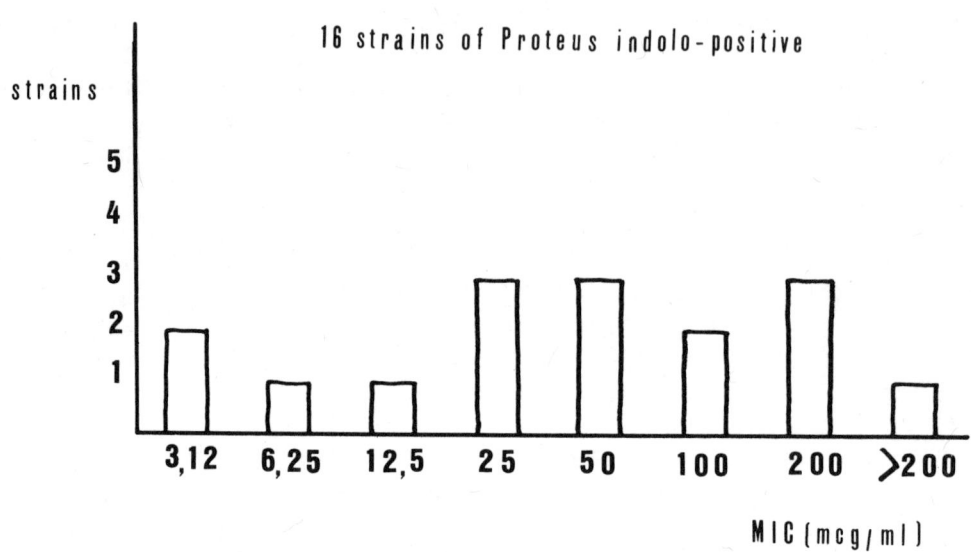

Table 3
Susceptibility to indanyl carbenicillin of:

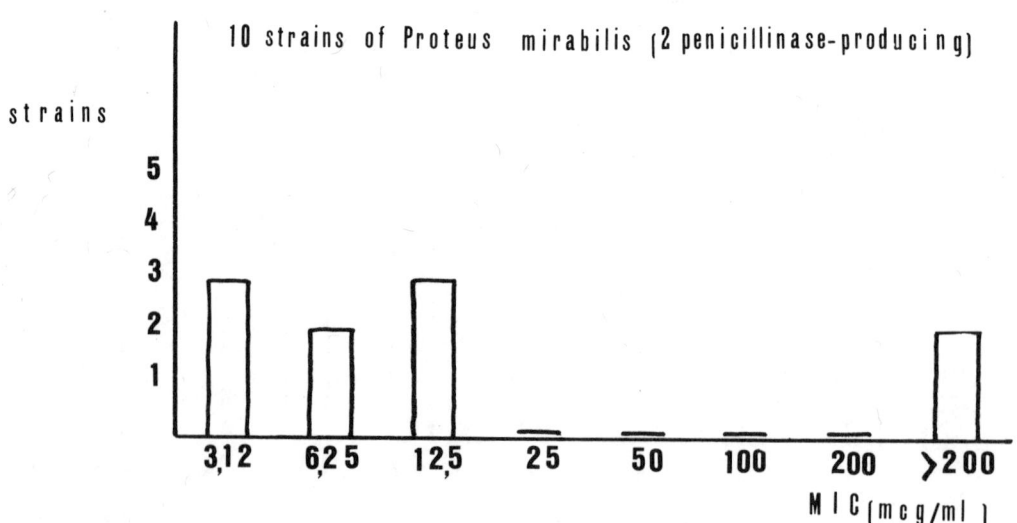

The clinical investigation was conducted in 40 patients whose age varied from 20 to 84 years; the 32 males and 8 females presented the following nosological distribution:

- renal neoplasia (with a septic picture)   5 patients
- lithiasic hydropyonephrosis   6 patients
- cystopyelitis   5 patients
- vesical neoplasia (with cystitic process)   10 patients
- adenoma of the prostate (with inflammatory complications)   8 patients
- carcinoma of the prostate (with inflammatory complications)   6 patients

Indanyl carbenicillin was administered to the patients admitted to the trial in the average dose of 6 tablets a day (each tablet is dosed at 500 mg equal to 382 mg of carbenicillin base) for a period of 9 days.

The following parameters were taken into consideration to evaluate the drug's therapeutic effectiveness: thermic curve, subjective urination symptomatology (strangury, pollakiuria and dysuria), septic urinary picture.

Moreover, the product's eventual side effects were evaluated both from a subjective viewpoint and by means of the observation of the more important hematochemical constants (glycemia, BUN, hemochrome, liver function tests, etc.)

Thermic Curve

From the evaluation of this parameter (table 4) it appeared that in 25 patients (62%) a complete regularization of the thermic curve was obtained, 6 patients (15%) showed a partial regularization

Table 4

Indanyl carbenicillin's action on the thermic curve

	Complete resolution	Partial resolution	Persistence of hyperpyrexia
Fever	62%	15%	23%

Table 5

Indanyl carbenicillin's action on the
subjective urination symptomatology

Symptom	Complete resolution	Partial resolution	No resolution	Symptom not determinable
Pollakiuria	61%	12 %	12%	15 %
Strangury	63%	12.5%	17%	7.5%
Dysuria	60%	13 %	12%	15 %

and, lastly, in 9 patients (23%) a hyperpyretic state was maintained.

Subjective Urination Symptomatology

For this parameter, the difference between the initial extent of the symptom and that at the end of the therapy was taken into consideration.

The results are summarized in table 5. From the analysis of the data, it can be clearly seen that the results are almost identical as concerns pollakiuria, strangury and dysuria.

We wish to specify that in about 5% of the patients the subjective urination symptomatology could not be evaluated, in that 4 of them were subjects with an indwelling catheter and in 2 the symptomatology was already absent before the beginning of the therapy.

Antibacterial Action

The evolution of the septic urinary picture was evaluated by carrying out a uroculture with bacterial count at the beginning and end of the treatment. Patients in whom the bacterial count was higher than 10^6 cells per ml were admitted to the test.

The results summarized in table 6, to which the reader is referred, were evaluated as follows: sterilization, reduction in the number of bacteria to 10^5 cells/ml, number of bacteria unchanged.

Table 6

Indanyl carbenicillin's antibacterial action on strains of Pseudomonas aeruginosa, Escherichia coli, indole-positive Proteus, and Proteus mirabilis

Type and total number of strains	Sterilization	Reduction in the number of bacteria to 10^5/ml	Number of bacteria unchanged
8 Pseudomonas aeruginosa	5	–	3
13 Escherichia coli	13	–	–
11 indole-positive Proteus	4	4	3
8 Proteus mirabilis	2	4	2

COMMENTS AND CONCLUSIONS

As far as the side effects are concerned, no significant modifications of the hematochemical constants taken into consideration were noticed. Modest disorders from gastric intolerance were observed in 4 patients; the extent of them was never such as to require the withdrawal of the therapy.

Analyzing the data relative to the drug's action on the clinical symptomatology and on the evolution of the septic urinary picture, the overall results can be evaluated as follows:

    excellent results   – in 24 patients equal to 60%
    mediocre results   – in 8 patients equal to 20%
    insignificant results   – in 8 patients equal to 20%.

This evaluation agrees with both the data of the in vitro trials we carried out and the data reported by the literature. The mediocre and insignificant results are to be attributed not so much to a poor antibacterial action of the drug but rather, and to a considerable extent, to the presence of local factors (indwelling catheter, calculosis, neoplastic tissue) favoring the persistence of the infection and to the practical impossibility of reaching high dosages (greater than 10 g) with the oral administration.

Even with its natural limits, indanyl carbenicillin therefore places itself among the drugs of choice in the treatment of urinary tract infections sustained by germs susceptible to carbenicillin.

REFERENCES

1. Acred, P., Brown, D.M., Knudsen, E.T., Rolinson, G.N. and Sutherland, R. (1967), Nature, 215, 25.
2. Bastian, H.P. and Bruhl, P., Indanyl Carbenicillin, a Pfizer Symposium, London, April 12, 1973.
3. Brumfitt, W., Percival, A. and Leigh, D.A. (1967), The Lancet, 1, 1289.
4. Butler, K., English, A.R., Ray, V.A. et al (1970), J. Infect. Dis., 122 (Suppl.), S1.
5. Butler, K., English, A.R., Briggs, B. et al (1973), J. Infect. Dis., 127 (Suppl.), S97.
6. Butler, K., Indanyl Carbenicillin, a Pfizer Symposium, London, April 12, 1973.
7. English, A.R., Retsema, J.A., Ray, V.A. et al (1972), Antimicrobial Agents and Chemotherapy, 185.
8. Garcia Rodriguez, J.A. et al (1974), Medicina Clinica, October, numero extra, 9.
9. Grove, D.C. and Randall, W.A. (1955), Assay Methods of Antibiotics, A Laboratory Manual, Med. Enc. N.Y., 17.
10. Kayser, F.H., Hany, A. and Lupi, G.A., Indanyl Carbenicillin, a Pfizer Symposium, London, April 12, 1973.
11. Knudsen, E.T., Rolinson, G.N. and Sutherland, R. (1967), Brit. Med. J., 2, 75.
12. Mioli, V. and Tarchini, R., Indanyl Carbenicillin, a Pfizer Symposium, London, April 12, 1973.
13. Renzini, G. and Ferri, A. (1974), Medicina Clinica, October, numero extra, 7.
14. Robinson, O.P.W. (1967), Antimicrobial Agents and Chemotherapy, 614.
15. Rolinson, G.N. and Sutherland, R. (1967), Antimicrobial Agents and Chemotherapy, 609.

CLINICAL EXPERIENCE WITH GEOPEN (CARBENICILLIN)

Ž. IVIĆ

University Hospital "Dr. M. Stojanović"
Clinic of Otorhynolaryngology and Cervicofacial
Surgery, Vinogradska 29
41000 Zagreb, Yugoslavia

Carbenicillin is a semisinthetic penicillin known as a powerful agent against gram negative microorganisms such as Proteus vulgaris and Pseudomonas aeruginosa. Thus we decided to examine its effect in treating chronic middle and external ear infections, as well as oral, pharyngeal and laryngeal mucosa infections following irradiation therapy of malignant tumors of oral cavity, pharynx and larynx. The investigation was carried out in the Clinic of Otorhynolaryngology and Cervicofacial Surgery of the University Hospital "Dr. M. Stojanović."

Bacteriological examination of the middle ear secretions as well as a sputum examination of patients with mucosal infections, following irradiation and cytostatic therapy of malignant tumors, often revealed the presence of both microorganisms: Proteus vulgaris and Pseudomonas aeruginosa.

Available antibiotics usually failed to be effective in treating infections due to these microorganisms. During the first phase of examining the drug, Geopen was given to twenty patients. Twelve of them suffered from middle and external ear infections, and eight from mucosal infection, following radiotherapy and cytostatic therapy of malignant tumours in the oral cavity, pharynx and larynx.

These slides show the diagnosis, method of application, duration of treatment, and dosage. Twelve patients received the drug because of middle and external ear infections. There were 7 males and 5 females, ranging between 20 to 45 years of age. We were able to isolate Pseudomonas aeruginosa in all of the patients. Five of them had a mixed infection with two or more bacterial strains. All patients had intermittent secretion and were treated first with at least one antibiotic. Application was intramuscular and the treatment lasted 8 days.

In six of the twelve patients there was a complete subsidence of secretion and the bacteriological examination was negative. We only found saprophytes. Three months after therapy ended, there were no secretions nor clinical symptomatology.

In the four patients treated with Carbenicillin, secretion diminished. The bacteriological examination revealed that Pseudomonas aeruginosa was successfully eradicated. Using conservative treatment we were able to attain complete subsidence of secretion.

In only two of our patients, the application of Carbenicillin was unsuccessful, even after prolonged treatment.

Infection of the mucosa of the oral cavity, pharynx and larynx is greatly complicated following radiotherapy and cytostatic therapy of malignant tumors. In the sputum of those patients we were nearly always able to identify gram negative microorganisms: Pseudomonas aeruginosa and E. Coli. These patients usually suffered from a sore throat, painful mastication and difficulties in swallowing, not only because of the primary illness, but because of the superponed infection, ranging from mucositis to perichondritis of the laryngeal cartilages. All patients were treated by Carbenicillin given intramusculary. Mean duration of the therapy was 12 days, the dosage 4 X 2 gr for the first four days, then 4 X 1 gr until the end of treatment. All eight patients showed clinical improvement, manifested in diminished salivation and pain, and improved mastication and swallowing. It is quite understandable that this kind of treatment was ineffective regarding the primary illness.

CONCLUSION AND SUMMARY

We find Carbenicillin very effective in treating middle and external ear infections caused by gram negative microorganisms: Proteus vulgaris and Pseudomonas aeruginosa. The drug was less effective in treating mucosal infections of oro, hipopharynx and larynx following radiotherapy and cytostatic therapy. Nevertheless in these patients we observed clinical improvement due to subsidence of the superponed infection.

No side effects were recorded nor were there disturbance in liver functions and blood picture. Tolerance of the drug was excellent.

This article is to be considered a preliminary report. The results obtained have encouraged us to continue the investigation of this drug. We hope to inform you soon of the results tested on a larger number of patients.

NUMBER OF PATIENTS	DIAGNOSIS	CURED	IMPROVED
12	OTITIS MEDIA CHRONICA SUPPURATIVA ET EXTERNA	7	5

Figure 1

NUMBER OF PATIENTS	DIAGNOSIS	IMPROVEMENT OF SECONDARY INFLAMATION IN THE MOUTH AND THROAT
8	NEOPLASMA LINGUAE ET HYPOPHARYNGIS	

Figure 2

INDANYL CARBENICILLIN AND URINARY INFECTIONS

R. Pedrotti and V. Forte

Urological Department

Ospedale Regionale di Trento, Italy

Indanyl carbenicillin's activity is widely known. Carbenicillin indanyl sodium is a derivative of alpha-carboxybenzylpenicillin (carbenicillin) that in its turn is a new broad-spectrum semisynthetic penicillin to which a considerable effectiveness against Pseudomonas and Proteus is attributed (English and Evangelisti 1973, Standiford et al 1968). Indanyl carbenicillin is stable in an acid environment and can therefore be used by oral route; it is rapidly absorbed and metabolized, causing the formation of carbenicillin and indanyl metabolites (Bo et al 1972, Kayser et al 1973). The spectrum of action of carbenicillin, and therefore also of its indanyl ester, is vast and takes in Gram-positive and Gram-negative bacteria from Escherichia to Clostridium including Proteus, Pseudomonas, etc. (Berrill et al 1973, Cox 1973). After oral administration of 1 g of indanyl carbenicillin every 6 hours, very high urinary concentrations (more than 1 mg/ml) are obtained; said concentrations are many times greater than the MIC's relative to the germs most involved in urinary infections (Knirsch 1972).

METHODS AND RESULTS

Fifty patients, chosen from among those who presented urinary infection - without obstruction or other associated pathology - and admitted consecutively to our Hospital, were treated with indanyl carbenicillin for 7 days, at the dose of 0.5 grams 4 times a day. Of these cases, 28 were males and 22 females, all between 18 and 61

TABLE 1

Basic parameters observed in the 50 UTI patients

Before treatment

Clinical – Soft Parameters	Laboratory – Hard Parameters
Dysuria	Leukocyturia
Pain	Uroculture
Fever	Antibiogram
Leukocytosis	
Erythrocyte sedim.	

After treatment

Clinical – Soft Parameters	Laboratory – Hard Parameters
Dysuria	Uroculture
Pain	Antibiogram
Fever	
Leukocytosis	
Erythrocyte sedim.	

TABLE 2

Side effects consequent on the indanyl carbenicillin treatment

Disorder	Slight	Moderate	Severe
Nausea	4	–	–
Gastric pain	1	1	–
Diarrhea	2	–	–
Cutaneous allergy	1	–	–
TOTAL	8	1	0

years old, with an average age of 31. Our group of patients was studied before the treatment from the clinical and bacteriological points of view, according to the two groups of parameters reported in some German literature, as table 1 shows.

The individual tolerance to the drug seemed to be more than satisfactory. Table 2 indicates the trifling extent of side effects of indanyl carbenicillin.

Out of the whole group of 50 patients, 44 obtained complete re-

TABLE 3

Analysis of the failures of the indanyl carbenicillin treatment from a bacteriological viewpoint

	Type of infection		No. of failures
(1)	Multiple-germ infections (12 cases)		1
(2)	Single-germ infections (32 cases)		4
	a) E. coli:	9 cases, 2 failures	
	b) Klebsiella:	7 cases	
	c) Enterococcus:	7 cases	
	d) Staphylococcus:	4 cases, 1 failure	
	e) Pseudomonas:	3 cases	
	f) Proteus:	2 cases, 1 failure	
(3)	Sterile uroculture	(6 cases)	1
		TOTAL 50	6

covery after treatment. The criteria of recovery were based upon the same two parameters: disappearance of clinical symptomatology (observed in 49 subjects) and sterilization of urine (observed in 44 subjects).

We now want to analyze from different points of view the relationship between failures and some parameters. From the clinical viewpoint, in terms of a subdivision of the cases according to their type of infection, the poor results in the small number of cystoprostatitis subjects (2 failures out of 3 patients) were not surprising, after only 7 days of treatment. The different proportion of negative results among the groups of cystitis (3 failures out of 29 patients) and cystopyelitis (1 failure out of 18 cases) seems to be not significant.

From the bacteriological point of view (see table 3), the highest percentage of successful treatments seemed to be in the group of multiple-germ infections. It is interesting to note that the infections due to E. coli, as per the initial culture, showed in some cases another kind of germ at the end-control.

All of the antibiograms we carried out before the treatment showed varying degrees of susceptibility to carbenicillin, except of course the "sterile culture". Also in the cases where the in vitro tests indicated a greater susceptibility to other chemoantibiotic

TABLE 4

Drug of choice according to in vitro sensitivity test (disks method)

Antibiotic	No. of patients	Clinical failures
Carbenicillin	24	0
Rifampicin	8	1
Gentamicin	4	2
Ampicillin	3	0
Chloramphenicol	2	0
Tetracycline	2	1
Nalidixic acid	1	1
TOTAL	44	5

N.B. In 6 cases (1 clinical failure), sterile cultures were observed.

TABLE 5

Analysis of the failures observed in 50 indanyl carbenicillin-treated patients

Type of infection	Treated previously	Germ responsible before treatment	Antibiogram results	Germ observed after treatment
Cystopyelitis	No	E. coli	Gentamic+++ Carbenic ++ Furadant ++	Enterococcus
Cystitis	No	Staphylococcus	Rifampic+++ Carbenic ++ Tetracyc ++	Staphylococcus
Cystitis	Yes	Sterile	—	Pseudomonas
Cystitis	No	E. coli	Nalid ac+++ Carbenic ++ Furadant ++	Proteus
Cystoprostatitis	Yes	Multiple-germ	—	E. coli Enterococcus
Cystoprostatitis	No	Proteus	Gentamic+++ Carbenic ++	Proteus

N.B. ++ = germ susceptible to the drug
      +++ = germ very susceptible to the drug

agents, we always treated the patients with indanyl carbenicillin. Table 4 gives the "drug of choice" according to the antibiogram results. From a clinical point of view, the negative results obtained with indanyl carbenicillin seem to be fairly uniformly distributed.

Thirty-two patients of our group had been previously treated with one or more different antibiotics; 18 had never been treated. It seems to be important to stress that the percentage of failures is lower in the group of previously treated patients (2 cases of failure) compared with those who had never been treated (4 cases of failure). Indanyl carbenicillin also showed a very high activity against germs clinically resistant to other drugs.

The small group of patients in which carbenicillin failed is summarized in table 5. We believe that the failure in cases 1, 2 and 6 may be attributed to the administration of indanyl carbenicillin instead of the drug indicated by the antibiograms as being more active.

CONCLUSIONS

Indanyl carbenicillin is a very effective antibiotic in urinary tract infections. We saw the best results of its activity among the infections already treated with other antibiotics and resistant to them. For the treatment of these "clinically resistant" cases, the antibiogram should always be performed. In cases of infection with "sterile urine culture", indanyl carbenicillin can be given with a satisfactory percentage of success on the clinical symptomatology.

REFERENCES

1. Berrill, W.T., Maskell, R., Pead, L. and Polak, A., Indanyl Carbenicillin, a Pfizer Symposium, London, April 12, 1973.
2. Bo, A.V., Renzini, G. and Ricci, P. (1972), Advances in Antimicrobial and Antineoplastic Chemotherapy, I/1, 41.
3. Cox, C.E., Indanyl Carbenicillin, a Pfizer Symposium, London, April 12, 1973.
4. English, A.R. and Evangelisti, D., Indanyl Carbenicillin, a Pfizer Symposium, London, April 12, 1973.
5. Kayser, F.H., Hany, A. and Lupi, G.A., Indanyl Carbenicillin, a Pfizer Symposium, London, April 12, 1973.

6. Knirsch, A.R. (1972), Advances in Antimicrobial and Antineoplastic Chemotherapy, I/2, 1337.
7. Standiford, H.C., Kind, A.C. and Kirby, W.M.M. (1968), Antimicrobial Agents and Chemotherapy, 286.

ORAL TREATMENT WITH CARINDACILLIN IN PATIENTS SUFFERING FROM URINARY TRACT INFECTIONS

L. Cioni, N. Pilone and L. Moriconi

Nephrological Department

Spedali Riuniti di S. Chiara, Pisa, Italy

INTRODUCTION

As is well known, the antibiotic carbenicillin has been used for some time in the treatment of urinary tract infections supported by Escherichia coli, Proteus and especially by Pseudomonas aeruginosa. However, up till now this drug could not be administered by oral route because it was available only in its sodic form which is unstable at acid values of pH (Renzini and Ferri 1974, Butler et al 1970). The relatively recent synthesis of an acid-stable indanyl ester of carbenicillin has made it possible to administer the antibiotic orally, in that this compound (indanyl carbenicillin) is readily absorbed from the gastroenteric mucous membrane (Bailey 1972, Butler et al 1973).

We therefore wished to test, by means of clinical trials, the therapeutic effectiveness of the new product in patients with urinary sepsis.

MATERIAL AND METHODS

Twenty-five patients of both sexes (11 males and 14 females), between 6 and 65 years of age, were treated with indanyl carbenicillin. The patients, affected with various kidney diseases, were carriers of urinary tract infections supported by E. coli, Proteus, Pseudomonas aeruginosa or other Enterobacteriaceae which were quantitatively present in the order of at least 10^5–10^6 germs/ml. Some of the patients had a variously impaired renal function, as appeared from the blood creatinine values.

Indanyl carbenicillin was administered in doses of 2 to 4 grams daily, according to the patients' body weight, at regular intervals during the 24 hours, for periods of time ranging from 8 to 10 days. In establishing the dosage, a possible impairment of the kidney function was not taken into account, since it is known that indanyl carbenicillin is not toxic either at the systemic level or, specifically, at the renal level (Butler et al 1973, Butler 1973, Gould and Gould 1973, Westenfelder and Madsen 1973). However, in order to verify the eventual appearance of side effects, controls of the hemochromocytometric examination, transaminases and creatininemia were carried out before and after the treatment (Boxerbaum et al 1968).

The therapeutic response was evaluated on the basis of the urine culture, performed before and after the treatment. The urine culture was considered positive when the bacterial concentration was above 10^5 microorganisms/ml and negative when such concentration was below 10^2 microorganisms/ml.

In evaluating the therapeutic response, the criterion of all or nothing was adopted, that is to say the responses with negative urine culture were considered positive and all the others, negative.

RESULTS

The results obtained are presented schematically in tables 1 and 2. As appears from these tables, the subjects examined were, for convenience's sake, grouped either on the basis of the disease from which they were suffering or on the basis of the microorganisms found in the urine. In table 1, the appearance of side effects is also reported.

Table 1 indicates that 6 patients out of the 10 affected with chronic pyelonephritis from urolithiasis showed a positive response, and 4 a negative response, to the treatment. In one case, a slight gastric intolerance appeared.

Out of the 8 patients suffering from chronic pyelonephritis without urolithiasis, 2 gave a positive response and 5, a negative

TABLE 1

Results (in terms of the type of infection) of the indanyl carbenicillin treatment in 25 UTI patients.

Disease	Number of cases treated	Results Positive	Results Negative	Side* effects	% of positivity
Chronic pyeloneph. from urolithiasis	10	6	4	1	60%
Chronic pyeloneph. without urolithia.	8	2	5	1§	25%
Urinary sepsis of varying origin	7	6	1	0	87%

* cases of gastric intolerance
§ treatment interrupted on the 4th day

TABLE 2

Results (in terms of the microorganisms found in the urine) of the indanyl carbenicillin treatment in 25 UTI patients.

Microorganism	Number of cases treated	Results Positive	Results Negative	% of positivity
Pseudomonas aeruginosa	9*	7	1	77.7%
Escherichia coli	8	3	5	37.5%
Proteus	6	3	3	50 %
Providencia stuarti	2	1	1	50 %

* In one patient, the treatment was stopped on the 4th day because of marked gastric intolerance.

one. The treatment was stopped on the 4th day in one of the patients because of the appearance of marked gastric intolerance.

Six patients out of the 7 with urinary sepsis of varying origin reacted positively to the treatment.

The treated cases have been grouped in table 2 according to the microorganisms found by means of the urine culture test.

Out of the 9 patients affected with urinary sepsis caused by Pseudomonas aeruginosa, 7 reacted positively, and one negatively, to the therapy. In only one of them, the treatment was interrupted because of gastric intolerance.

Three out of the 8 patients with infection from E. coli showed a positive response and 5, a negative one.

Three of the 6 patients affected with Proteus gave a positive response and 3, a negative one.

Of the 2 patients with infection caused by Providencia stuarti, one responded to the treatment positively and the other, negatively.

The controls, performed after the treatment, of the transaminases, creatininemia and hemochromocytometric examination did not reveal toxic effects in any case. Only 2 patients manifested gastric intolerance, owing to which in one of them it was necessary to withdraw the treatment, as mentioned above.

CONCLUSIONS

The results obtained show that the therapeutic effectiveness of indanyl carbenicillin (carindacillin) in the urinary tract infections which we tested is somewhat variable.

Within the limits of our case histories, we think we can state that the therapeutic activity of indanyl carbenicillin is carried on prevalently against Pseudomonas aeruginosa. Moreover, the results seem to indicate that the antibiotic is generally more effective in patients not suffering from a very complex renal pathology; this would be in agreement with our previous experience concerning the use of carbenicillin administered parenterally and with what is asserted by many other authors.

Furthermore, in evaluating these data it should certainly be borne in mind that often our patients had been treated previously, and sometimes repeatedly, with other antibiotics, so that even very extensive bacterial resistances could frequently be present.

In conclusion, in our opinion indanyl carbenicillin represents without any doubt a quite useful tool in medical practice for treating urinary tract infections, owing also to the absence of noticeable side effects. In particular, this antibiotic proves to be very helpful in urologic patients subjected to instrumental maneuvers, either for immediate therapy or for prophylaxis. More specifically, indanyl carbenicillin may be used beneficially in subjects with important previous renal diseases, in whom the superimposition of pyelonephritis would prove to be disastrous from a functional point of view.

Lastly, the clinical results obtained later, and not reported here, suggest that the drug considerably reduces the acute episodes of urinary sepsis, when administered in monthly cycles of 7-10 days.

REFERENCES

1. Bailey, R.R. (1972), Canad. Med. Ass. J., 107, 316.
2. Boxerbaum, B., Doershuk, C.F., Pittman, S. and Matthews, L.W. (1968), Antimicrobial Agents and Chemotherapy, 292.
3. Butler, K., Indanyl Carbenicillin, a Pfizer Symposium, London, April 12, 1973.
4. Butler, K., English, A.R., Briggs, B., Gralla, E., Stebbins, R.B. and Hobbs, D.C. (1973), J. Infect. Dis., 127 (Suppl.), S97.
5. Butler, K., English, A.R., Ray, V.A. and Timreck, A.E. (1970), J. Infect. Dis., 122 (Suppl.), S1.
6. Gould, J.D.M. and Gould, J.C., Indanyl Carbenicillin, a Pfizer Symposium, London, April 12, 1973.
7. Renzini, G. and Ferri, A. (1974), Medicina Clinica, October, numero extra, 7.
8. Westenfelder, M. and Madsen, P.O. (1973), J. Infect. Dis., 127 (Suppl.), S154.

CARINDACILLIN IN THE THERAPY OF URINARY TRACT INFECTIONS

T. Germinale and C. Giglio

Urology Department

Ospedale Civile, Genoa, Italy

The use of antibiotics in urinary tract infections should always be effected on the basis of the knowledge of the microbial agents involved; in fact, in our practice, we always utilize urine cultures before the decision is taken on the type of antibiotic to be employed.

The germs we observe in UTI are especially Gram-negative rods, particularly E. coli, indole-positive Proteus and Pseudomonas aeruginosa; during the last two years, the frequency of the observation of Proteus and Pseudomonas strains has been considerably increasing.

For these reasons, the choice of the antibiotic to be used should consider some characteristics of the various drugs currently available. In brief, the drug of choice should (Germinale and Giglio 1975)
(1) have a spectrum of antibacterial activity as broad as possible;
(2) be eliminated by the urine in an active form and in the greatest amount possible in relation to the sensitivity of the bacteria;
(3) be active in a vast pH range;
(4) be well tolerated, from both a general and a local point of view.

We perfectly agree with the opinion of Shubin et al. (1975) when they consider – in the absence of lab tests – gentamicin as the first drug of choice in UTI but, due to our routine use of the urine culture, we believe that carbenicillin better corresponds to the previously indicated points. Carbenicillin, in fact (as carbenicillin sodium parenterally or as indanyl carbenicillin by oral route), presents a broad spectrum of activity including Pseudomonas strains, is eliminated with the urine in a very large amount, is active in a pH range from 4 to 8 and shows the lack of toxicity characteristic of the penicillins.

OUR CASE HISTORIES AND COMMENTS

At the last International Congress of Chemotherapy, in Athens, we reported (Germinale and Giglio 1974) the data on our use of carbenicillin and gentamicin in 30 patients with UTI. We now wish to report on the use of carbenicillin — as indanyl carbenicillin by oral route — in a group of 40 other patients suffering from UTI due to E. coli, Proteus spp and Pseudomonas strains. The daily dosage was always between 2 and 4 g, divided into 4 administrations; the duration of the treatment was generally 15-20 days.

TABLE 1

Semiquantitative* evaluation of the symptomatology (A) and global results (B) in 40 indanyl carbenicillin-treated, UTI-affected patients.

(A)

	Total Score	Average Score
Before treatment	335	8.4
After treatment	110	2.7

(B) Global Clinical Results**

Good 28 (70%)	Fair 10 (25%)	Negative 2 (5%)

* Symptoms considered: pollakiuria; fever; shivers; tenesmus; frequency of urination; dysuria; muscular, abdominal, and costovertebral pains.
Values attributed to each symptom: 0 = absent, 1, 2 and 3 = slight, moderate and marked intensity.
** According to the criteria indicated by Germinale and Giglio (1974).

The results are expressed in a semiquantitative manner in table 1. In a very few cases, we also obtained — with the collaboration of Prof. G. Renzini — the urinary levels of the drug; the levels obtained — in the presence of "normal" kidney function and for the 6 hours after the administration — were always higher than 500 mcg/ml after a 1 g dose.

On the basis of these results, we confirm indanyl carbenicillin's great safety and very good clinical activity. In our opinion, however, this drug should be used only in the UTI from E. coli, Proteus spp and Pseudomonas aeruginosa; against this last rod, indanyl carbenicillin represents — as far as we know — the only drug active by oral route which is available in Italy.

REFERENCES

1. Germinale, T. and Giglio, C. (1974), Progress in Chemotherapy, II, 714.
2. Germinale, T. and Giglio, C., "Uno sguardo alla terapia delle infezioni urinarie": paper read at the "Convegno di Chemioterapia — Tavola Rotonda su Chemioterapia delle infezioni Urinarie", Turin, June 19–20, 1975.
3. Shubin, H., Weil, M. and Nishijima, H. (1975), in Gram-Negative Bacterial Infections (edited by B. Urbaschek, R. Urbaschek, and E. Neter); 411. Wien: Springer-Verlag.

URINARY LEVELS OF CARINDACILLIN IN THE PEDIATRIC AGE

A. Ferro, G. Ceccarelli and G.R. Burgio

Istituto di Clinica Pediatrica

Università di Pavia, Italy

From an etiological viewpoint, urinary tract infections — which are often, especially in the pediatric age, associated with or favored by morbid situations that constitute either an obstacle to the urinary flow or lesion of the kidney or of the same urinary tract — are prevalently due to Gram-negative bacteria, in particular to germs of the coliform group (E. coli in particular but also Aerobacter aerogenes and Klebsiella pneumoniae), of the Proteus group, particularly Proteus vulgaris and Proteus morganii, and to Pseudomonas aeruginosa. According to some authors (Hradec et al 1972), about two thirds of the urinary infections are due to Gram-negative germs, with a large prevalence of E. coli, Proteus and Pseudomonas. According to Sanna (1975), who reported on more than 8,000 strains isolated from urinary infections, E. coli is in question in 17% of the cases, Proteus in 20%, and Pseudomonas pyocyanea in 13.5%.

Enterococcus and Staphylococcus predominate among the Gram-positive germs even though in the various case histories Streptococcus and pneumococcus can also be found, with a frequency that varies according to the type of patients concerned.

In view of this, the medical therapy of urinary tract infections in infancy avails itself not only of general measures — generous intake of liquids, rest in bed even if not very protracted — but also of chemoantibiotics whose use must not prescind from the clinical consideration based above all on the kind of infection (initial acute attack, acute but recurrent infection, chronic infection).

Among the antibiotic drugs that find use in urinary tract infections, the group of the semisynthetic penicillins is widely employed in pediatrics, especially owing to their exceptionally trifling toxicity which is only partly compensated negatively by the possibility of the well-known phenomena of hypersensitivity. Of this group, ampicillin is a remarkable drug not only for its tolerance but also for the good levels which it reaches in both the plasma and the urine. Nevertheless, ampicillin's antibacterial spectrum does not include Pseudomonas aeruginosa which, on the contrary, is affected − granted at high concentrations − by the activity of another derivative of the same group, carbenicillin.

As a matter of fact, at high concentrations carbenicillin is effective against many strains of Pseudomonas aeruginosa, Proteus and other bacterial species included in the penicillin spectrum.

Since carbenicillin causes high urinary concentrations, the best results with this antibiotic have been obtained in the treatment of urinary tract infections even though, during the treatment, it is possible to observe the appearance of highly resistant strains whose importance, nonetheless, must not be too overrated (Bodey 1974). In particular, in cases of serious infection from Pseudomonas strains, the use of carbenicillin can be associated with that of gentamicin; this combination probably constitutes (Gardner 1974) the most effective therapy for these serious situations.

Nevertheless, in addition to being − like ampicillin − penicillinase-sensitive, carbenicillin is also acid-labile, and its use is therefore obligatorily to be effected by parenteral route. The relatively recent availability of an acid-resistant derivative (indanyl carbenicillin) of carbenicillin has made it possible to employ this antibiotic per os, granted limitedly to use in urinary tract infections since only at the urine level does the antibiotic reach sufficient concentrations.

Indanyl carbenicillin's hygroscopicity and its particularly bitter taste, on the other hand, have made it impossible to formulate the substance in solususpension which is suitable for pediatric use. This has led to the ascertainment that, even though the urinary levels of carbenicillin after oral administration of indanyl carbenicil-

TABLE

Case no.	Age in years	Base Diagnosis	Amount in ml of urine eliminated during the 6 hours	Indanyl carbenicillin administered in mg	Urinary level (mcg/ml) of carbenicillin
1	4 11/12	Rheumatic fever	208	1.000	600 mcg/ml
2	2	Rhinopharyngeal sarcoma	230	500	160 mcg/ml
3	7	Cooley's disease	120	1.000	270 mcg/ml
4	4 8/12	Hypophysial dwarfism	180	1.000	122 mcg/ml
5	9 6/12	Hypophysial dwarfism	210	1.000	180 mcg/ml
6*	4	Rheumatic fever	200	500	50 mcg/ml

* Creatinine clearance = 20 ml/min.

lin in adults are available in the literature (Butler 1973, Fabre et al 1972, Kayser et al 1973, Wallace et al 1970), no datum pertinent to the pediatric age is available in the literature. In view of this, we recently thought it interesting to evaluate in some children – who were to undergo antibiotic treatment owing to the presence of a urinary tract infection – the urinary levels of carbenicillin obtainable after a single administration of indanyl carbenicillin per os. For this purpose, 6 young children between 2 and 9 6/12 years of age, hospitalized in our clinic for various base affections (see the table), were treated with indanyl carbenicillin tablets (first appropriately broken to bits in order to allow their ingestion). The urine eliminated during the 6 hours following administration of the drug was collected, and the urine's carbenicillin content was dosed with the microbiological method, using a strain of Sarcina lutea ATCC 9341 as the test microorganism (Bo et al 1972).

The results obtained (see the table) show that in children, too, provided that their renal function is not impaired, the per os administration of indanyl carbenicillin allows reaching high urinary levels of carbenicillin which are sufficient for antibacterial action against the most common germs in question in urinary infections.

It is therefore to be hoped that the utilization of this carbenicillin ester in urinary tract infections in the pediatric age will be made possible through the formulation of microtablets suitable for pediatric use, once the causal agent and its susceptibility – in respect of the urinary concentrations – to carbenicillin have been determined.

REFERENCES

1. Bo, A.V., Renzini, G. and Ricci, P. (1972), Advances in Antimicrobial and Antineoplastic Chemotherapy, I/1, 41.
2. Bodey, P. (1974), Antibiotics and Chemotherapy, 18, 49.
3. Butler, K., Indanyl Carbenicillin, a Pfizer Symposium, London, April 12, 1973.
4. Fabre, J., Burgy, C., Rudhardt, M. and Herrera, A. (1972), Chemotherapy, 17, 334.
5. Gardner, P. (1974), Pediatric Clinics of North America, 21 (3), 617.
6. Hradec, E., Komarek, O. and Rosova, V. (1972), Advances in Antimicrobial and Antineoplastic Chemotherapy, I/2, 1297.

7. Kayser, F.H., Hany, A. and Lupi, G.A., Indanyl Carbenicillin, a Pfizer Symposium, London, April 12, 1973.
8. Sanna, A., "Microbiologia delle infezioni delle vie urinarie": paper read at the "Convegno di Chemioterapia – Tavola Rotonda su Chemioterapia delle infezioni Urinarie", Turin, June 19–20, 1975.
9. Wallace, J.F., Atlas, E., Bear, D.M., Brown, N.K., Clark, H. and Turck, M. (1970), Antimicrobial Agents and Chemotherapy, 223.

CLINICAL PHARMACOLOGICAL STUDIES WITH BACAMPICILLIN

L. Magni, B. Sjöberg, J. Sjövall and J. Wessman

Research and Development Laboratory, Medical Department

Astra Läkemedel AB, S-151 85 Södertälje, Sweden

Ampicillin is a widely used semisynthetic penicillin with a high activity in vitro against Gram-positive and Gram-negative bacteria. A disadvantage, however, is its incomplete oral absorption, 30-50 % of the drug being excreted unchanged in the urine (Rolinson et Sutherland 1973). In attempts to improve absorption, derivatives which are hydrolysed to ampicillin in vivo have been made. Metampicillin and hetacillin, condensation products of ampicillin with formaldehyde and acetone respectively, were reported to give superior blood levels of ampicillin (Franchi et Perraro 1967; Bunn et al. 1966) but this has later been questioned (Sutherland et al. 1972; Sutherland et Robinson 1967). Certain ampicillin esters, such as pivampicillin and talampicillin, are orally well absorbed giving serum levels of ampicillin higher than those obtained with ampicillin itself (Daehne et al. 1970; Clayton et al. 1974; Shiobara et al. 1974). In comparative trials between ampicillin and pivampicillin upper gastrointestinal discomfort appears to be more troublesome while the frequency of diarrhoea seems to be less pronounced with pivampicillin (Wilcox et al. 1973). Preliminary reports from Japan on talampicillin indicate a higher frequency of upper gastrointestinal side effects than normally seen with ampicillin (Gomi et al. 1975).

Bacampicillin is a new semisyntnetic aminopenicillin that has been synthetised at the Research Laboratories of Astra Läkemedel AB.

It differs from ampicillin by an ethoxycarbonyloxyethyl group attached to the carboxyl group of the penicillin nucleus thus forming an ester. The transformation into ampicillin in vivo is so rapid that no unchanged compound could be detected in the blood after oral administration of bacampicillin to animals and man. On oral administration to animals, bacampicillin was better and more rapidly absorbed than ampicillin giving higher levels in blood and tissues (Bodin et al. 1975).

MATERIAL AND METHODS

The purpose of the present studies was to investigate the basic pharmacological behaviour of bacampicillin in man. Each study has been carried out in a cross-over fashion, all preparations being given on the same day to different subjects in a randomized order and then alternated randomly at intervals of at least one week. No food was allowed from midnight until 2-3 hours after administration of the test dose. The studies were performed in 10-12 healthy volunteers in each study with a general age distribution of 20-40 years. All were shown to have normal liver and kidney function.

The concentrations in serum and urine were determined using the cylinder plate method with Micrococcus luteus (Sarcina lutea ATCC 9341) as test organism according to the method described by Grove et Randall (1955). The samples were frozen at the end of each experimental day and stored at $-20°C$ together with reference solutions of ampicillin until analysed. Serum was diluted in pooled human serum while the diluent for the urine samples was Sörensen´s phosphate buffer of pH 7.0.

RESULTS AND DISCUSSION

Figure 1 shows the serum levels after oral administration of bacampicillin 400 mg and the corresponding equimolar amount of oral ampicillin (278 mg). The results confirm the earlier findings in animals showing that bacampicillin gives higher serum levels of ampicillin more rapidly than oral ampicillin. The mean individual peak serum level ($\pm$ standard error of the mean) after administration of ampicillin was 3.4 ± 0.40 µg/ml and the corresponding level achieved with bacampicillin was 8.7 ± 0.62 µg/ml. An increase of approximately 2.5 times the peak serum level reached with oral ampicillin ($t_{dep.} = 7.04$, $p < 0.001$). The more complete and faster absorption of bacampicillin is also reflected by the area under the serum concentration time curve (AUC) during the observation time which was 81 ± 30 % greater with bacampicillin ($p < 0.05$), thus illustrating a totally higher bioavailability of bacampicillin (figure 1).

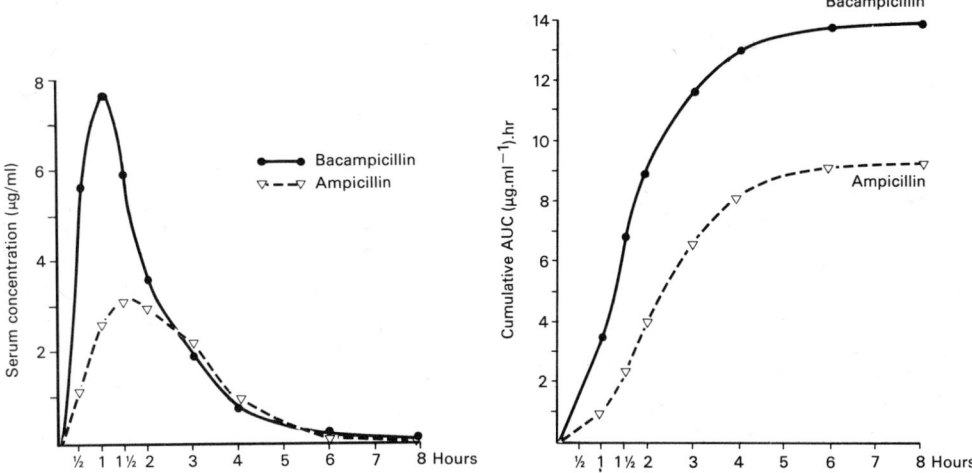

Figure 1. Mean serum levels and cumulative bioavailability (AUC) in 12 volunteers after oral administration of bacampicillin 400 mg and an equimolar amount of ampicillin (278 mg).

The urinary recovery of ampicillin during 0-8 hours was 43 ± 4.2 % of that ingested. This was about 3/5 of the 70 ± 3.2 % urinary recovery of ampicillin following bacampicillin. The slower absorption of ampicillin compared to bacampicillin is also reflected in a slow urinary excretion with 18 % and 47 % respectively excreted during the first 2-hour interval. Furthermore, this difference is not compensated by a substantially higher excretion after this time. Thus the higher bioavailability of bacampicillin is also reflected in a higher urinary excretion of ampicillin.

The relationship between dose and bioavailability following oral administration of bacampicillin was studied with 200 mg, 400 mg and 800 mg, the results of which are presented in figure 2. The mean individual peak serum values were with increased doses 5.3 ± 0.39 µg/ml, 8.9 ± 0.64 µg/ml and 16.5 ± 0.93 µg/ml. These results also indicate an almost perfect linear relationship between dose and mean maximum serum concentration, the correlation coefficient for the individual regression lines varying between 0.96 and 1.00.

From the area under the serum concentration time curve (AUC) in the observed interval it seems that the relative bioavailability is equal for the three doses used. This is illustrated by the linear relationship between dose and area in figure 2. The urinary recovery of ampicillin during 0-8 hours may be taken to suggest a somewhat higher excretion for a low than for a high dose (77-71-66 %). However these differences were not significant on the 5 % level.

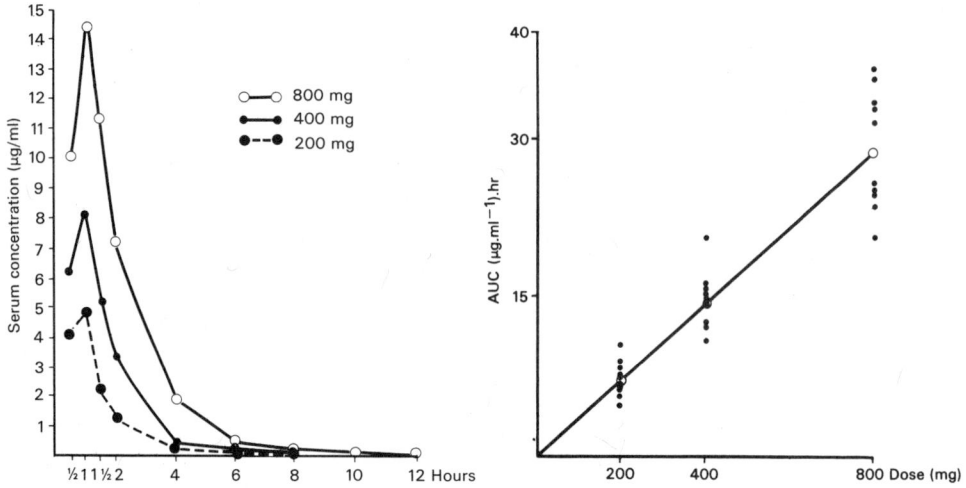

Figure 2. Mean serum levels of ampicillin and area under the serum concentration time curve (AUC) in 10 volunteers after single oral doses of bacampicillin.

There was a tendency towards higher peak serum concentrations, larger area under the serum concentration time curve (AUC), and a higher urinary excretion rate when the tablets were taken with food than in a fasting state. This was valid both for the 400 and the 800 mg doses given. The mean individual peak serum level after administration of 400 mg was 8.0 ± 0.96 µg/ml in the fasting state and 8.4 ± 0.73 µg/ml taken with food. The corresponding values after administration of 800 mg were 12.1 ± 0.50 and 13.3 ± 0.67 µg/ml, respectively. However, none of these differences were significant on the 5 % level.

Bacampicillin thus combines the high antibacterial activity of ampicillin in vitro with a more complete oral absorption leading to an enhanced activity in vivo reflected in higher serum concentration and higher urinary excretion. The better oral absorption of bacampicillin may also reduce the incidence of drug-related gastrointestinal side effects occurring in patients receiving oral ampicillin.

SUMMARY

Bacampicillin is a new penicillin that is absorbed more rapidly and more completely than ampicillin. It is rapidly transformed in vivo to ampicillin giving peak serum levels approximately 2.5 times

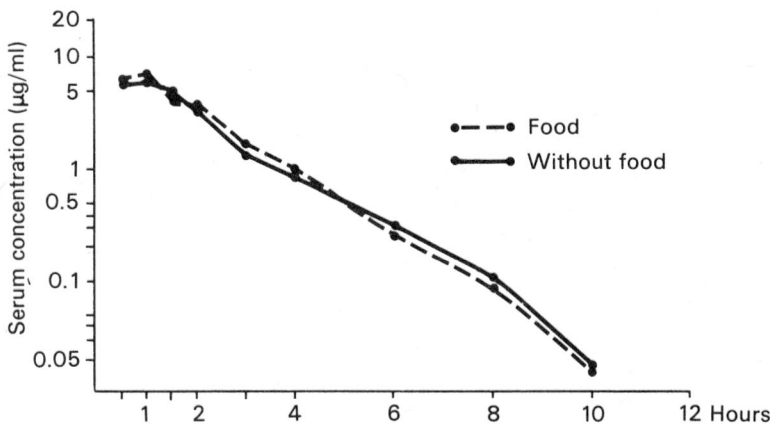

Figure 3. Mean serum levels of ampicillin in 12 volunteers after single oral doses of 400 mg bacampicillin with or without food.

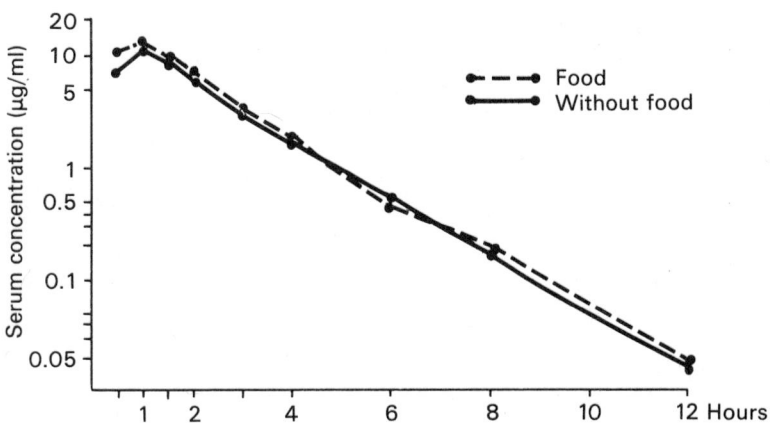

Figure 4. Mean serum levels of ampicillin in 12 volunteers after single oral doses of 800 mg bacampicillin with or without food.

as high as those of an equimolar oral dose of ampicillin. There was a linear relationship between dose and area under the serum concentration-time curve (AUC) after administration of bacampicillin in doses of 200, 400, and 800 mg. No significant influence on absorption was seen when bacampicillin was taken together with food.

REFERENCES

BODIN, N.-O., EKSTRÖM, B., FORSGREN, U., JALAR, L.-P., MAGNI, L., RAMSAY, C.-H. and SJÖBERG, B., (1975), 9th International Congress of Chemotherapy, London. To be published.
BUNN, P.A., MILICICH, S. and LUNN, J.S., (1966), Antimicrobial Agents and Chemotherapy, p. 947.
CLAYTON, J.P., COLE, M., ELSON, S.W. and FERRES, H., (1974), Antimicrobial Agents and Chemotherapy, p. 670.
DAEHNE, W., FREDERIKSEN, E., GUNDERSEN, E., LUND, F., MORCH, P., PETERSON, H.J., ROHOLT, K., TYBRING, L. and GODTFREDSEN, W.O., (1970), J. Med. Chem. 13, 607.
FRANCHI, R. and PERRARO, F., (1967), Atti Accad. Med. Lomb., 22, 543.
GOMI, K., HAYAKAWA, H., KOHNO, M., KATAYAMA, T., FUJIMORI, I. and KATSU, M., (1975), 23rd Congress of Chemotherapy, Kobe.
GROVE, D.C. and RANDALL, W.A., (1955), Assay methods of antibiotics: a laboratory manual. Medical Encyclopedia, New York.
ROLINSON, G.N. and SUTHERLAND, R., (1973), In S. Garattini (ed.) Advances in pharmacology and chemotherapy vol. 11 Academic Press Inc., New York, p. 151-220.
SHIOBARA, Y., TACHIBANA, A., SASAKI, H., WATANABE, T. and SADO, T., (1974), J. Antibiotics, 27, 665.
SUTHERLAND, R., ELSON, S. and CROYDON, E.A.P., (1972), Chemotherapy (Basel) 17, 145.
SUTHERLAND, R. and ROBINSON, O.P.W., (1967), Brit. med. J. 2, 804.
WILCOX, J.B., BROGDEN, R.N. and AVERY, G.S., (1973), Drugs, 6, 94.

CLINICAL AND BACTERIOLOGICAL STUDY ON BACAMPICILLIN IN SKIN AND SOFT TISSUE INFECTIONS

Erik Skog, Erik Sandström and Gösta Wallmark

Södersjukhuset

100 64 STOCKHOLM 38, Sweden

In the clinical evaluation of antibiotic treatment it is preferable to study the effect of well defined infections caused by susceptible bacteria. Streptococcal skin infection seem to be a good clinical model for such a study as it allows continuous visual evaluation and good standardization of the conditions.

Bacampicillin is a new semisynthetic penicillin belonging to the ampicillin group of drugs. It is rapidly and more completely absorbed than ampicillin after oral administration, resulting in a rapid liberation of active ampicillin. Oral bacampicillin gives serum levels about 2-3 times as high as an equivalent dose of ampicillin.

The objective of this limited study was to test the usefulness of the above mentioned model in an evaluation of the therapeutic efficacy and tolerance with bacampicillin in streptococcal skin infections.

MATERIAL AND METHODS

Patients

Twenty-one adult patients, fourteen men, mean age 50.9, SD $\pm$ 10.1 and seven women, mean age 57.3 SD $\pm$ 13.0, were included in this study on the basis of proven or presumed streptococcal skin infection. They had no clinical disease that could influence the evaluation of the drug treatment, such as penicillinallergy, or kidney or liver disturbances. None of the patients was pregnant. All were well informed and consented to the trail.

Laboratory Investigations

Samples for bacteriological culture were taken from wound secretion and skin before, during, and after treatment. The samples were sent to laboratory within the hospital by means of standard bacteriological technique and processed the same day. Clinical chemistry including haematology, liver and renal tests as well as urine analysis were performed before and with weekly intervals until one week after termination of the treatment.

Treatment

Bacampicillin (batch F53) was supplied in tablets of 400 mg. One tablet was given three times daily. The aim was to treat the patient for at least ten days or until complete resolution of their symptoms. The treatment was interrupted in two patients, MR because of presence of penicillinase-producing Staph. aureus and SS as an initial good response was followed by a sudden bullaformation. Topical treatment was limited to solutio alsoli 1 % cum spiritus 10 %.

Clinical and Bacteriological Evaluation

The clinical effect was assessed daily with the parameters erythema, secretion, pus, oedema and general impression as compared to the day before.

The clinical effect was evaluated as:

<u>Good</u>   Clinical findings subsided completely during therapy in a time comparable to standard treatment and no sign of infection was present at the follow-up.

<u>Moderate</u>   Clear improvement but not complete healing while on treatment or markedly slower resolution than on standard treatment.

<u>Poor/nil</u>   Little or no clinical response to therapy. The bacteriological effect was evaluated by the presence or absence of pathogens, β-hemolytic streptococci group A or B, and/or Staphylococcus aureus.

Table 1

Diagnosis	Pat.	Age	Sex	Treatment days	Effect
Erysipelas	AR	69	M	10	good
"	VE	63	M	11	"
"	ES	63	F	11	"
"	SH	40	M	11	"
"	EE	70	F	10	"
"	EF	57	F	10	"
"	GP	49	M	12	"
"	JK	39	M	12	"
"	BM	33	M	11	"
"	HS	48	F	18	"
"	GM	61	F	16	mod.
"	MR	44	M	3	"
"	SS	50	M	4	"

Evaluation of tolerance

All patients were initially informed about the drug and were asked to report any discomfort. They were subsequently asked every day about their well-being with active questions, at least once while on treatment about pruritus, bowel disorders, nausea and skin rashes.

RESULTS

Clinical and Bacteriological Effect

Table 1 includes all patients admitted under the diagnosis of erysipelas. Hemolytic streptococci group A are the known etiology of this disease but unfortunately hard to isolate from the lesion. Therefore the results in this group rests on clinical observations alone except in two cases. In ten patients the disease was cured at a similar rate as with our standard therapy, penicillin V.[*] Fig. 1 and 2 illustrate the time the parameters erythema and swelling were judged to be completely normalized in the ten patients showing a good response. The treatment was prolonged in one patient, HS, with the disease located to the face. Of the three patients classified to respond moderately, GM had a bullous erysipelas which initially showed a good response but on day 11 developed

[*] 0.65 g t. i. d.

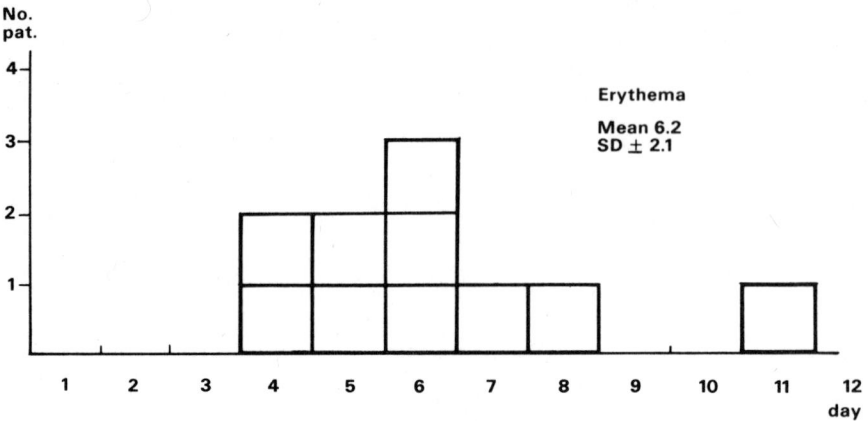

Fig. 1. Patients with erysipelas.
Day symptom was normalized. N = 10.

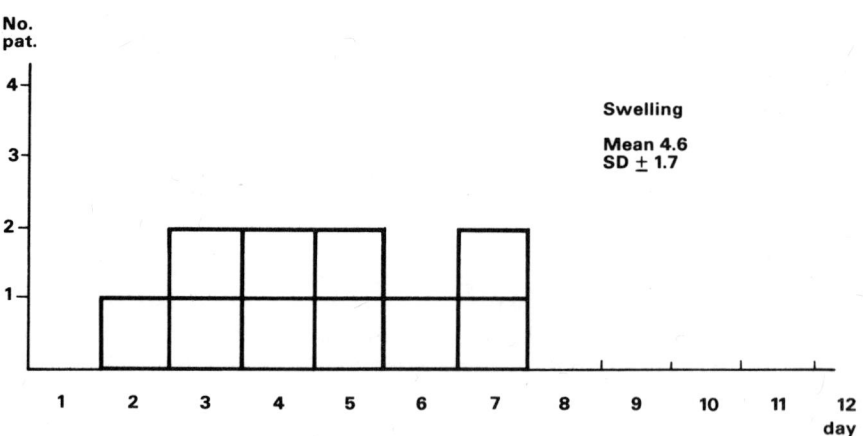

Fig. 2. Patients with erysipelas.
Day symptom was normalized. N = 10.

a necrosis with growth of two phage types of penicillinase-
producing Staph. aureus not initially present. As the condition
did not improve further, the therapy was altered on day 16.
MR had his therapy interrupted after 3 days in spite of good
clinical effect as soon as penicillinase-producing Staph.
aureus were cultured because of the above mentioned experience
with case GM. This might not have been necessary as will be
shown later. In SS the therapy was interrupted after 4 days
because a large bulla arouse on day 3 after an initial good
improvement. With previous observations of large areas of
necrosis after erysipelas with concomitant penicillinase-
producing staphylococci it was not felt justified to continue
a therapy not directed against penicillinase-producing
staphylococci.

Table 2 shows the results in eight patients with other
streptococcal infections where it could be seen that initially
positive cultures of β-streptococci turned negative. PL and
ED had infections with both hemolytic streptococci group A
and penicillinase-producing Staphylococcus aureus. The β-streptococci were eliminated under the therapy in both. AS had
invers psoriasis with a prior positive skin culture from the
groin showing hemolytic streptococci group A, which was not
present at the onset of therapy. The patient is included for
the sake of completeness. In ÅM, hemolytic streptococci were
eliminated slowly, still being culturable after 2 weeks.

Table 2

Diagnosis	Pat.	Age	Sex	Treatment days	Effect
Impetigo	ÅH	47	M	10	good
"	BW	50	M	10	"
Pyodermia	KG	34	F	11	"
"	PL	53	M	13	"
Impetigo	ED	56	M	17	"
Tonsillit.	AS	65	M	10	"
Pustul.pl.	GP	68	M	13	"
Eczema mic.	ÅM	50	M	22	mod.

To summarize out of the nine patients with cultured hemolytic streptococci in the skin all had negative cultures at the follow up, in three cases in spite of concomitant penicillinase-producing Staph. aureus. Of the twenty patients with skin infections caused by hemolytic streptococci, sixteen showed a good response and four a moderate response, two of these might well have turned out to show a good response if therapy had not been interrupted, one further case was probably complicated by super infection of penicillinase-producing Staph. aureus probably from the ward.

SIDE-EFFECTS

No patient reported any adverse reactions related to the drug, except that one patient had a slight headache on day 2 and another developed a small eczematous patch which rapidly disappeared with hydrocortisone creame while on treatment. This patient did not have reagins against penicilloyl. The symptoms in these two patients were probably not related to the bacampicillin treatment.

Laboratory Analysis

No patient developed any abnormal haematological or renal laboraratory findings during or after treatment which could be referred to bacampicillin. A slight elevation in SGOT or SGPT was seen in four patients, maximally 60 units which could be explained by alcohol intake. A slight elevation in alcaline phosphatase was seen in one patient with rheumatoid arthritis since 20 years, she was also treated with furosemid (Lasix®), chlorzoxazon (Paraflex®), and acetylsalicylic acid (Magnecyl®).

DISCUSSION

In this series a new ampicillin, bacampicillin, was studied on patients with skin infections, definitely and probably caused by hemolytic streptococci group A. It must be pointed out that penicillin V or bensylpenicillin but not ampicillin is the drug of choice in such infections. Streptococcal skin infections were chosen solely because such infections constitute a fairly homogenous group of infections, suitable for an evaluation of the clinical efficacy of an antibiotic.

It was found that the proposed model allowed good control over the clinical course with easy visual evaluation of the effect from day to day. Data obtained using different parameters offers opportunity to compare different antibiotics or different doses of a given antibiotic in larger studies.

In this study bacampicillin was given in an oral dosage of 400 mg t. i. d. for about 10 days to 20 patients with erysipelas or other streptococcal skin infections. The clinical and bacteriological effect was good in 16 and moderate in 4 cases. The results are comparable to those obtained with penicillin V according to earlier experience.

Bacampicillin was well tolerated. No side effects attributable to the treatment were observed.

BACAMPICILLIN IN RESPIRATORY TRACT AND URINARY TRACT INFECTIONS

B. Ursing, M. Lindroth, and C. Kamme

Department of Infectious Diseases
Department of Medical Microbiology
University Hospital
Lund, Sweden

INTRODUCTION

Bacampicillin is a new antibiotic within the amino penicillin group. Studies in both animals and human volunteers have shown that ampicillin is quickly liberated as an antibacterially active metabolite after absorption. Compared to oral ampicillin, bacampicillin in an equimolar dose gives considerably higher serum and urinary concentration of active antibiotic.

The aim of this open study was to investigate the clinical tolerance of bacampicillin in hospitalized patients. Furthermore, the serum concentrations achieved were studied.

MATERIAL AND METHODS

Patients

The study included 24 patients, 13 males and 11 females. Seventeen were treated for respiratory infections and seven for urinary tract infections. The mean age was 67 years (range 24-87 years). All patients were hospitalized at the Department of Infectious Diseases in Lund, Sweden (Table 1).

Table 1. Patients according to diagnosis and sex

Diagnosis	Male	Female	Total
Repiratory tract infections	7	10	17
Urinary tract infections	6	1	7
Total	13	11	24

Patients with microorganisms resistant to ampicillin were excluded as well as patients with known malignant diseases, or confirmed allergy to penicillins and/or cephalosporins.

Patient Examination

The registration of medical history was made initially. The patients were observed daily during the treatment. After treatment a final clinical and bacteriological evaluation was made.

The following laboratory tests were performed before, during and after therapy: urine analysis (albumin, glucose, sediment); hematology (ESR, haematocrit, haemoglobin, RBC, platelets, WBC with differential count); blood chemistry (serum creatinine, bilirubin-total, alkaline phosphatase, SGOT, SGPT).

Before treatment started specimens for culture were taken from the nasopharynx, the throat, sputum, and urine. When possible, specimens were taken also during and after treatment. To avoid contamination, midstream specimens of urine were collected. Serological tests for influenzae virus and mycoplasma pneumoniae were made.

Treatment

The dosage schedule was chosen according to the severity of the disease. Ten and fourteen patients were treated with bacampicillin 600 mg and 800 mg respectively, three times daily. The patients were treated until three days after normalization of body temperature and always for at least ten days.

Assay of Bacampicillin

The serum levels of ampicillin after single doses of bacampicillin were assayed in the beginning of the treatment period, in general on the first morning at start of the treatment. In order to achieve a virtually complete excretion of the last dose, this was given not less than fourteen hours before the test dose. Blood samples were obtained by venepuncture before intake of the test dose and after 0.5, 1, 1.5, 2, 4, and 6 hours. Serum was separated and kept at $-20°C$ until analyzed.

The concentration of ampicillin was measured with the agarwell method. Diagnostic sensitivity test agar base (Oxoid), pH 7.2, was used as medium and Sarcina lutea ATCC 9341 as the test organism.

RESULTS

Serum Concentration

The serum levels of ampicillin after administration of bacampicillin 800 mg and 600 mg were studied in all 24 patients and are given in Figs. 1 and 2. The mean individual peak serum level ± SE independent of time was $9.9 ± 0.9$ µg/ml and $9.2 ± 1.1$ µg/ml after administration of bacampicillin 800 mg and 600 mg respectively.

Therapeutic Effect

The clinical evaluation was made according to the following criteria: <u>Good</u> - clinical findings subsided in a few days with no evidence of infection at the time the drug was discontinued nor during the follow-up; <u>Moderate</u> - clinical findings subsided significantly in a few days but signs of incomplete resolution were observed; <u>Poor</u> - no apparent response to therapy; <u>Unassessable</u> - efficacy was impossible to evaluate.

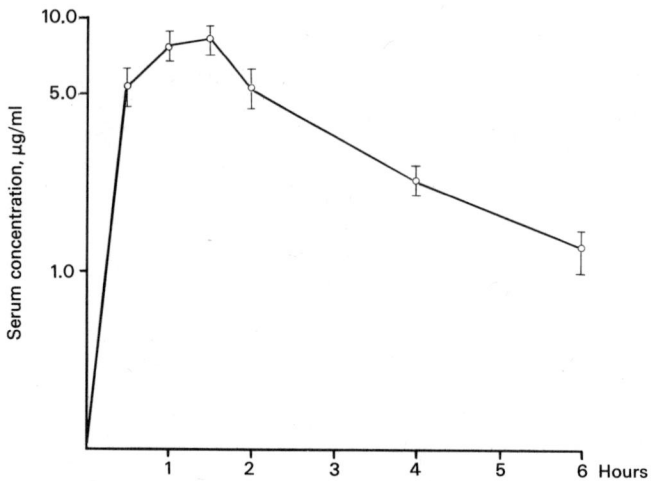

Fig. 1 Bacampicillin 800 mg: mean serum concentration ± standard error of the mean

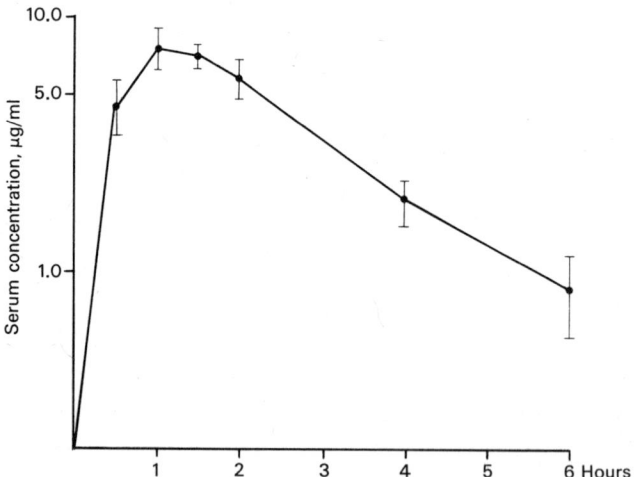

Fig. 2 Bacampicillin 600 mg: Mean serum concentration ± standard error of the mean.

Table 2. Bacampicillin: clinical results in respiratory tract infections

Diagnosis	Clinical Effect				
	Good	Moderate	Poor	Unassessable	Total
Acute bronchopneumoniae	5	1		1*	7
Pneumoniae	1	2		2*	5
Bronchitis	2	1		1	4
Acute sinusitis	1				1
Total	9	4	–	4	17

* mycoplasma pneumoniae

Respiratory Tract Infections

Seventeen patients were treated for acute respiratory tract infections. Six received 600 mg and eleven patients received 800 mg bacampicillin. The treatment period was 3-21 days.

Good or moderate clinical effect was seen in thirteen patients (Table 2). The clinical response was unassessable in four patients. Two of these cases were proved to be a mycoplasma pneumoniae infection. In another case the treatment was interrupted because of exanthema and in a further case due to nausea, which was probably caused by intensive treatment of asthma bronchiale with other drugs.

Urinary Tract Infections

Four patients treated for acute or recurrent urinary tract infections showed a good clinical response. One patient was treated with 600 mg and the others with 800 mg for 11-14 days.

The clinical efficacy could not be evaluated in three cases. One of these patients was treated for prostatitis, but the treatment was considered inadequate and was interrupted after ten days. The final evaluation was also unassessable in a case with clinical signs of pyelitis and negative bacteriological findings, later complicated by a concurrent Herpes Zoster. A patient with fever of uncertain origin was also unassessable.

Microbiological Evaluation

Diplococcus pneumoniae was initially isolated in six patients and Haemophilus influenzae in two patients with respiratory tract infections. At the time of the follow-up, these pathogens were not isolated again. In the other cases with clinical signs of respiratory tract infections, initial bacteriological findings showed a non-pathogen flora.

The clinical diagnosis of urinary tract infection was supplemented with finding of pathogenic bacteria (Escherichia coli) in one case. The initial pathogen could not be isolated again after therapy.

Laboratory Findings

No evidence of hematologic, renal, or liver toxicity was seen. Two patients treated with bacampicillin 800 mg and one with 600 mg showed a slight elevated eosinophil count during treatment. In one of these cases the eosinophil count was still elevated three days after the treatment had been completed.

Side Effects

Two patients developed exanthema during treatment with bacampicillin 800 mg after nine and twelve days and the treatment was discontinued. One patient treated with 600 mg had mild loose stools during two separate days and the treatment was fulfilled.

CONCLUSION

Bacampicillin has shown good clinical results in this material of hospitalized patients with respiratory and urinary tract infections. Bacampicillin was well tolerated with mild lower and no upper gastro-intestinal disturbances seen. Two patients developed rash during treatment. No evidence of hematologic renal or liver toxicity was seen. High serum concentrations of ampicillin were achieved both after 600 and 800 mg bacampicillin.

CLINICAL STUDY OF BACAMPICILLIN IN URINARY TRACT
INFECTIONS - A COMPARISON WITH AMPICILLIN

Wilhelm J. Kaipainen, Timo Timonen,
and Veijo Raunio
Departments of Internal Medicine and
Medical Microbiology
University Central Hospital, Oulu, Finland

SUMMARY

The purpose of the present study was to compare the clinical efficacy and tolerance of bacampicillin given in a twice daily dosage to ampicillin given in the normal three times daily dose to patients with urinary tract infection. Twenty three patients with an urinary tract infection were given either bacampicillin 400 mg. or 800 mg. x 2 or ampicillin 556 mg. x 3 in double blind technique for ten days. In this study bacampicillin given twice daily in equimolar or 1/2 equimolar doses to ampicillin gave as good clinical effect as ampicillin given three times daily. Many of our patients had predisposing factors like anatomical abnormalities, functional disturbancies and contributing diseases for urinary infections. No side effects were seen in the bacampicillin group but in one given ampicillin and iodine contrast an exanthema was seen.

MATERIAL AND METHODS

Patients

All the patients in this study were hospitalized in the internal medical ward of the University Central Hospital of Oulu, Finland because of an urinary tract infection and judged to need oral therapy with ampicillin. Patients with known allergy to penicillins, malignancy, indwelling catheter, urinary stones, neurogenic bladder and micro-organism not sensitive to ampicillin were excluded.

Material

Twenty-three patients, 20 women and three men aged from 18 to 84 years – mean 50.4 years were included. Ten of these patients were febrile on admission. Many patients had underlaying conditions and functional disturbancies predisposing to urinary tract infections:

Underlaying conditions

Anatomical	Hyperplasia prostatae	2
	Degeneratio polycystica renum	2
	Pelvis et ureter duplex	1
Functional	Creatinine clearance below 1, 4 ml/s	6
Other Diseases	Hypertonia arterialis	6
	Diabetes mellitus	4
	Arthritis urica	1
	Hypokalemia	1
	Total	23

Diagnosis

The diagnosis was confirmed in addition to positive anamnesis and microscopical examination of the sediment by bacteriological assessment of more than 10^5 bacteria per ml/urine– midstream samples before start of treatment.

Treatment

One of the following three regimens was given for ten days by double blind technique according to randomised blocks of three:

Bacampicillin 400 mg. x 2
Bacampicillin 800 mg. x 2
Ampicillin 556 mg. x 3

Laboratory tests

The following laboratory tests were taken in addition to anamnesis and status before treatment, during treatment on the 7th day and after treatment on the 14th and 30th day:

Haematology
: ESR, Haemoglobin
PCV, RBC, Platelets
WBC including differential count

Blood chemistry
: S-Creatinine
S-bilirubin total and direct
S-Alkaline phosfatase
S- GOT, S- GPT

Urine analysis
: Creatinine clearance
Albumine, Glucose
Sediment, Culture
PH, Specific gravity

Therapeutical evaluation

The clinical effect was evaluated after treatment as follows:

<u>Good</u>: Clinical symptoms disappeared. No significant bacteriuria and not more than 5 leucocytes/field in the sediment.

<u>Improvement</u>: No significant bacteriuria during treatment but with incomplete resolution of evidence of infection.
<u>Failure</u>: No apparent response to therapy and bacteria not eliminated during treatment. <u>Unassessable</u>: Efficacy was impossible to evaluate. The reason was stated.

RESULTS

The results are given in tables 1-4.

Good or improved clinical effect was seen in all patients treated with bacampicillin 400 mg. x 2. E. coli was isolated from all patients before treatment but no pathogens were isolated again during and after treatment. The creatinine clearances were diminished below 1 ml/s in the two patients who had pyuria after treatment.

Diagnosis	Clinical Effect			Bacteriological Findings		
	Good	Improvement	Failure	Before	During	After
Recurrent	X			E.coli+	−	−
Acute	X			E. coli	−	−
Chronic	X			E.coli+	− +	−
Chronic		X		E.coli+	− +	− +
Acute on chr.	X			E.coli+	−	−
Acute	X			E.coli+	−+	−
Acute		X		E.coli+	−+	−+
Acute	X			E.coli	−	−

Table 1 Results of therapy: Bacampicillin 400 mg. x 2 in pyelonephritis, += more than 5 leucocytes/field in sediment.

Diagnosis	Clinical Effect			Bacteriological Findings		
	Good	Improvement	Failure	Before	During	After
Acute			+	E.coli +	−+	E.coli+
Acute	+			Enteroc. −		−
Acute	+			Enteroc.+	−	−
Chronic		+		−	+ −	Klebsiella
Acute on chr.		+		E.coli +	−+	E.coli
Acute	+			E.coli +	−	−
Acute 1)	+			−	+ −	−

Table 2 results of therapy: Bacampicillin 800 mg. x 2 in pyelonephritis and cystitis
+ = more than 5 leucocytes/field in sediment
1) = cystitis

Good or improved clinical effect was seen in 6 patients and failure in one. Bacteriuria and pyuria became negative in 4 patients both during and after treatment. One patient dropped out because he was not supplied with enough medicine by mistake. In one patient with acute pyelonephritis E.coli was eliminated during treatment, while after treatment there was a relapse with E. coli and pyuria continued. This patient had prostatic hypertrophy.

Another patient with chronic pyelonephritis had pyuria before treatment which was eliminated during treatment, but after treatment Klebsiella appeared without pyuria. This patient aged 84 and her S- creatinine was elevated to 118 mol/1. E. coli was found before treatment in a third patient with acute on chronic pyelonephritis, but was eliminated during treatment while pyuria continued. After treatment she was reinfected with E.coli not sensitive to ampicillin (group 4), but there was no pyuria. No underlying condition could explain her urinary infection.

Diagnosis	Clinical Effect			Bacteriological Findings		
	Good	Improvement	Failure	Before	During	After
Recurrent	+			E.coli +	−	−
Acute		+		E.coli +	−+	−+
Chronic	+			E.coli +	−	−
Recurrent			+	−	+ −+	−+
Chronic	+			−	+ −	−
Recurrent	+			−	+ −	−

Table 3 Results of therapy: <u>Ampicillin 556 mg. x 3</u> in pyelonephritis, + = more than 5 leucocytes/field in sediment.

The bacteria were eliminated in all patients treated with ampicillin. Pyuria however continued in two cases during and after treatment. One of these patients had diabetes mellitus and the other arterial hypertonia. One patient developed an exanthema on the third day and ampicillin had to be withdrawn.

		Clinical Effect			
Drug	Total	Good	Improved	Failure	Unassessable
Bacampicillin 400 mg. x 2	8	6	2		
Bacampicillin 800 mg. x 2	8	4	2	1	1
Ampicillin 556 mg. x 3	7	4	1	1	1
Total	23	14	5	2	2

Table 4 Results of therapy - all patients.
In the total material good clinical effect was seen in 14 patients, 5 improved, two failed and two were unassessable. There was no statistical difference between the groups.

Side Effects

The patients were asked for any side-effects, which they could refer to the antibiotic treatment during and after therapy. Except for exanthema in one patient treated with ampicillin no side effects were noticed. This patient was cholecystographied with iodine contrast on the second day of treatment and developed rash the following day. So both ampicillin and iodine could be the provoking factor. No evidence of hematologic, renal or liver toxicity was seen which could be related to the tested drugs.

CONCLUSION

Bacampicillin given twice daily in equimolar or 1/2 equimolar doses to ampicillin has in this difficult material given as good clinical effect as ampicillin given three times daily. Many of our patients had predisposing factors for urinary tract infections. No side effects were seen in the bacampicillin group, but in one case given ampicillin and iodine contrast an exanthema was seen.

BACAMPICILLIN IN ACUTE TONSILLITIS

Pål-Henry Jeppsson, Olle Nylén, Sven Jönsson and
Paula Branefors-Helander

Sahlgrenska sjukhuset, University of Gothenburg
413 45 Gothenburg, Sweden

ABSTRACT

Bacampicillin was evaluated in 58 patients with acute tonsillitis. Patients were assigned randomly to receive either 200, 400, 600 or 800 mg three times daily for 10 days. Initial cultures were positive for β-haemolytic streptococci in 32 of 57 cases (56 %). The cure rate was 97 % at follow-up after three weeks. Two patients were considered as therapeutic failures clinically. In one of them all bacteriological cultivations yielded indigenous growth. In the other patient the initial cultivation yielded β-haemolytic streptococci, which, however, could not be isolated at control after one and three weeks.

The aim of this investigation was to gain information of the dose-response relationships regarding efficacy and tolerance in treatment with bacampicillin administered orally.

Bacampicillin is an ester of ampicillin (fig. 1) which is resorbed rapidly and almost completely (fig. 2) and is retransformed to ampicillin at absorption.

These circumstances diminish to a high degree the risk for gastro-intestinal disturbances and also give a higher concentration in serum than that achieved with non-esterified ampicillin.

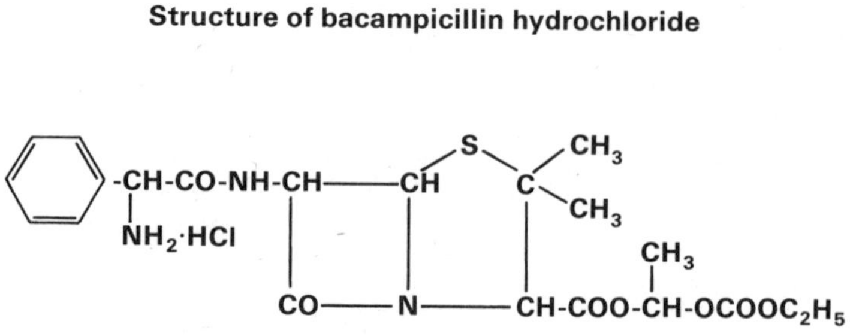

Structure of bacampicillin hydrochloride

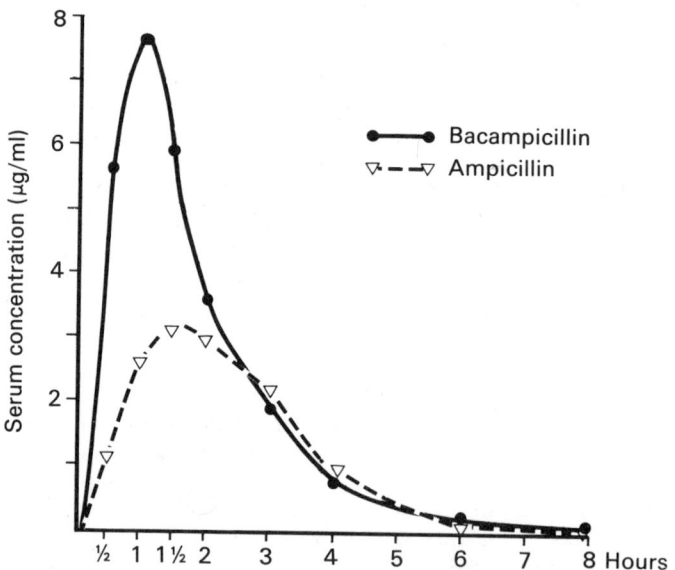

Fig. 1

Fig. 2 Mean serum levels of ampicillin in 12 volunteers after oral administration of bacampicillin 400 mg and an equimolar amount of ampicillin, 278 mg.
(Clinical Pharmacological studies of bacampicillin, L. Magni, B. Sjöberg, J. Sjövall, J. Wessman, 9th Int. Congress of Chemotherapy, London 1975, (press)

MATERIAL – METHODS

Acute tonsillitis was chosen as suitable experimental model because it is a well defined and confined bacterial infection. Patients with the following criteria were included in the study: reddened, swollen tonsils with exudate, no clinical signs of mononucl. inf. and a negative serotest for this disease (Monosticon). Patients with the following remarks were excluded: known progressive disease, kidney or liver function disturbances, allergy to penicillin and/or cephalosporins, suspicion of pregnancy. Children under seven years of age were excluded too.

The time schedule of the investigation is illustrated in fig. 3. A clinical examination was made at the first visit, after 7 - 10 days and after 21 - 23 days. Samples for bacterial cultivation were taken from the tonsils on all three occasions. The samples were inoculated on the same day as collection. A sero-test to exclude mononucleosis infectiosa was performed at the first visit.

Patients included in the study were treated with oral bacampicillin three times daily in equal portions with either of the following dosages: 200 mg, 400 mg, 600 mg or 800 mg fourteen days. The tablets were administered in accordance with a code list drawn up with the aid of a random number table. Clinical and microbiological evaluations were made independently to determine the therapeutic effect.

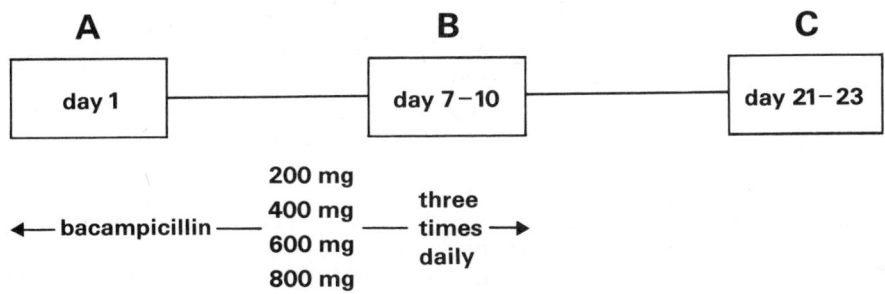

Clinical examination (A-B-C)

Samples for bacterial cultivation from the tonsils (A-B-C)

Serotest for Mononucleosis (A)

Fig. 3

The following criteria were used for clinical evaluation of efficacy:
Good - no signs of infection.
Improved - remaining redness and intermittent irritations.
Failure - remaining signs of tonsillitis.
Not assessable - patients who did not fulfil the treatment or did not return for control.

BACTERIAL CULTIVATION TECHNIQUE

The following media were used for primary cultivations: (1) blood agar (placenta-pepton agar with 5 % of horse blood); (2) gentian-violet agar (placenta-pepton agar with 5 % of horse blood and gentan-violet 1/80,000); (3) haematin agar (tryptone-yeast extract agar with 10 % of horse blood, heated to 80°C for 20 min. before the addition of gentian-violet 1/80,000).

After the inoculation, a strip containing XV factor was placed on the blood agar plates. For selection of H. influenzae colonies, a disc containing 50 mg oleandomycin was placed on the haematin agar plates, which were incubated in 5 - 6 per cent CO_2 atmosphere at 37°C. The blood agar and the gentian-violet agar plates were incubated in air at 37°C. All plates were incubated for at least 18 h before the first reading and then for another 24 h before the final reading. The preliminary identification of the different bacterial species was based on colonial characteristics and microscopic examination. For confirmation of the preliminary diagnosis, additional tests were performed for the following bacterial species: for the haemophilus group, dependece on X, V or XV factors; for Streptococcus pyogenes group A, sensitivity to bacitracin and ability to produce soluble streptolysin; for Staphylococcus pyogenes (var, aureus), ability to produce coagulase and to ferment mannitol.

The following bacterial species were denoted as potentially pathogenic: Str. pyogenes group A, H. influenzae and Staph. aureus. In the samples, diphtheroids, Neisseria, α-streptococci, Staph. albus, H. parainfluenzae and H. parahaemolyticus were labelled as indigenous growth. Single colonies of Staph. aureus were also considered non-pathogenic.

The amount of growth on the primary plates for each one of the aforementioned bacterial species was graded as heavy, moderate or sparse.

RESULTS

The material included 58 patients, 29 men and 29 women. The age and sex distribution is shown in fig. 4. The results of the initial bacterial cultivations are demonstrated in table 1. From 32 of the 57 patients (56 %) β-streptococci were isolated initially. The initial sample from one patient was lost. Four of the isolated strains were of a potentially nephritogenic sero-type (type 12). In one patient Haemophilus influenzae was found as the sole pathogenic species and in another patient only Staphylococcus aureus was found. In both patients the growth was recorded as heavy. From 23 patients no pathogenic bacteria could be isolated.

In table II the clinical effect at the control after three weeks is related to the given dosage of bacampicillin. 48 patients were considered healed at this control. Two patients, 16 years of age, were considered as therapeutic failures. The bacterial cultivations from the first patient yielded β-streptococci, which, however, could not be re-isolated after treatment. Eight patients were unassessable. Six did not return for follow-up. One patient had an acute biliary disease without correlation to the treatment but did not fulfil the therapy. The last patient did not fulfil the medication because of urticaria, the cause of which might be the treatment with bacampicillin. No differences in clinical effect could be demonstrated with regard to given dosages.

The result of the bacterial cultivations at the control after one week from the 32 patients with initial growth of β-streptococci is demonstrated in table III. Those cultivations showed that the β-streptococci were eradicated in 30 patients. In one patient β-streptococci not belonging to group A were re-isolated. One patient was unassessable. The cultivations after three weeks showed that two patients in the 400 mg

Table 1. Results of initial bacterial cultivations from 57 patients

	200	400	600	800	total
β-streptococci (group A)	8	7	9	8	32(56%)
H.influenzae				1	1
Staph. aureus		1			1
non-path. culture		6	6	5	6	23(40%)
total	14	14	14	15	57

Table II. Clinical effect related to dosage (control 3 w.)

	200	400	600	800	total
good	10	12	14	12	48
failure	1	1			2
unassessable	3	1	1	3	8
total	14	14	15	15	58

Table III. Results of the bacterial cultivations after 1 week in 32 patients with initial positive culture of β-streptococci

	200	400	600	800	total
eliminated	7	6	9	8	30(97%)
reisolated	1*				1
unassessable		1			1
total	8	7	9	8	32

*A strain of β-streptococci not belonging to group A. This strain was isolated on all three occasions.

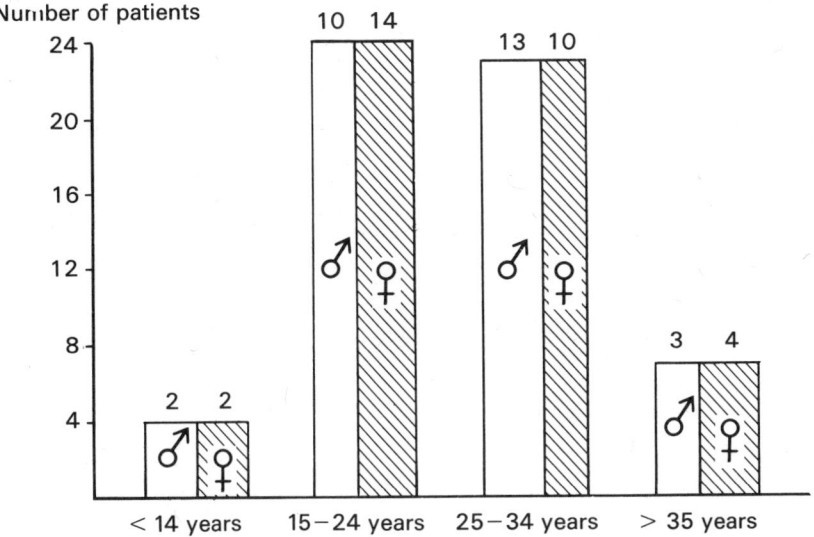

Fig. 4 Age and sex distribution

group and one in the 600 mg group had been reinfected during the ten days after termination of therapy. The four patients in whom a potentially nephritogenic streptococcal serotype was found were considered healed and the bacteria were eradicated at the control after three weeks.

The incidence of side-effects could be evaluated in 50 patients. Suggestive drug-related reactions occurred in 7 patients: urticaria (1), loose stools (3), pruritus genitalis (1) and heartburn (2). The reactions were mild or moderate and did not interfere with the therapy except in the patient with urticaria. All patients but one with side-effects were treated with either 600 or 800 mg three times daily. Thus the side-effects might be related to the higher dosages given.

CONCLUSION

58 patients with acute tonsillitis were treated with bacampicillin administered orally. β-haemolytic streptococci were found in 32 of these patients. 97 % of the latter patients were cured.

CLINICAL STUDY ON BACAMPICILLIN IN OTITIS MEDIA ACUTA AND
SINUSITIS ACUTA

        Olle Olsson   Claes Henning

        Departments of Oto-Rhino-laryngology and Microbiology

        Hospital of Sundsvall, Sundsvall, Sweden

Introduction

The aim of this study was to compare the clinical efficacy and tolerance of bacampicillin in a twice daily dosage with ampicillin given three times daily.

Most strains of Haemophilus influenzae and Gram-positive bacteria are sensitive to ampicillin. They are also frequently found in acute otitis and sinusitis. Thus patients with these diagnosis were selected for the study.

Material and methods

Patients

Totally 52 patients attending the ENT-Department in the Hospital of Sundsvall have been included in the trial, 30 patients with clinical evidence of acute otitis media and 22 with acute sinusitis. The patients ranged from 6-67 years of age. Only patients over the age of 5 were included as a paediatric suspension was not available. Patients with know allergy to penicillins and cephalosporins as well as malignant diseases were excluded.

Bacteriological diagnosis

Samples for bacteriological culturing were taken before treatment and at follow-up visits. In patients with acute otitis media all specimens were taken from nasopharynx. In patients with acute sinusitis specimens before treatment were taken both from irrigation fluid and nasopharynx. After treatment, specimens were only taken from nasopharynx in these cases as pus was not present in the maxillary sinus.

Treatment

The patients were treated orally with either bacampicillin 400 mg twice daily or ampicillin 500 mg three times daily. The study was performed in a double-blind fashion and the patients were allocated to the two different treatment regimens according to a code-list drawn up with a random number table.

Treatment

Drug	Dosage		
	Morning	Day	Night
Bacampicillin	400 mg	placebo	400 mg
Ampicillin	500 mg	500 mg	500 mg
Duration of therapy: 10 days			

Table 1   (Olsson et Henning 1975)

Both drugs were given as tablets of identical shape and colour and the treatment period was 10 days.

Patients with sinusitis were irrigated initially and all patients were given nasal decongestants.

Evaluation of efficacy

The clinical evaluation was made at the final follow-up visit, 2 or 3 weeks after start of treatment as good – improvement or failure according to the following criteria.

Otitis media

Good:	Normal hearing and a normal and mobile ear drum
Improvement:	Persisting hearing impairment but no sign of acute infection
Failure:	Persisting infection

Sinusitis

Good: Symptom-free. Pale and clean inside nose. X-ray negative or with only slight mucous membrane swelling.

Improvement: Nasal catarrh and serous secretion from the nose

Failure: Persistent trouble with purulent secretion from the nose

The bacteriological evaluation was made separated from the clinical evaluation.

Results

Fifty patients are included in the final clinical evaluation. The results from initial microbial cultures in 52 patients are presented.

Initial bacterial findings

Acute otitis media

Pathogenic bacteria were isolated in 21 of 30 patients with otitis media. In thirteen cases Haemophilus influenzae were isolated and in 10 patients pneumococci (table 2).

Initial findings	Bacampicillin	Ampicillin	Total
Pneumococci	3	5	8
Pneumococci + H. influenzae	2		2
H. influenzae	4	6	10
H. influenzae + H. parainfluenzae		1	1
Normal flora	8	1	9
Total	17	13	30

Table 2. Acute otitis media: Initial microbiological findings in nasopharynx.

Acute sinusitis

Of 22 patients with acute sinusitis 12 patients had pathogenic bacteria isolated initially.
Haemophilus species were seen in 5 cases, pneumococci in 3 cases, and Gram-negative rods in 3 cases (table 3).

Initial findings	Bacampicillin	Ampicillin	Total
Pneumococci		2	2
Pneumococci + H influenzae	1		1
H. influenzae	2	1	3
H. parainfluenzae		1	1
E. coli	1		1
Coliformae	1		1
E. coli + coliformae		1	1
β-streptococci		2	2
Normal flora	4	6	10
Total	9	13	22

Table 3. Acute sinusitis: Initial microbiological findings in irrigation fluid or nasopharynx.

Clinical evaluation

Acute otitis media

Of 16 patients treated with bacampicillin for acute otitis media 15 patients showed a good clinical response and of 13 patients treated with ampicillin a good clinical response was seen in 11 patients. One patient treated with ampicillin discontinued the treatment because of diarrhoea. One patient in each group developed otosalpingitis during treatment and the effekt was judged as improvement (table 4).

	N	good	improvement	failure	unassessable
Bacampicillin 400 mg b.i.d.	16	15	1[1]		
Ampicillin 500 mg t.i.d.	13	11	1[1]		1[2]

1) otosalpingit   2) discontinued treatment, diarrhoea

Table 4. Acute otitis media: Clinical effect.

Sinusitis acuta

Twenty-two patients with sinusitis acuta have been includes in the study, 9 treated with bacampicillin and 13 with ampicillin. Eigh patients treated with bacampicillin showed a good clinical response while an improvement was seen in 1 patient with allergic rhinitis. In the ampicillin group there were 12 patients with good effect while 1 patient discontinued the treatment because of diarrhoea (table 5).

	N	good	improvement	failure	unassessable
bacampicillin 400 mg b.i.d.	9	8		1[1]	
ampicillin 500 mg t.i.d.	13	12			1[2]

1) allergic rhinitis   2) discontinued treatment, diarrhoea

Table 5. Acute sinusitis: Clinical effect

The therapeutic effect was also judged in all patients with a X-ray point-system according to Axelsson. A quite healthy maxillary sinus was given 0 points and a complete opacity of the sinus on X-ray was given 6 points. The mean points before treatment were 5.4 and after treatment 1.1 in the group of patients treated with bacampicillin (figure 1). The points for ampicillin were 4.5 and 0,9 respectively. No statistical difference in the decrease of points were however seen between the two drugs (T-test).

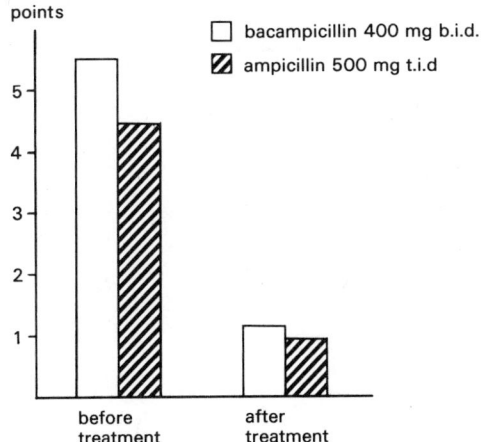

Figure 1. X-ray of sinus maxillaris means points before and after treatment.

Bacteriological evaluation

There was no definite difference between the treatment groups in the bacteriological evaluation. The pneumococci were eliminated after treatment in all 11 cases. E. coli and coliform bacteriae were eliminated in 2 out of 3 cases. Haemophilus species were initially isolated in 17 cases, most of them in the otitis media group of patients. After treatment Haemophilus influenzae was isolated from nasopharynx in 14 cases although these patient showed a good clinical response.

Side-effects

At the final visit the patients were asked for any side-effects they could relate to the antibiotic therapy. Seven (27%) of the 26 patients treated with ampicillin developed diarrhoea. In 2 of these cases the diarrhoea was severe and necessitated treatment to be interrupted. One of these patients also developed an urticaria after 11 days. One patient with vomiting and one with exanthema were also seen in the ampicillin group. The patient with exanthema had β-haemolytic streptococci group A before and after treatment and Scarlatina could not be excluded in this case. The only side-effect reported in the patients treated with bacampicillin was one case who developed loose stools. Thus the side-effects in the bacampicillin group were very few (table 6) compared to those in the ampicillin group. The difference in side-effect between the two drugs is statistically significant ($p = 0.004$, Fisher's two-tail test)

Side-effects	Bacampicillin N = 26	Ampicillin N = 26
Diarrhoea		7
Loose stools	1	
Vomiting		1
Urticaria		1
Exanthema		1

$P = 0.004$ (Fisher's two-tail test)

Table 6. Side effects in 52 patients treated with bacampicillin 400 mg b.i.d. or ampicillin 500 mg t.i.d.

Summary

Bacampicillin 400 mg given twice daily in acute otitis media and sinusitis has shown as good clinical effect as ampicillin given 500 mg three times daily. Bacampicillin was very well tolerated giving significantly fewer side-effects than ampicillin.

CLINICAL, BACTERIOLOGICAL, AND PHARMACOLOGICAL STUDY OF BACAMPICILLIN IN CHRONIC MAXILLARY SINSUSITIS

Veijo Raunio, Kalevi Jokinen, and Seppo Karjalainen

Department of Medical Microbiology and Otolaryngology
University Hospital, Oulu, Finland

This is a preliminary report of a study which is going on. As high peak serum concentrations are considered to be of importance for the distribution of penicillin into sinussecretion and sinusmucosa (Lundberg & Malmborg 1974) and thus clinical response in the treatment of sinusitis it was of interest to investigate if dose/re-response relationships regarding therapeutic efficacy and tolerance exist with bacampicillin in treatment of acute sinusitis. Furthermore a pharmacological study of absorption of bacampicillin was performed.

Material and methods

The present material is an interim report of a clinical investigation started during August-December 1974 at the Departments of Otolaryngology and Clinical Microbiology at the University Hospital of Oulu, Finland.

Patients

Totally 31 patients have completed the antibiotic treatment and have returned for a final follow-up visit about 3 weeks after start of treatment. Patients with known allergy to penicillins and/or cephalosporins, mononucleosis infectiosa, severe progressive affection, kidney and/or liver function disturbances, as well as patients older than 70 years and children under the age of 10 are excluded.

Diagnosis

All patients had an anamnesis and clinical signs of chronic maxillary sinusitis.

Treatment

Bacampicillin was available in tablets of 400 mg and ampicillin in tablets of 278 mg, i.e. equimolar to 400 mg bacampicillin. The patients were in a doupleblind fashion allocated to one of the following treatment groups according to a code-list drawn by means of a random number table. Bacampicillin was given twice daily and ampicillin three times daily.

Tablets given

Dosage schedule	Morning	Day	Night
Bacampicillin			
400 mg x 2	400+placebo	placebo+placebo	400+placebo
800 mg x 2	400+400	placebo+placebo	400+400
Ampicillin			
556 mg x 3	278+278	278+278	278+278

The bacampicillin, ampicillin and placebo tablets were of identical shape and colour and packed in a strip-pac, labelled morning, day, night.

Radical sinus maxillaris surgery was performed in all patients according to Caldwell-Luc. They were treated for 10 days with either antibiotic. Mucosa sample was taken.
If the required therapeutic effect had not been reached at follow-up, other antibiotics were instituted according to sensitivity tests of the bacteria isolated. If necessary the patients were also given decongestine nose drops.

Patients examination

Medical history and clinical status were initially registered. Follow-up was carried out daily during the four first days and after 7 and 21 days.

The following laboratory tests were carried out daily on day 0 (before start of treatment), after 1 week and after 3 weeks.

Haematology   EST, haematocrit, haemaglobin, erythrocytes
                           platelets, WBC including differential
                           count.

Blood chemistry: Serum creatinine, bilirubin-total,
                     alkaline phosphatase, GOT, GPT

Urine analysis: Albumin, glucose, sediment

Evaluation of efficacy

The evaluation of the clinical and bacteriological results was done independently. Thus the clinical effect could be judged as good even if pathogenic bacteria were reisolated.

The bacteriological results were evaluated according to the following criteria:
- Initial pathogen eliminated, now normal flora (no pathogen)
- Same pathogen isolated
- Initial pathogen eliminated, now new pathogen
- Partially the same pathogen isolated (at least one pathogen eliminated)
- Still normal flora
- Initially normal flora, now pathogen flora
- Initial pathogen isolated, plus new pathogen
- No assessable (one assay etc.)

The following criteria for evaluation of the clinical result were used:

Good   Symptom-free, pale and clean inside nose and no pus.

Moderate Nasal catarrh and serous secretion from the nose

Poor   Persistent discomfort with purulent secretion from the nose

Determination of drug concentration

Blood specimens were drawn immediately before the first administration of the drug (zero sample) and at 0.5, 1, 1.5, 2, 4, 6 and 8 hours after the intake.

All blood samples were separated by centrifugation and the serum was stored at $-40°C$ until the assays were performed.

Microbiological assay

Ampicillin concentrations were determined by the microdisc method designed by Jalling et al. (1972). Sarcina lutea ATCC 9343 was used as the tese organism.

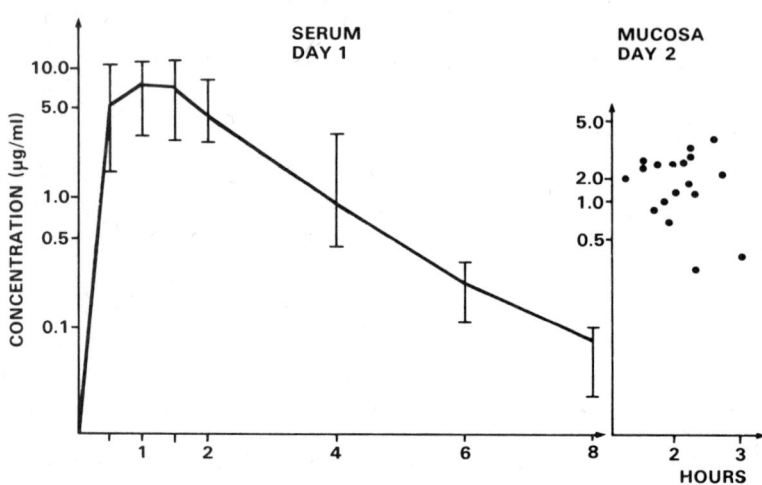

Fig. 1. Bacampicillin 800 mg: concentration of ampicillin in serum and mucosa in µg/ml.

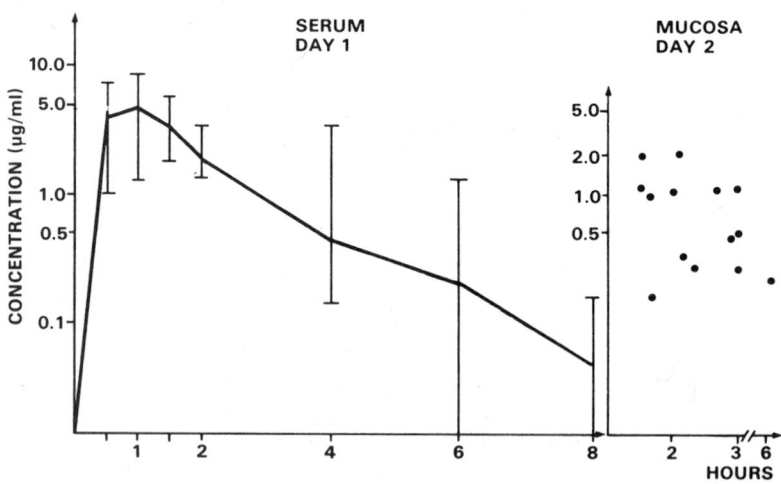

Fig. 2. Bacampicillin 400 mg: concentration of ampicillin in serum and mucosa in µg/ml.

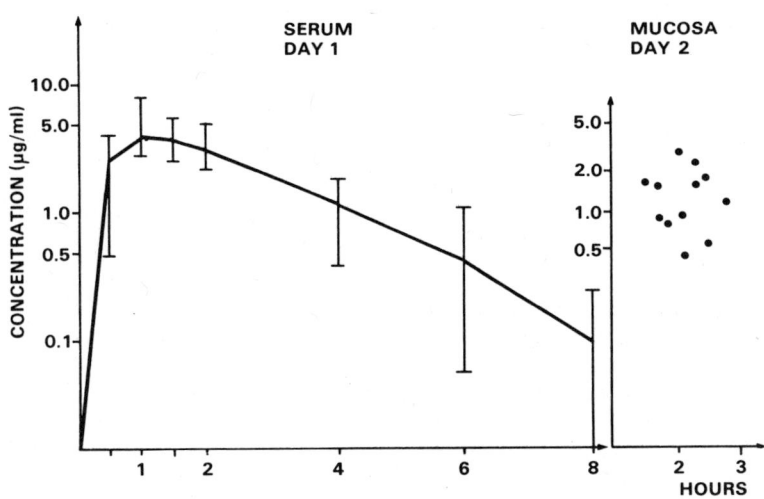

Fig. 3. Ampicillin 556 mg: concentration of ampicillin in serum and mucosa in µg/ml.

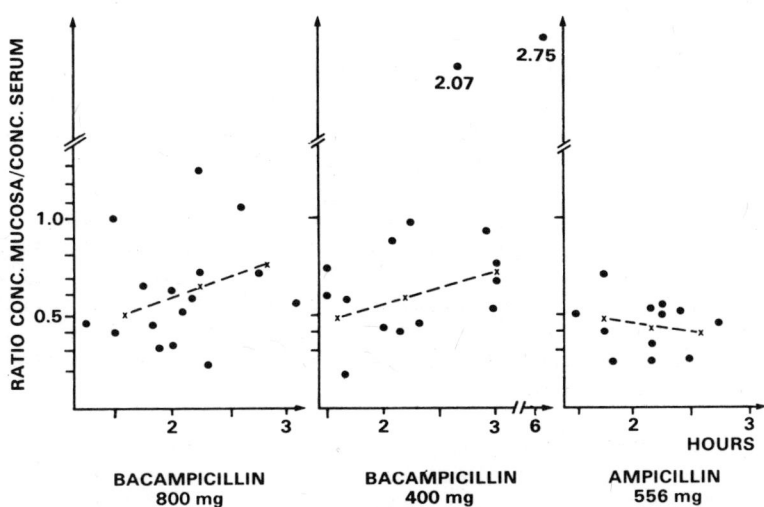

Fig. 4. Ratio tissue concentration/serum concentration after administration of bacampicillin 800 mg and 400 mg and ampicillin 556 mg.

Bacteriological analyses

Bacteriological examination was performed on secretion samples obtained from the sinus pre-operatively by puncture, during operation, and postoperatively by irrigation. Bacteriological cultivations were made on the following media: blood agar, chocolate agar, lactose agar plate and thioglycolate broth.

Results

Antibiotic assay

In all patients determinations of antibiotic concentration in serum was made on the first day of the treatment.

Bacampicillin was better and faster absorbed than ampicillin, mean peak values independent of time of 800 and 400 mg bacampicillin and 556 mg ampicillin was 7.54, 6.37 and 4.65 ug/ml respectively. The peak concentration was achieved within 2 hours.

Chemically 556 mg ampicillin is equivalent to 800 mg bacampicillin. In this study bacampicillin 800 mg gave approximately 60 % higher peak value and the 400 mg dose approximately 30 % higher peak value compared to ampicillin 556 mg.

Clinical effect

The clinical effect was judged as good or improved in all patients. Of the 10 patients treated with 800 mg bacampicillin, 7 showed a good response. Patient 9 with a moderate response, had an allergic rhinitis which made the clinical assessment difficult.

Six patients in the 400 mg bacampicillin group (11 patients) responded good to the treatment. One of these patients was reinfected with β-streptococci at home 20 days after start of treatment. After completed treatment this patient had cultures of normal flora in the maxillar sinuses and the clinical effect was judged as good. The moderate effect in patient 2 was explained by a concurrent allergic rhinitis.

In the ampicillin-treated group three patients responded more slowly and the clinical effect was judged as moderate. All these patients were cured within one month after stop of treatment without any other antibiotic treatment.

Bacteriological evaluation

In 30 patients the antibiotic treatment had started before the bacteriological samples from sinus maxillaris were taken. Pus was present in 22 cases thus indicating a purulent infection, but only in four cases bacteria were isolated. This could be explained as the penicillin present in the samples was enough to kill the bacteria. These cases are considered due to bacterial pathogens of unknown origin.

In the 800 mg bacampicillin group Haemophilus influenzae was isolated before treatment in one patient and the bacteria were eliminated after treatment. Three patients with bacteriological finding after treatment also had secretion and thus, the clinical result was rated as moderate.

After completed treatment, the bacteria were eliminated in four patients treated with 400 mg bacampicillin twice daily. Patient 22 was reinfected at home with β-hemolytic streptococci ten days after completed treatment. Four patients treated with ampicillin showed positive cultures after treatment. In three of these cases, two pathogens were found at the same time. All three patients also had secretion and were evaluated moderate or poor in response. In the other six patients, the bacteria were eliminated.

Side-effects

All patients were asked for any adverse reaction during and after the therapy. No patient treated with bacampicillin developed any adverse reaction. Patient 2 treated with ampicillin complained of gastrointestinal pain during 7 days on therapy and this reaction was evaluated as a probable combination of ampicillin and other drug therapy.

The general impression was that bacampicillin was very well tolerated.

Laboratory analysis

No abnormal values were found that could be correlated to the penicillin therapy. No toxic effect on liver as seen in SGOT-, SGPT-, alkalinephosphatase- and bilirubin values was found.

MECILLINAM AND PIVMECILLINAM – NEW BETA-LACTAM ANTIBIOTICS WITH HIGH ACTIVITY AGAINST GRAM-NEGATIVE BACILLI

F. Lund, K. Roholt, L. Tybring and W.O. Godtfredsen[*]

Leo Pharmaceutical Products

2750 Ballerup, Denmark

A common structural feature of all penicillins used in medicine is the presence of an acylamido group in the 6β-position of penicillanic acid, (cf. fig.1) and it has been generally assumed that this grouping is a prerequisite for antibacterial activity of β-lactam antibiotics.

However, in 1972 Lund and Tybring reported that a new type of penicillanic acid derivatives which do not possess this structural feature, namely 6β-amidinopenicillanic acids – are antibacterially active and that their antibacterial properties differ fundamentally from those of the penicillins.

The general structure of these antibiotics is shown in fig. 1. It will be seen that the usual acylamido grouping in the 6-position of penicillanic acid has been replaced by an amidino grouping. Chemically, these compounds can be described as substituted formamidines.

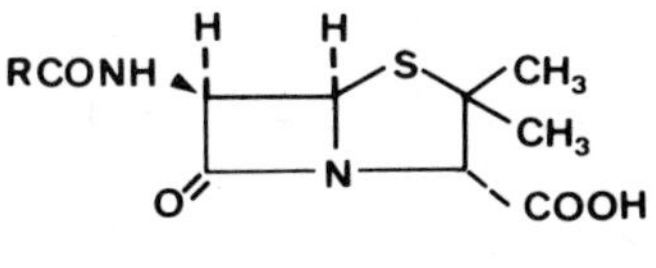

Penicillin 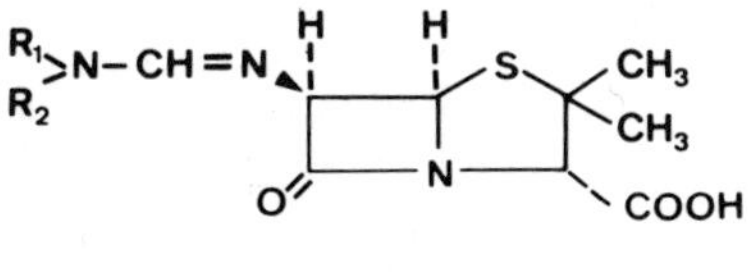   **6-Amidinopenicillanic acid**

Fig. 1

One of the more interesting of the many compounds of this type which have now been synthesized is the one shown in fig. 2. This compound was originally designated FL 1060, but has now been given the generic name mecillinam. The present and the following papers in this section will deal with the properties of this semi-synthetic antibiotic and its pivaloyloxymethyl ester, which is called FL 1039 or pivmecillinam.

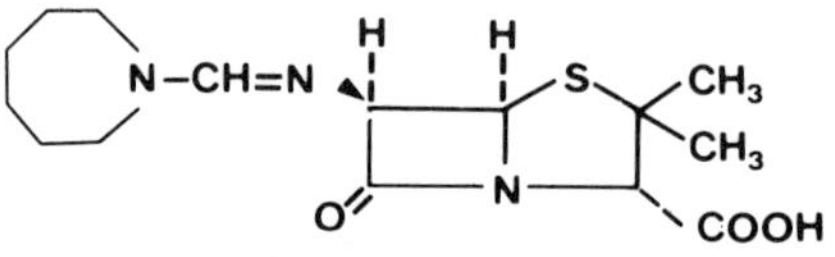

Mecillinam (FL 1060)

Fig. 2

ANTIBACTERIAL ACTIVITY IN VITRO

The antimicrobial spectrum of mecillinam as compared to that of ampicillin is shown in table 1. The figures indicate the IC_{50}-values – e.g. the concentrations required for a 50% inhibition of growth.

Table 1

Antibacterial Spectrum of Mecillinam and Ampicillin

	IC_{50} (µg/ml)	
	Mecillinam	Ampicillin
Staph. aureus	5.0	0.016
Streptococcus pyogenes	0.50	0.006
Streptococcus faecalis	>100	0.20
Neisseria gonorrhoea	0.16	0.005
Haemophilus influenzae	16	0.16
Escherichia coli	0.015	1.3
Enterobacter cloacae	0.16	>100
Klebsiella pneumoniae	0.10	0.32
Proteus vulgaris	0.16	40
Proteus mirabilis	0.10	0.50
Salmonella typhimurium	0.10	1.0
Shigella dysenteriae	0.050	1.0
Serratia marcescens	0.10	32
Pseudomonas aeruginosa	160	500

You will note that the most striking property of mecillinam is a remarkably high activity against Enterobacteriaceae, including E.coli, Enterobacter, Klebsiella, Proteus, Salmonella and Shigella species as well as some strains of Serratia marcescens.

The activity against Gram-positive bacteria like staphylococci and streptococci is lower and this is also true for the Gram-negative species Neisseria and Haemophilus influenzae. Organisms like Streptococcus faecalis and Pseudomonas aeruginosa are practically resistant to mecillinam. Particularly impressive is the strong activity against E.coli which to my knowledge is unsurpassed by any antibiotic.

Mecillinam is inactivated by β-lactamases, but is generally more stable than ampicillin and penicillin G.

MODE OF ACTION

The unusual structure of mecillinam in connection with its unique antimicrobial spectrum raised of course the question whether its mode of action is similar to or differs from that of the usual penicillins.

Certain peculiarities of the morphologic changes of coli cells exposed to mecillinam suggested that its mode of action is not the same as that of the penicillins. Whereas low but growth-inhibiting concentrations of ampicillin cause E.coli to form long rod-shaped cells in which bulges appear at the end or at the septum of the cell mecillinam at concentrations of 0.1 µg/ml or higher causes the cells to enlarge and gradually become spherical. The end product is superficially similar to the spheroplasts produced when E.coli is exposed to penicillins under conditions of high osmolality. However, in contrast to such spheroplasts these large spherical cells still seem to have an intact cell wall and they are osmotically stable. The suspicion of a different mode of action has been confirmed by biochemical investigations performed in Professor Parks and Professor Stromingers laboratories. These investigations have shown that mecillinam like the penicillins interferes with the biosynthesis of the cell wall, but that the target of the inhibition is different. Thus, none of the three enzymatic activities in E.coli that have been reported to be sensitive to penicillins are inhibited by mecillinam at concentrations up to 1000 times the growth inhibiting concentration.

SYNERGY WITH OTHER ANTIBIOTICS

The fact the mecillinam has shown to be an inhibitor of cell wall biosynthesis in a manner different from that of the penicillins suggest of course that combination of mecillinam with a penicillin like ampicillin could give rise to a synergic action. That this is the case has been demonstrated both in vitro and in vivo.

In table 2 are shown examples on synergy between ampicillin and mecillinam in vitro. In the two first columns are shown the MIC-values for mecillinam and ampicillin, respectively, and in the next column the amounts of a 1:1 mixture of the two compounds necessary for inhibition of growth. The figures in the last column indicate how many times more active the mixture is than it would have been if the combined effect of the two compounds was merely additive.

Table 2

In vitro Activity of Mecillinam and Ampicillin Alone and in Combination

Microorganism	MIC (µg/ml)			f
	Mecillinam	Ampicillin	Mecillinam + Ampicillin 1:1	
E. coli	1	10	0.05 + 0.05	18
E. coli	>100	10	1.5 + 1.5	>6
Klebsiella pneumoniae	100	3	0.15 + 0.15	19
Proteus vulgaris	100	30	0.15 + 0.15	154
Salmonella typhi	10	3	0.15 + 0.15	15
Shigella flexneri	3	3	0.15 + 0.15	10
Haemophilus influenzae	>10	0.3	0.1 + 0.1	>3

It will be seen that synergy is not limited to organisms sensitive to both compounds, but can also be demonstrated in cases where the organisms is more or less resistant to one of the two antibiotics. An interesting example of such an organism is Hemophilus influenzae which is sensitive to ampicillin, but rather insensitive to mecillinam. Nevertheless, a 1:1 combination is more active than ampicillin alone.

The synergy demonstrated in vitro has been confirmed by numerous experiments in mice.

PHARMACOKINETICS

As will appear from fig. 3 which compares the serum levels observed after administration of mecillinam to volunteers by the oral and the intramuscular route, respectively, the drug is poorly absorbed when given by mouth.

It was therefore desirable to develop an orally active derivative, and as we shall see this objective has been achieved with the preparation of the corresponding pivaloyloxymethyl ester, called pivmecillinam.

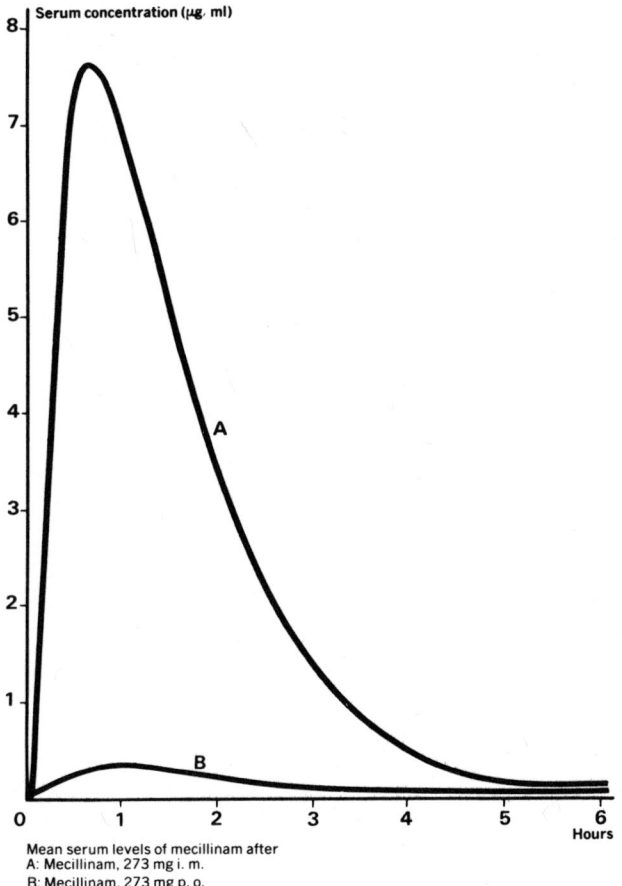

Mean serum levels of mecillinam after
A: Mecillinam, 273 mg i. m.
B: Mecillinam, 273 mg p. o.

Fig. 3

The structure of this ester is shown in fig. 4. Pivmecillinam has no antibacterial activity _per se_, but it is very well absorbed from the gastro-intestinal tract, and after the absorption it is rapidly hydrolyzed with liberation of the antibacterially active compound mecillinam.

The hydrolysis is catalyzed by enzymes present in blood and many tissues – including the intestinal mucosa – and is assumed to take place as outlined in fig. 4: First pivalic acid is split off enzymatically with formation of the unstable hydroxymethyl ester which subsequently decomposes spontaneously into mecillinam and formaldehyde.

Fig. 5 depicts the results of a cross-over study where equimolar amounts of pivmecillinam and mecillinam were given to a group of healthy volunteers by the oral and intramuscular routes, respectively. It will be seen that oral administration of pivmecillinam results in serum levels of mecillinam which – although somewhat lower than those obtained when the latter compound is injected intramuscularly – are quite satisfactory. The urinary recovery of mecillinam amounts to abt. 60% after intramuscular or intravenous injection of mecillinam and to abt. 45% after oral administration of pivmecillinam indicating that abt. 75% of orally administered pivmecillinam is absorbed.

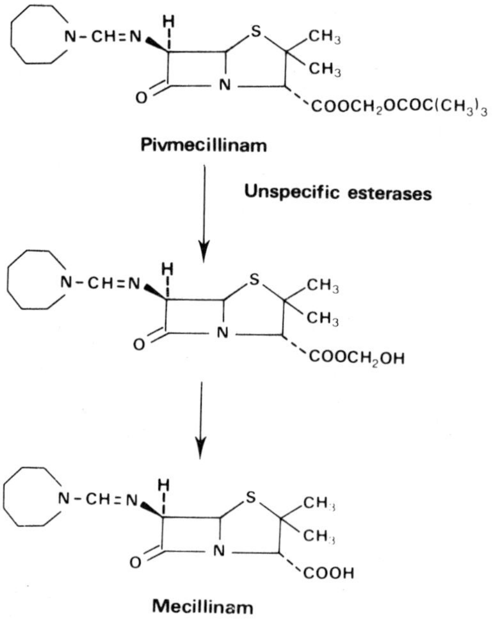

Fig. 4

It is worth emphasizing that the pharmacokinetic properties of mecillinam and pivmecillinam are very similar to those of ampicillin and pivampicillin, respectively, a fact which of course will be of importance in connection with a possible concomitant use of the two antibiotics in order to utilize the synergism clinically.

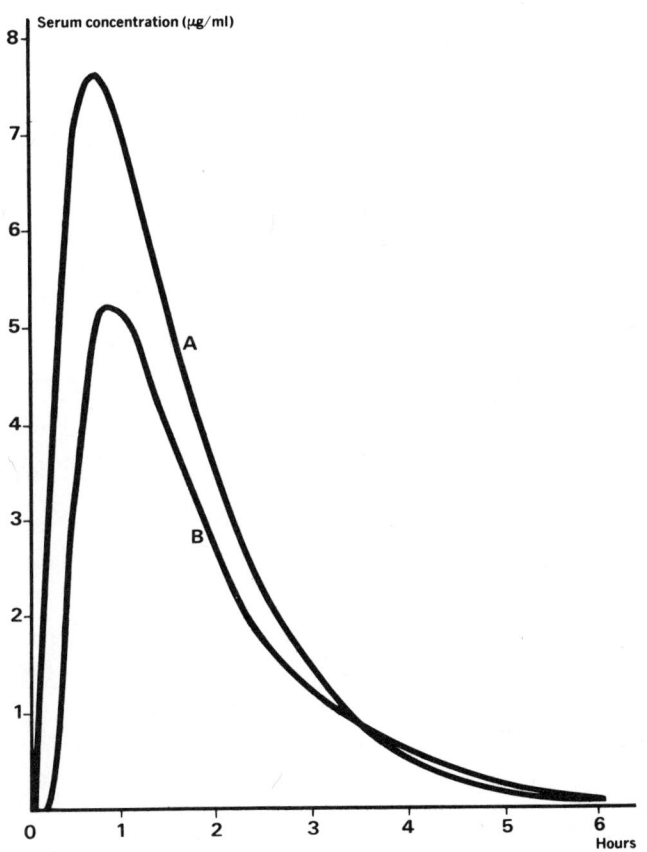

Mean serum levels of mecillinam after
A: Mecillinam, 273 mg i. m.
B: Pivmecillinam, 400 mg p. o. (~273 mg of mecillinam)

Fig. 5

THE DISPOSITION OF MECILLINAM AND PIVMECILLINAM IN MAN

J.Andrews, M.J.Kendall, and M.Mitchard

Department of Therapeutics and Clinical Pharmacology
Birmingham University, Medical School

Peak serum mecillinam concentrations of 5-6 µg/ml were obtained after an intramuscular injection of mecillinam and concentrations of about 2 µg/ml and 3 µg/ml after capsules containing doses of 200 mg and 400 mg of pivmecillinam respectively in volunteers lying supine in beds. A six day course of two 200 mg capsules of pivmecillinam taken four times a day did not significantly alter the plasma mecillinam concentration/time profile. Two 500 mg probenecid tablets taken before 400 mg of pivmecillinam reduced the urinary clearance of mecillinam and increased the peak serum concentrations to between 4 and 5 µg/ml. Moderate activity resulted in higher serum mecillinam concentrations probably due to an increase in absorption efficiency.

INTRODUCTION

Mecillinam is a novel amidinopenicillanic acid derivative which although being superficially similar to the penicillins, has an important structural difference and a different spectrum of antibacterial activity.

Preliminary studies in animals and man have demonstrated that mecillinam is poorly absorbed from the gastro intestinal tract and is therefore given parenterally. However, as for ampicillin the pivaloyl ester is efficiently absorbed after oral administration.

This paper reports disposition studies carried out in six volunteers which attempt to evaluate the effect of two dose levels, probenecid, a five day course of treatment with the antibiotic and the effect of bed rest on plasma mecillinam levels.

VOLUNTEER STUDIES AND METHODS

Subjects

Studies were carried out in six healthy university students aged between 20 and 25 who were not taking other drugs. All subjects were required to fast for twelve hours before the beginning of each study and food was subsequently allowed four hours after taking the antibiotic.

Procedure

Studies commenced at 9 to 9.30 a.m. on the same day of consecutive weeks. Subjects were admitted to a hospital side ward and a plastic intravenous cannula connected to a normal saline drip through a three-way tap was inserted into a forearm vein: the saline was allowed to drip in slowly to prevent clotting in the cannula. The bladder was emptied and a blood sample (5 ml) was collected immediately prior to the drug dose. Blood samples were then collected at 5, 10, 15, 30 and 60 mins and then at $1^1/_2$, 2, $2^1/_2$, 3, 4, 5, 6 and 8 hours: the 5 and 10 mins samples were omitted when the antibiotic was taken orally. In each case a 2 ml blood sample was collected and discarded before collecting the sample for analysis. A six hour urine was collected.

Antibiotic Assay

Blood samples were allowed to clot. Serum and urine mecillinam concentrations were assayed using the agar cup plate method with the Leo HA^2 Escherichia coli as test organism. Mecillinam hydrochloride dihydrate was used as reference standard but the results are expressed as μg/ml of anhydrous mecillinam/ml serum or as per cent of the administered dose.

Antibiotic Studies

i. Intra muscular. Mecillinam hydrochloride dihydrate (335 mg) was injected into the deltoid muscle.

ii. Oral. A 200 mg dose was given as a capsule containing pivmecillinam hydrochloride (200 mg). Two capsules were given for a 400 mg dose and this dose was repeated after a six day interval during which the subjects took two 200 mg capsules of pivmecillinam hydrochloride qds. The effect of probenecid was investigated by giving probenecid (2 x 500 mg tablets) half an hour before two 200 mg capsules of pivmecillinam hydrochloride. Two 200 mg capsules of pivmecillinam hydrochloride were given to the subjects when lying supine in bed and on another occasion when the subjects were walking about and sitting down. In this latter case the cannulae were not connected to a drip but were flushed with saline after each sample had been collected.

RESULTS AND DISCUSSION

The mean peak serum mecillinam concentrations obtained after one and after two 200 mg capsules of pivmecillinam hydrochloride were 1.75 and 2.98 µg/ml respectively. Absorption and disposition characteristics for the studies are presented in Table 1. The mean serum mecillinam half life after the single 200 mg capsule was 1.26 hours and the AUC was 3.71: unfortunately some of the urine samples from this study were incorrectly stored before analysis under conditions which allowed the drug content to deteriorate. The per cent of the dose recovered in the 6 hour urines are therefore not quoted.

Pivmecillinam is rapidly absorbed producing peak plasma concentrations about 1.5 hours after oral administration. The antibiotic is efficiently absorbed from the capsule formulation of the hydrochloride in terms of the amount of mecillinam reaching the systemic circulation as can be seen from the AUC data presented in Table 1. The AUC after the 400 mg capsule was 80% of that obtained after the intramuscular injection. In both studies the volunteers were supine in bed and under these conditions it would normally be assumed that clearance of a drug would be the same irrespective of the route of administration. However, the $t_{\frac{1}{2}}$ after the oral dose was longer at 1.5 hours than the 1.15 hours after the injection. In view of this there is a larger pre systemic loss of mecillinam after oral administration of pivmecillinam than is suggested by the 20% decrease in the AUC. The pre systemic loss, i.e. losses due to metabolism in the intestinal mucosa and liver, appears to be a first order process at least up to a dose of 400 mg of pivmecillinam as, although the peak plasma concentration of 2.98 µg/ml after the 400 mg dose is less than twice that of 1.75 µg/ml obtained after a 200 mg dose, the AUC is almost exactly double at 7.6 and 3.7 respectively.

Although the six day course of treatment did not influence the amount of drug absorbed from a 400 mg capsule there did appear to be a small consistent increase in peak serum mecillinam concentration which occurred more quickly than after a single dose. The reasons for this are not clear; it may be partly due to small amounts of the previous, overnight dose remaining in the blood.

Probenecid decreases the urinary clearance of mecillinam as is shown by the increase in half life to 1.84 hours and the reduced amount of mecillinam recovered in the 6 hour urine. This

Table I. Mean (± S.E.M.) absorption and disposition characteristics of mecillinam in six volunteers after two x 200 mg capsules of pivmecillinam hydrochloride by mouth and 335 mg of pivmecillinam hydrochloride dehydrate by intramuscular injection.

	Peak serum concentration µg/ml	Peak time, hr.	$t_{\frac{1}{2}}$ + hr.	AUC #	6 hr urine % dose
Supine	3.0 (0.24)	1.7 (0.17)	1.5 (0.07)	7.6 (0.34)	25 (2.0)
After 400 mg pivmecillinam for 6 days.	3.35 (0.27)	1.5 (0.18)	1.15 (0.12)	7.7 (0.26)	25 (2.2)
After 2 x 500 mg probenecid tablets.	4.6 (0.39)	1.7 (0.18)	1.84 (0.17)	14.0 (0.84)	19 (3.7)
Ambulent.	3.8 (0.36)	1.3 (0.18)	1.09 (0.09)	8.6 (0.26)	23 (4.3)
Intra muscular mecillinam.	5.7 (0.7)	0.43 (0.12)	1.15 (0.06)	9.5 (0.54)	15 (4.6)

+ $t_{\frac{1}{2}}$ is the serum mecillinam half life.

\# AUC is the area under the serum mecillinam concentration/time curve.

means that the time for which the plasma mecillinam concentrations remain above a given value are increased by at least one hour.

Pivmecillinam appears to be efficiently absorbed in ambulent subjects as indicated by the higher peak serum concentrations and larger AUC's than obtained in the same subjects when in bed as shown in Table 1. A comparison of the AUC with that obtained after intramuscular injection shows that over 90% of the antibiotic reaches the systemic circulation: in this case the clearances as indicated by the $t_{\frac{1}{2}}$ values appear to be similar. Therefore, moderate physical activity appears to promote the absorption of pivmecillinam from the gastro intestinal tract and reduces the amount destroyed before it reaches the general circulation.

In the above discussion the serum mecillinam concentration half life values ($t_{\frac{1}{2}}$) have been assumed to be a measure of drug clearance. This is justified because of the close agreement obtained between the computer generated curves and the experimental data which suggests that the distribution of mecillinam could be described by a one compartment model.

PLASMA PROFILE & URINARY EXCRETION of MECILLINAM after PIVMECILLINAM

R.L. PARSONS, Gillian M. HOSSACK & Gillian M. PADDOCK

Dept. Clinical Pharmacology

Guy's Hospital Medical School. London. SE1.9RT

Introduction Pivmecillinam (F.L. 1039. Leo) is the pivaloyloxymethyl ester of mecillinam (F.L. 1060. Leo). Like the related pivampicillin, which is the pivaloyloxy methyl ester of ampicillin, pivmecillinam is biologically inactive until in-vivo hydrolysis to its biologically active constituent mecillinam. These reactions are shown in Fig. 1.

Our interest in this 6 β amidinopenicillanic acid ester was stimulated by finding significant malabsorption of pivampicillin in adult patients with coeliac disease (1.2). We wondered whether pivmecillinam, which is also hydrolysed by non-specific gastrointestinal esterases to its biologically active constituent mecillinam, would be abnormally absorbed in this condition.

Subjects & methods 13 normal subjects (mean ± SEM age 24.77 ± 1.22 years, height 172.94 ± 2.92 cm, weight 67.23 ± 3.20 kg.) and 12 adult patients with coeliac disease (mean ± SEM age, 47.08 ± 3.73 years, height 164.84 ± 3.05 cm, weight 55.81 ± 3.38 kg.) who had had the diagnosis of coeliac disease confirmed by small intestinal biopsy, and had received a gluten free diet for periods ranging from 11 months to 10 years were studied.

Both groups received ampicillin (500 mg.), or pivmecillinam (400 mg.) after an overnight fast. The normal subjects were studied on other occasions after

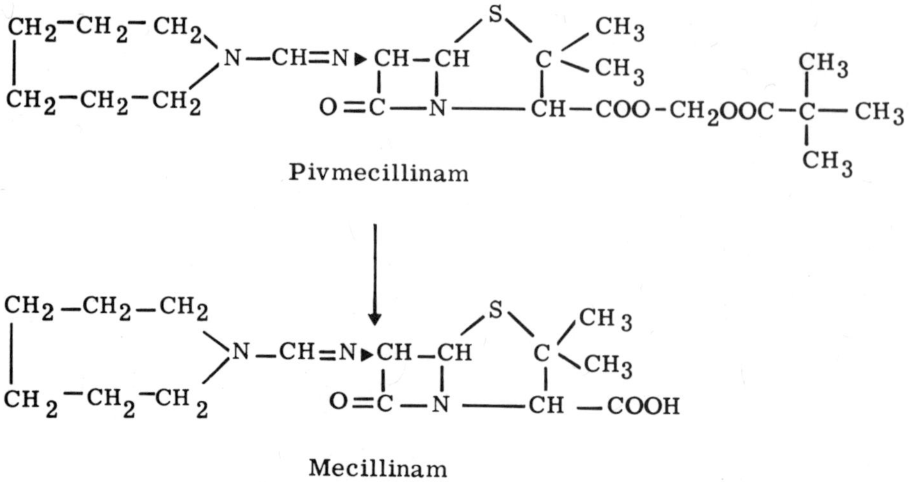

Figure I. Hydrolysis of pivampicillin & pivmecillinam to their active constituents.

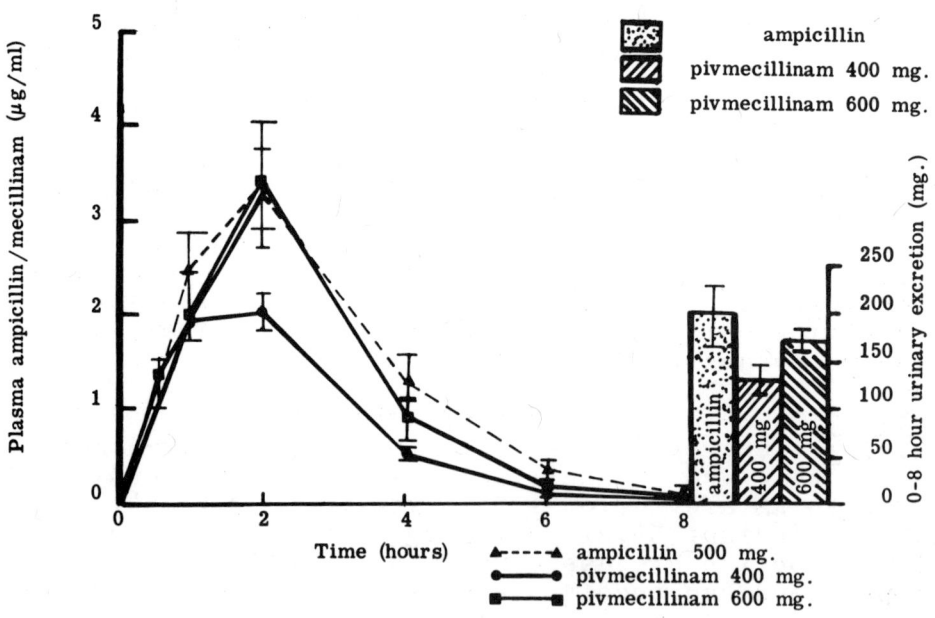

Figure 2. Plasma profile & 0-8 hour urinary excretion of mecillinam after pivmecillinam 400 mg./compared with that after 500 mg. of ampicillin & 600 mg.

administration of pivmecillinam (400 mg.) with a Lundh test meal (3) and 600 mg. (starved).

Blood samples were collected prior to dosing and again at 30 minutes, 1, 2, 3, 4, 6 & 8 hours later. Two hourly fractionated urine collections (0-2; 2-4; 4-6; & 6-8 hours) were made during the four studies.

Fluids were permitted after collection of the 1 hour samples & food after the 2 hour samples.

During the higher dose study of pivmecillinam (600 mg.) duplicate blood & urine samples were collected. One of each pair of blood samples was centrifuged immediately and frozen at $-20°C$. The other sample of the pair remained at room temperature on the bench throughout the day. The samples that had been frozen immediately after collection were thawed immediately prior to plating all the samples at the end of the study. The samples collected during the first three studies were all left at room temperature until the end of the day. All samples were plated on the same day as the study.

The concentration of mecillinam was measured by small plate microbiological assay based on the method of Grove & Randall (1955) (4), using E. coli as the test organism.

The appropriate concentration range of standard solutions of ampicillin trihydrate & mecillinam hydrochloride dihydrate were diluted in a mixture of dipotassium hydrogen phosphate & dihydrogen potassium phosphate buffer. The concentrations of ampicillin and mecillinam in the unknown samples were then calculated from the standard curve of zone size plotted against concentrations of the standards. All results are expressed as the anhydrous salt.

Results

Ampicillin (500 mg.)/Pivmecillinam (400 & 600 mg.)

Fig. 2 shows the plasma concentration/time profile after ampicillin (500 mg.) which is compared with the two doses (400 & 600 mg.) of pivmecillinam. The mean $\pm$ SEM plasma concentration of mecillinam after 600 mg. was almost identical to that after ampicillin (500 mg.) for the whole of the eight hours. The peak after 400 mg. of pivmecillinam (2.03 ± 0.19 µg/ml) was significantly ($P<0.05$) less than that after ampicillin (500 mg.).

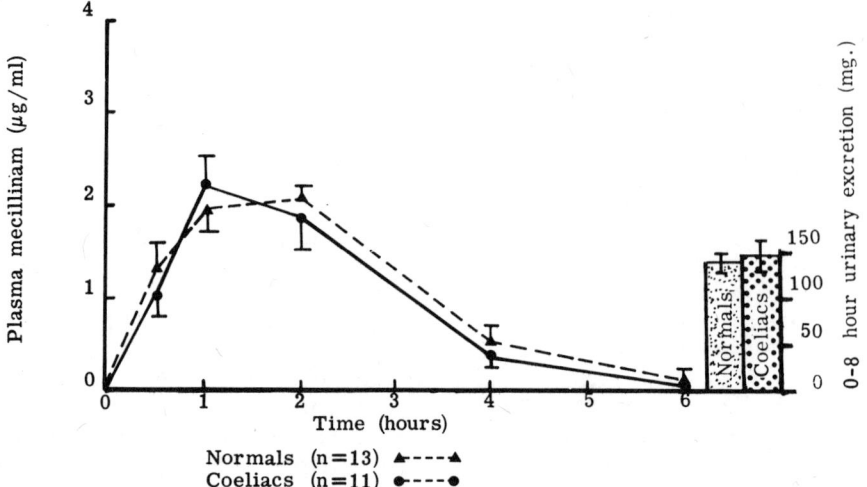

Figure 3. Mean plasma & 0-8 hour urinary mecillinam in normal subjects & Coeliac disease after 400 mg. pivmecillinam.

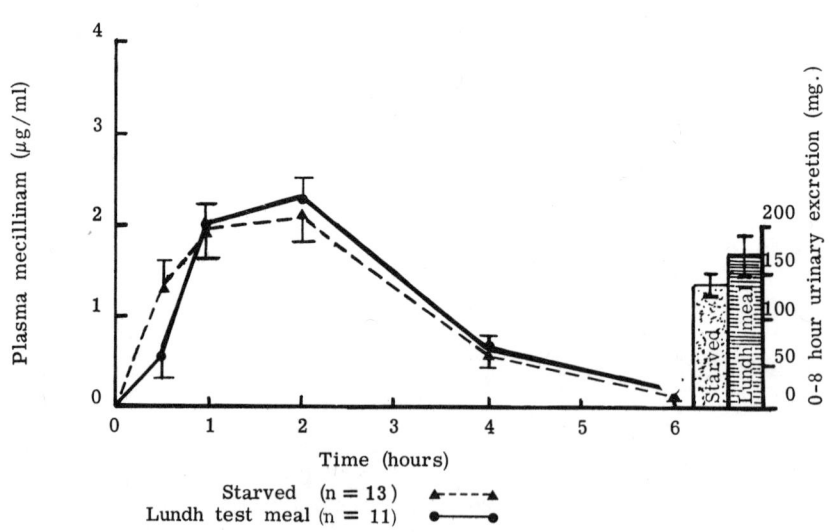

Figure 4. Mean plasma & 0-8 hour urinary excretion of mecillinam in normal after Lundh test meal.

Pivmecillinam (400 mg.) Adult coeliac disease (Fig. 3)

Fig. 3 shows the plasma concentration/time profile after pivmecillinam (400 mg.) in the starved normal & coeliac subjects. There was no significant difference in the mean ± SEM plasma concentration or in the total 0-8 hour urinary excretion of mecillinam (Fig. 6), between the normal & coeliac patients.

Apart from the final 2 hours (6-8 hours), there was no significant difference between the normal & coeliac subjects in the fractionated urine collections. The 6-8 hour urinary excretion of mecillinam was significantly ($P<0.01$) greater in the coeliacs (5.48 ± 2.66 mg.) than in the normal subjects (2.38 ± 0.29 mg.).

Pivmecillinam (400 mg.) + Lundh test meal (Fig. 4 & 7)

The mean ± SEM plasma concentration after simultaneous administration of a Lundh meal (3) and pivmecillinam (400 mg.) is shown in Fig. 4. This reproducible test meal did not alter the mean ± SEM plasma conentration of mecillinam. The 0-8 hour urinary excretion after the meal (166.42 ± 22.72 mg.) was not significantly greater than that in the starved state (135.74 ± 22.72 mg.).

Pivmecillinam (600 mg.)

Figure 5 shows that the mean ± SEM plasma concentration & total 0-8 hour urinary excretion of mecillinam after 600 mg. of pivmecillinam was higher in all the frozen samples than in duplicates which had been left at room temperature on the bench. These differences were not statistically significant.

Discussion

The absorption pattern of pivmecillinam in coeliac disease did not mirror that which we have previously demonstrated in this condition after pivampicillin. This suggests that the site for hydrolysis of pivmecillinam differs from that for pivampicillin. Both compounds are lipid soluble esters which require hydrolysis by non specific esterases to their active constituents. These esterases are situated within the intestinal mucosa, in the liver, or in the tissues. Absorption of these drugs is due to their highly lipid soluble nature.

An alternative explanation of the results is that the esterase content of the intestinal mucosa of the coeliac patients studied on this occasion was higher than

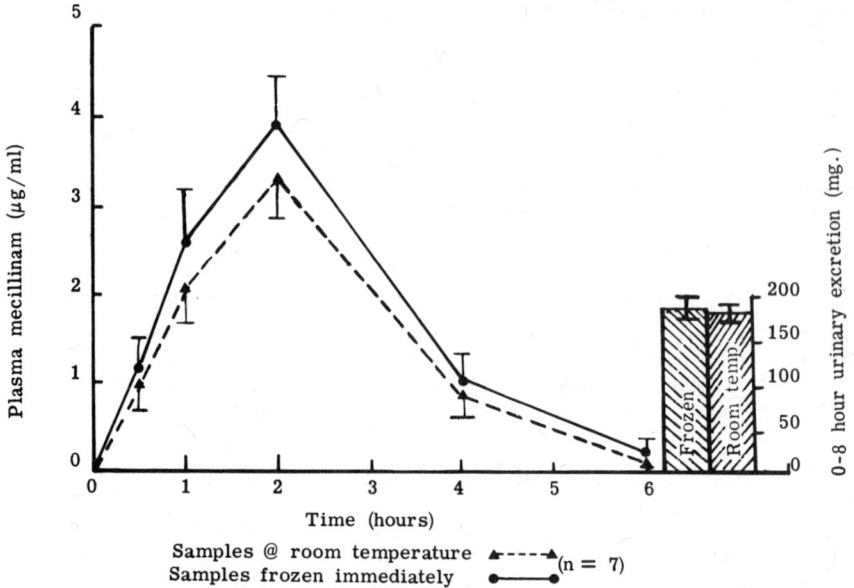

Figure 5. Mean plasma & 0-8 hour urinary excretion of mecillinam in normal subjects after pivmecillinam 600 mg.

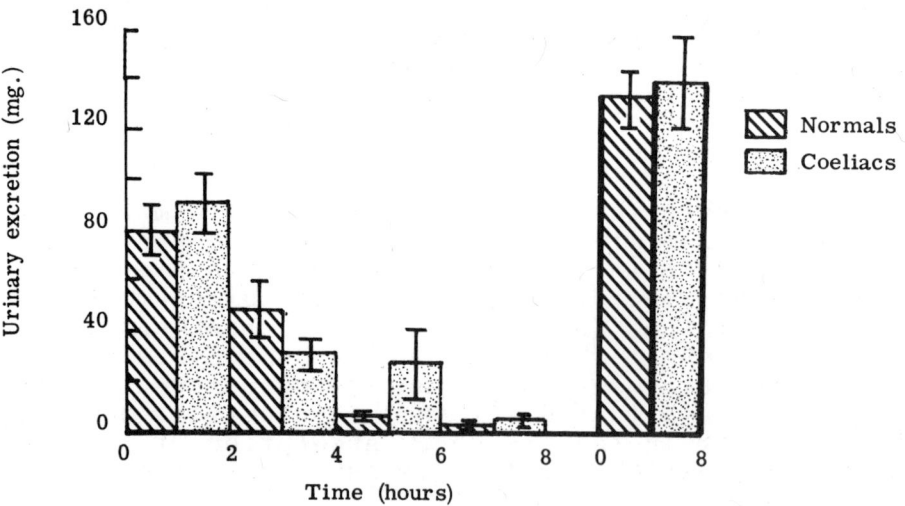

Figure 6. Mean Fractionated urinary excretion of mecillinam after pivmecillinam. 400 mg. to normals & coeliacs.

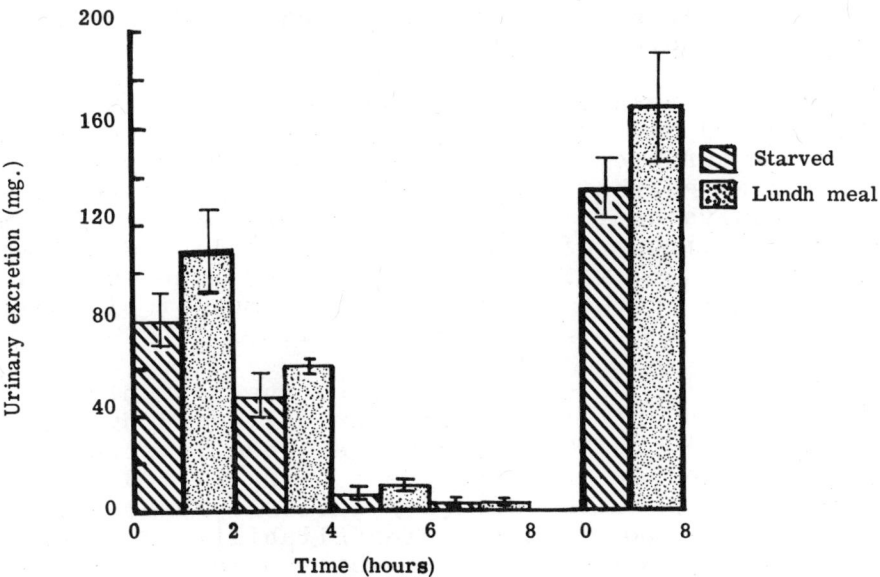

Figure 7. Mean Fractionated urinary excretion of mecillinam after pivmecillinam 400 mg. to normals ± Lundh. test meal.

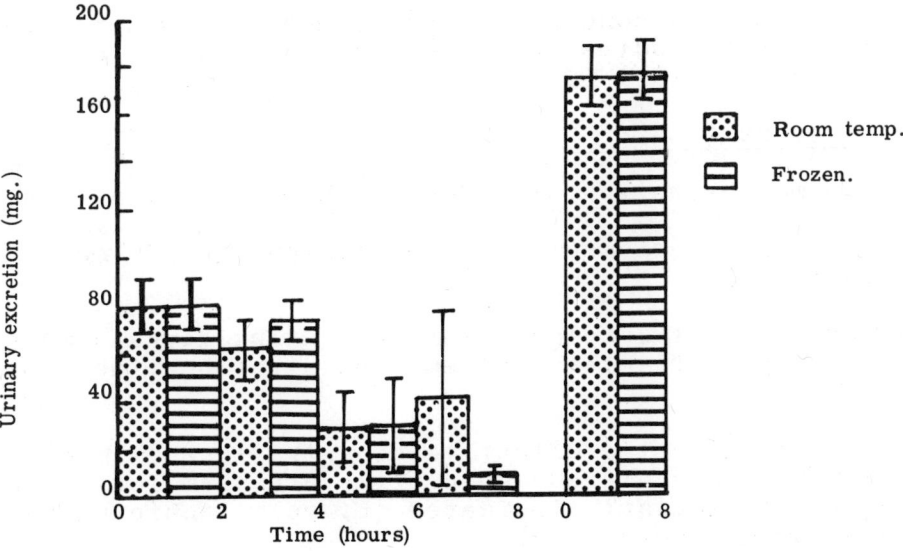

Figure 8. Mean Fractionated urinary excretion of mecillinam after pivmecillinam 600 mg. to starved normal subjects.

that of the patients who participated in the absorption study of pivampicillin.(1.2).

In choosing a dose of pivmecillinam that was equivalent to 500 mg. of ampicillin, we were guided by the results of our previous studies (1.2.5) with pivampicillin. These suggested that 400 mg. of pivmecillinam would produce equivalent plasma conentrations of mecillinam to the concentrations of ampicillin that followed 500 mg. of ampicillin or 350 mg. of pivampicillin. The results of the two dose studies suggest that 600 mg. of pivmecillinam is equivalent to 500 mg. of ampicillin.

The 600 mg. dose study doubled the peak plasma mecillinam concentration over that estimated by leaving the samples of the 400 mg. study at room temperature throughout the day prior to their being plated. This finding emphasises the need for careful preservation of plasma samples taken during bioavailability studies, so that the estimated results reflect the actual plasma concentration achieved, rather than the lower concentrations which result from deterioration during storage.

The Lundh meal did not impair the absorption of pivmecillinam. This mirrors our previous findings with the other 6 aminobenzylpenicillins and cephalexin (5).

The plasma concentrations of mecillinam achieved during these studies were above the M.I.C. of this antibiotic against E. coli (0.016 - 1.0 µg/ml).

Conclusions

1). No malabsorption of pivmecillinam in coeliac disease.

2). 600 mg. of pivmecillinam equivalent to 500 mg. of ampicillin.

3). Freezing of samples prior to plating gives a more accurate picture of the plasma conentration/time profile of mecillinam.

4). Therapeutically effective conentrations of mecillinam in the plasma achieved against the organism for which the drug is particularly indicated (E. coli) achieved by both 400 & 600 mg. doses.

References

1). Parsons, R.L., Bywater, M.J. & Marshall, M. (1974) The absorption of cephalexin and three aminobenzylpenicillins in adult coeliac disease. Progress in Chemotherapy. Proceedings of the 8th International Congress of Chemotherapy. (1973). Vol 1. 534 - 542. Edit. G. Daikos. Published by the Hellenic Society for Chemotherapy. Athens.

2). Parsons, R.L. Hossack, G. & Paddock, G. (1975) The absorption of antibiotics in adult patients with coeliac disease. Journal of Antimicrobial Chemotherapy. 1, 39 - 50.

3). Lundh, G. (1962) Pancreatic exocrine function in neoplastic and inflammatory disease, A simple & reliable new test. Gastroenterology. 44, 588 - 597.

4). Grove, D.C. & Randall, W.A. Assay methods of antibiotics. A laboratory manual. Medical Encyclopedia Inc. New York. (1955).

5). Parsons, R.L. Hossack, G.M. & Paddock, G.M. (1975) Absorption of aminobenzylpenicillins and cephalexin in normal subjects whilst starved and with a Lundh test meal. Journal of Antimicrobial Chemotherapy. 2, in press.

MECILLINAM: FACTORS AFFECTING IN VITRO ACTIVITY

D.S. REEVES, R. WISE, M.J. BYWATER*, S.R. STERN

DEPARTMENT OF MEDICAL MICROBIOLOGY

SOUTHMEAD HOSPITAL, WESTBURY-ON-TRYM, BRISTOL BS10 5NB

Mecillinam (FL.1060, Leo Laboratories; 6B-(hexahydro-1H-azepin-1-yl)-methyleneamino-penicillanic acid) is a new class of semi-synthetic penicillin derivatives characterised by the presence of a 6B-amidino substitution in the penicillanic acid nucleus. Preliminary studies indicated a high degree of activity against Gram negative bacteria (Lund and Tybring, 1972). It was decided therefore to assess the activity of mecillinam in the laboratory particularly with a view to its use in infections of the urinary tract.

An initial evaluation of activity was made in comparison with that of ampicillin and cephaloridine against a wide range of urinary and other clinical isolates. Factors affecting in vivo activity such as pH, inoculum size and the presence of serum were investigated. In view of the suggestion by Greenwood and O'Grady (1973) and Tybring and Melchior (in press) that the osmolarity or conductivity of a nutrient medium may have a marked effect on the activity of mecillinam, an in vitro study was made of the effect of urine osmolarity and conductivity on the activity of mecillinam against a strain of the common urinary pathogen Escherichia coli.

METHODS

The organisms used were in the main recent clinical isolates chosen to have a variety of resistances to ampicillin and cephaloridine. For the experiments with urines Esch. coli (N.C.T.C.10418) was used.

Minimal Inhibitory and Bactericidal Concentrations

Dilutions of antibiotics were prepared in Oxoid Diagnostic Sensitivity Test agar. Inoculation was with a multi-point method giving a colony count of 30 – 40 colonies in each inoculum area.

For experiments on the effect of pH, serum and inoculum-size, and on bactericidal activity dilutions of antibiotic were prepared in nutrient broth, normally at pH 7.4, in 1 ml amounts. The final inoculum was 1×10^3/ml as given by surface viable count except where stated. Variations to pH and inoculum size were made by appropriate adjustments to this method. All minimal inhibitory concentrations (m.i.c.'s) were read after 18 hours incubation at 37°C except where stated. The m.i.c. was taken as tubes showing only a slight growth or no growth. Minimum bactericidal concentrations (m.b.c.'s) were determined by the growth on blood agar of a 50 ul sub-culture after 18 hours incubation. A growth of 2 colonies or less was taken as the end point of bactericidal activity, which represented a 95% reduction in viable count.

Stability of mecillinam in test media. Solutions of mecillinam at 10 mg/l were prepared in 4 different fresh human serum each diluted 1 in 2 with phosphate buffer to ensure the starting pH was 7.3. A similar solution was also prepared in phosphate buffer alone. After taking an aliquot from each solution for storage at -20°C they were incubated at 37°C for 24 hours, aliquots being taken at intervals for storage at -20°C. All aliquots were assayed by a large-plate microbiological method using Difco Penassay agar with Esch. coli (N.C.T.C.10418) as indicator organism.

Protein binding. Two methods were used:- (i) 0.5 ml of ultra-filtrate of 5 ml pooled human serum containing 10 mg/l of mecillinam was prepared by centrifugation in an Amicon Centriflo Cone (M.W. exclusion 50,000). The ultrafiltrate was assayed as above against phosphate buffer standards pH 7.4. (ii) the supernatant from the same lot of pooled human serum containing mecillinam 10 mg/l as in (i) was assayed after centrifugation at 200,000 G at 4°C for 12 hours.

Activity of mecillinam in urine. The activity of mecillinam against Esch. coli (N.C.T.C.10418) was determined by preparing 2-fold dilutions of the antibiotic in the urine under examination and adding standard inoculum of the indicator organisms to each dilution. After incubation at 37°C for 8 and 18 hours the growth end-points were read. To maintain the constancy of inoculum found to be essential the organism was prepared in a large batch in 10% glycerol broth and stored as 1.5 ml aliquots in liquid nitrogen. For the experiment the inoculum was adjusted to give a final count of 1×10^3/ml. or 1×10^6/ml. The urines used were from healthy male volunteers. After adjustment of pH to 6.5 and cooling to 4°C with centrifugation to remove precipitate, they were sterilized by filtration. Dilutions of mecillinam from 16 to 0.015 mg/l in 2-fold steps were prepared by a master dilution technique. With each batch or urines a set of dilutions in nutrient broth acted as a control for reproducibility of technique. The conductivity of the urines were measured using an alternating current bridge, and the osmolarities determined using a Fisk QF osmometer.

RESULTS

The bacteristatic activity of mecillinam against 200 clinical isolates of varying bacterial species are shown in the table. Figure 1 gives the results for individual strains of Esch. coli in comparison with the activity of ampicillin and cephaloridine against the same strains.

Effect of inoculum size. Increasing the inoculum from 1×10^3/ml to 1×10^7/ml had a marked effect on the activity of mecillinam, particularly with Klebsiella spp. and Proteus mirabilis. The m.i.c.'s increased by as much as 100-fold typical values being 1 - 10 fold. The inoculum effect was smaller with some strains of Esch. coli and all strains of Salmonella spp. In a few instances using fully sensitive strains of Esch. coli simultaneous comparison with ampicillin and cephaloridine showed a much smaller inoculum effect.

There was also a fall in the bactericidal activity of mecillinam with increased inoculum size. The calculated ratio of MBC/MIC for each strain produced a wide variation in results. For an inoculum of 1×10^3 organism/ml, the ratio was usually 1 - 5, while for an inoculum of 1×10^7 organism/ml it was usually in the range of 4 - 40.

Organism	Number of Strains	Typical MIC (range) ug/ml	
Esch. coli (ampicillin sensitive)	32	0.25	(<0.1 - 1.0)
Esch. coli (ampicillin resistant)	22	1.0	(0.1 - 50)
Klebsiella spp.	29	1.0	(0.25->100)
Enterobacter spp.	3	0.5	(0.5 - 1.0)
Proteus mirabilis	39	25	(0.5 - 50)
Proteus spp. (indole + ve)	9	>50	(10 - >50)
Salmonella spp.	40	0.25	(<0.25-0.5)
Staph. aureus (penicillin sensitive)	21	50	(25 - >50)
Strep. faecalis	5	>50	(>50 only)

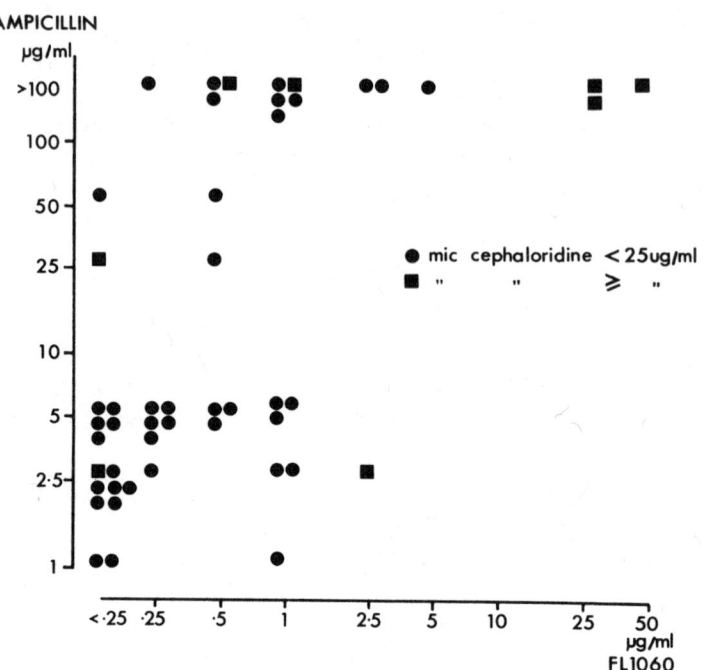

Fig.1: Activity of mecillinam (FL.1060), ampicillin and cephaloridine against individual strains of Esch. coli.

Effect of serum. Only changes in bactericidal activity were recorded since the serum (50%) obscured the reading of inhibitory activity. The m.b.c.'s increased in all but 3 instances. The median increase was 10-fold but some increases were 50-fold or more.

Effect of pH. Against a selection of Esch. coli and Klebsiella spp. the activity of mecillinam decreased by about 4-fold for an increase of pH from 6.4 to 7.4, and by about 10-fold between 7.4 and 8.4 (figure 2). A change was present with all 10 strains tested.

Stability of mecillinam in serum. After 24 hours at 37°C in pH 7.3 buffer the residual activity was 31% of initial concentration and in serum diluted with buffer the fall was to 13%.

Serum binding. In a number of experiments the results ranged from 15 to 25%.

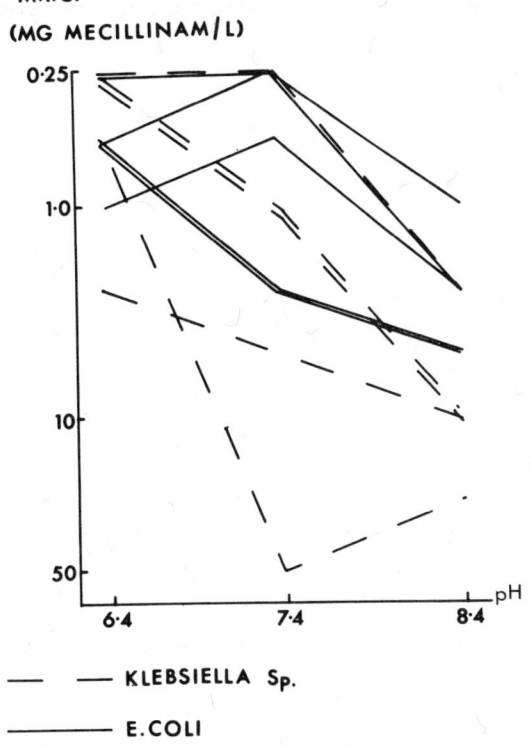

Fig.2: Effect of pH on the activity of mecillinam.

Activity in urine. The activity of mecillinam was increased by decreasing osmolarity and by decreasing conductivity, i.e. by dilute urine. This held good whether a single urine was diluted with sterile water or when individual specimens of urine of varying concentrations were compared. The increase in activity was approximately parallel to the degree of dilution. Correlations of 8-hour m.i.c. with both osmolarity and conductivity are significant at the $p < 0.01$ level.* The correlations m.b.c. at 8 hours and m.i.c. at 18 hours were less good but still significant at the $p < 0.05$ level. No correlation existed for the m.b.c. at 18 hours. The correlation with osmolarity and conductivity held good for the 8-hour m.i.c. when the inoculum was increased to 1×10^6/ml.

* See Fig. 3 and 4.

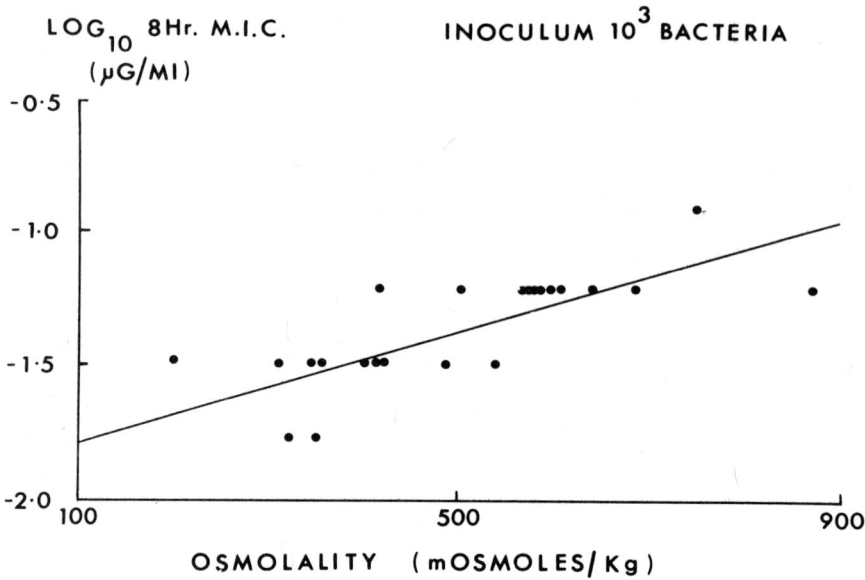
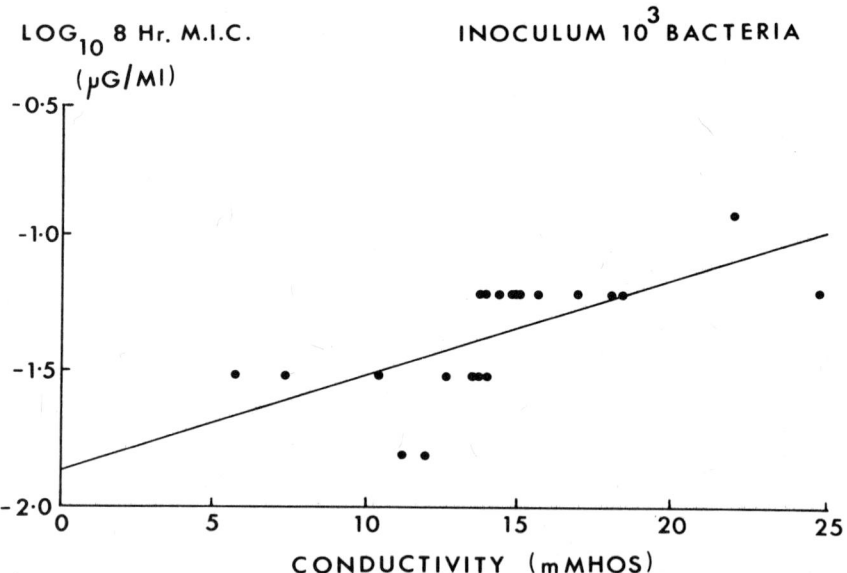

Fig.3 (above) Fig.4 (below). Correlation between urine osmolality/conductivity and the 8 hr. m.i.c. of mecillinam against Esch. coli (N.C.T.C.10418).

DISCUSSION

The high activity of mecillinam against Esch. coli and other Enterobacteria has been confirmed by work published before and after the experiments described here (Lund and Tybring, 1972; Greenwood and O'Grady, 1974). Species usually resistant to ampicillin (e.g. Klebsiella spp.) and cephaloridine (i.e. Enterobacter spp.) were also inhibited by mecillinam, although to a lesser degree than Esch. coli. This alone suggests that its mode of activity differs from these drugs, as does the virtual absence of useful activity against Gram positive species, and the very marked inoculum effect.

Although mecillinam is rather unstable in the presence of serum and in the presence of growing bacteria in culture media (Reeves et al, 1974), the relevance of these findings to therapy where the drug is continually being replaced by dosing is conjectural. The increase of activity in urine with dilution is of direct interest to the therapy of urinary infections. Although there is usually a large excess of antibiotic compared to its m.i.c. for the urinary pathogen, there is always the worry that encouraging a diuresis will dilute the antibiotic. Since the activity of mecillinam seems to increase in proportion to the degree of dilution use could be made of the hydrodynamic advantages of diuresis without fear of antibiotic dilution.

REFERENCES

Lund, F., and Tybring, L. Nature New Biology 236, 135-136 (1972).
Greenwood, D., and O'Grady, F. J. Clin.Path. 26, 1-6 (1973).
Greenwood, D., Brooks, H.L., Gargan, R., and O'Grady, F. J. Clin. Path. 27, 192-197 (1974).
Reeves, D.S., Wise, R., and Bywater, M.J. Journal of Antimicrobial Chemotherapy, 1974 (in press).

THE ACTIVITY OF MECILLINAM (FL1060), IN COMBINATION WITH OTHER
ANTIBIOTICS, AGAINST H. INFLUENZAE AND STREPTOCOCCUS FAECALIS

R. Wise, G.A.J. Ayliffe, J.M. Andrews & K.A. Bedford

Department of Medical Microbiology

Dudley Road Hospital, Birmingham B18 7QH

INTRODUCTION

Mecillinam, a member of a new group of β-lactam antibiotics, the 6 - β amidinopenicillanic acids, has considerable activity against the Enterobacteriacae (Lund & Tybring, 1972). This drug has little activity against the Gram positive organisms and its activity against Haemophilus influenzae has not been fully explored. This study was designed to see if any clinically useful synergistic combinations of other antibiotics together with mecillinam could be found.

There is some evidence that mecillinam and ampicillin may show antibacterial synergy against the Enterobacteracae (Tybring & Melchior, 1975). Other combinations were mecillinam plus clindamycin, fusidic acid, tetracycline, rifampicin and erythromycin.

The strains of Streptococcus faecalis were tested against combinations of mecillinam together with ampicillin and gentamicin.

MATERIALS AND METHODS

(A) H. influenzae

A preliminary screening test for synergistic combinations of drugs with mecillinam and ampicillin, clindamycin, sodium fusidate, tetracycline or erythromycin was performed using 10 strains of H. influenzae. These strains were chosen for their range of resistance to ampicillin. A further 9 strains were used in the mecillinam - ampicillin combination study.

The method employed was an agar plate chequer board procedure in which the two antibiotics were each incorporated at differing dilutions. The dilutions of ampicillin were from 0.015 - 8 mg/l, and the mecillinam from 0.25 - 1024 mg/l. A 'Denley Multipoint' inoculator was used and 10^2 - 10^3 organisms were inoculated onto the plates. The media used was a Levinthals agar ('Oxoid D.S.T.' plus 10% human blood). The plates were incubated at 37°C in 10% CO_2 for 18 hours. The minimum inhibitory concentration (MIC) was defined as a 90% reduction in the colony count.

The minimum bacteriocidal concentration (MBC) of combinations of mecillinam and ampicillin or fusidic acid was studied on 3 strains by a similar method to the above, but employing a Levinthals broth tube dilution procedure and an inoculum of 1 x 10^4 organisms/ml and subculturing the tubes at 18 hours onto Levinthals agar.

(B) Streptococcus faecalis

Ten strains of Streptococcus faecalis (Lancefield Grp.D) were grown overnight in Todd - Hewitt broth and agar plate dilution studies performed with combinations of mecillinam with ampicillin or gentamicin as above. The media employed was 'Oxoid D.S.T.' with 10% whole human blood. The MBC of the combinations mecillinam plus gentamicin were studied in 2 strains in a similar method to that above, but using 'Oxoid Sensitivity Test Broth'. An inoculum of 10^4 organisms/ml was employed.

RESULTS

(A) H. influenzae

No synergy could be detected between combinations of mecillinam with tetracycline, clindamycin, erythromycin or rifampicin. Synergy was noted between mecillinam and ampicillin or fusidic acid.

Mecillinam - ampicillin combination. The mean MIC of mecillinam to the 19 strains of H. influenzae was 512 mg/l (range 1024 - 64 mg/l). The MIC of ampicillin can be seen in Table I.

At no concentration of ampicillin and mecillinam was synergy marked, but it was interesting to note that amongst the ampicillin sensitive strains a ratio of 1:2 or less of ampicillin:mecillinam there was a consistent decrease in the MIC of ampicillin by a factor of 2 fold or greater. In other words the presence of only a small amount of mecillinam (e.g. 0.25 mg/l) would at least halve the MIC

TABLE I. Sum of the FICs at ratio of ampicillin:mecillinam

H. influenzae No's	1:2 or less	1:8-1:16	>1:128->1:512	MIC Ampicillin
A271, 262, 222, 273, 272, 106, 315, Z134	0.501		0.62	0.25 - 0.5
E699	0.251		0.375	1.0
A285		0.27	0.53	4
A335, 341, 118			0.5	4
A294, 334		0.50	0.53	8
A339, 287	*			8 & 16
A340	0.5		0.625	4
A328	*			0.25

* synergy not demonstrated

of ampicillin. The ampicillin resistant strains did not exhibit this phenomenon to the same degree, ratios of 1:8 or greater being required before a decrease in the ampicillin MIC was observed. This raised ratio was due to the fact that the ampicillin MIC was raised.

In the bacteriocidal studies, synergy was less marked. A ratio of ampicillin:mecillinam of 1:32 or greater was needed before a decrease in the MBC of the ampicillin was noted. The phenomenon observed in the MIC study, that of the effect of a small amount of mecillinam regularly lowering the MIC of ampicillin, was not observed in the bacteriocidal studies.

Mecillinam - fusidic acid combination. The H. influenzae ranged in susceptibility to fusidic acid from 16 - 2 mg/l (mean 4 mg/l), and to mecillinam from 1024 - 64 mg/l (mean 512 mg/l). Although synergy was regularly observed using this combination, as can be seen from Table II there was no set pattern. Synergy occurred to some extent over a wide range of combinations of the two drugs from a ratio of fusidic acid:mecillinam of 4:1 - 1:>128. The effect was most marked when ratios of 1:32 or greater were employed. In Table III the effect of sub-inhibitory amounts of mecillinam are shown. If half the MIC of fusidic acid is added to a combination of the two drugs then the MIC of mecillinam will fall by a factor of between >256 to 8 times (with a median value of 64). If a $\frac{1}{4}$ the MIC of fusidic acid is added then the MIC of mecillinam will fall by a factor of 128 to 2 times (a median value of 8).

No bacteriocidal synergy was observed. It was difficult to demonstrate bacteriocidal activity of either drug acting alone. This may be due to the relatively high inoculum used.

(B) Streptococcus faecalis

Mecillinam - gentamicin combination. The MICs of mecillinam of all 10 strains were ≥256 mg/l and the MIC of gentamicin varied between 4 - 16 mg/l. No useful bacteriostatic synergy could be detected. For example to lower the mic of gentamicin to 1 mg/l or less, an amount of mecillinam greater than 64 mg/l was necessary in all cases. It was doubtful if synergy was occurring at all in most cases. No bacteriocidal synergy could be demonstrated.

Mecillinam - ampicillin combination. The MIC of mecillinam to all 10 strains was ≥256 mg/l and the MIC of ampicillin varied between 0.5 - 2.0 mg/l. No bacteriostatic or bacteriocidal synergy could be demonstrated and only in a few strains was there a minimum additive effect.

TABLE II. Synergistic activity of mecillinam and fusidic acid

H. influenzae No.	Sum of the fractionally inhibitory concentrations (FIC) at ratios fusidic acid:mecillinam						MIC	
	4:1	2:1	1:2	1:8	1:32-1:64	>1:128	fusidic acid	mecillinam
A106		0.504				0.625	4	256
A118					0.18		2	512
A134	0.507						4	64
A128		0.501		0.375	0.375	0.375	2	512
A338		0.258					8	128
A328				0.52	0.31		4	1024
A287				0.51	0.16	0.375	2	1024
A272					0.375		8	512
E699				0.375			16	256
A335			0.562				4	128

TABLE III. H. influenzae: combinations of fusidic acid and mecillinam

	H. influenzae No.										
	106	118	134	128	338	328	287	272	699	335
MIC fusidic acid	4	2	4	2	8	4	2	8	16	4
	MIC of mecillinam mg/l									
Addition of $\frac{1}{2}$ fusidic acid MIC	1	32	2	1	0.5	16	16	16	32	8
$\frac{1}{4}$ fusidic acid MIC	32	32	8	4	1	32	128	64	32	64
No fusidic acid i.e. mecillinam MIC	256	512	64	512	128	1024	1024	512	256	128

DISCUSSION

The observation and quantification of in vitro antibiotic synergy is not straightforward. We have employed the concept of the fractional inhibitory concentration (FIC) for each antibiotic at a known antibiotic concentration (Elion et al., 1954, Bushby, 1973) this being the decimal fraction of the MIC of the respective drug at a known ratio of the two drugs compared to the MIC when acting alone. If the sum of the FICs is less than unity, synergy is occurring and the lower the figure, the greater the synergy.

The combination of ampicillin with mecillinam when tested against all but 3 of the 19 strains of H. influenzae showed synergy at some ratio of the two drugs. It is interesting to note that two of the strains which did not show this were ampicillin resistant. Also the amount of mecillinam required to show synergy tended to be greater in the ampicillin resistant strains. Amongst the ampicillin sensitive strains, a reduction of the ampicillin MIC was noted when low amounts (down to 0.25 mg/l) of mecillinam were present. Such levels of mecillinam should be readily obtainable from even low oral doses of the ester, pivmecillinam. It is possible that this could be clinically important. It would not be expected that ampicillin resistant strains would be susceptible to a combination as, in the clinical situation, the peak serum levels of mecillinam obtained in the body after a dose of 400 mgs of pivmecillinam are between 3 - 5 mg/l (Wise et al., 1975) and therefore outside the range of synergistic activity.

Fusidic acid is not normally considered to be a drug useful against H. influenzae. Although bacteriostatic synergy was consistently noted this could not be considered useful in the clinical situation as the amount of mecillinam necessary to show such synergy was often outside the range which could be attained in the body. Strain numbers 106, 134, 128 and 338 did have MICs of mecillinam of $\leq$ 2mg/l in the presence of $\frac{1}{2}$ the MIC of fusidic acid and such synergy could be considered as possibly clinically useful.

It was interesting to note that when the faecal streptococci were investigated for possible synergy between mecillinam and gentamicin - that none was noted. This is surprising, as the phenomenon is well known between β-lactam antibiotics and the aminoglycosides. The different action of mecillinam on the bacterial cell wall (Melchior et al., 1973) may well explain this.

REFERENCES

Bushby, S.R.M. Trimethoprim - Sulphamethoxazole: In vitro Microbiological aspects. Journal of Infectious Diseases 128: S442-462 (1973).

Elion, G.B., Singer, S., Hitchings, G.H. Antagonists of nucleic acid derivative. Journal of Biological Chemistry 208: 477-488 (1954).
Wise, R., & Reeves, D.S. In Press (1975).
Tybring, L., Melchior, N.H. In Press (1975).
Lund, F. & Tybring, L. 6 β-amidinopenicillanic acid acids - a new group of antibiotics. Nature, New Biology 236: 135-137 (1972).
Melchior, N.H., Blom. J., Tybring, L. & Birch-Anderson, A. Light & Electron Microscopy of the early response of E. coli to a 6 β-amidinopenicillanic acid (FL1060). Acta. Path. Microbiol. Scand. 81B: 393-407 (1973).

LABORATORY AND CLINICAL STUDIES WITH MECILLINAM

D. McGHIE, M.J. ROBERTSON, A.M. GEDDES, K.C.L. LIM

REGIONAL PUBLIC HEALTH LABORATORY AND DEPARTMENT OF COMMUNICABLE AND TROPICAL DISEASE, EAST BIRMINGHAM HOSPITAL, ENGLAND

Mecillinam (FL 1060) is a new antibiotic derived from a new class of Antibiotics, the 6 β amidino penicillanic acids and despite a close structural similarity with other β lactam antibiotics, it has markedly different properties. It is much more active against gram negative organisms than gram positive organisms, and is more active than existing β lactam antibiotics in clinical use against Enterobacteriae in general, and Escherichia coli and Salmonella species in particular.

In this paper its activity against Escherichia coli and Salmonella spp. is studied and the possible use in urinary tract infections typhoid and paratyphoid fevers, and in the chronic carriage of Salmonella spp. is discussed and clinical results are presented.

MATERIALS AND METHODS

Mecillinam (FL 1060) powder was supplied by Leo Laboratories. Dilutions were made in sterile distilled water from freshly made solutions and were not stored.

Two hundred strains of Escherichia coli were examined. These were isolated from recent cases of urinary tract infection in both domicil iary and hospital practice. Nineteen strains of Escherichia coli selected for their increased resistance to FL 1060 or Ampicillin were tested for cross resistance patterns and possible synergistic effects.

One hundred and twenty five salmonella strains were examined, and of these 20 were Salmonella typhi and 5 S. paratyphi.

Minimum inhibitory concentrations, (M.I.C.) were estimated by the agar dilution method using a multipoint innoculation and sensitivity test Agar. (Wellcotest). The strains were maintained on Nutrient agar slopes and were inoculated from the slopes using a straight wire in 4 ml. of peptone water. They were then incubated at 37°C. for 6 hours and a dilution made in Ringer's solution to ensure that between 10^3 and 10^4 organisms/ml. were deposited on the antibiotic containing plate.

The plates were then incubated at 37°C. for 18 hours and any area which contained more than one colony and growth easily visible to the unaided eye was noted.

Synergy tests were performed in the same way by incorporating equal amou nts of Mecillinam and Ampicillin in the agar plates.

SENSITIVITY OF ESCHERICHIA COLI

The M.I.C.'s. of Mecillinam for 100 strains of Escherichia coli from hospital urinary tract infections and 100 strains from domiciliary infections are shown in figure 1 and 2.

The comparative sensitivity to Ampicillin is also shown. As can be seen the activity of Mecillinam is generally much higher than that of Ampicillin, and whereas many hospital strains are resistant to Ampicillin there is no difference between hospital and domiciliary strains as regards the high degree of sensitivity to Mecillinam of the Escherichia coli strains studied.

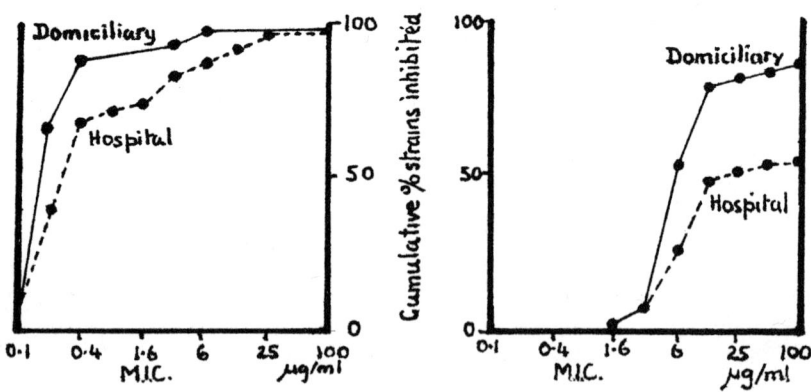

Sensitivity of Escherichia coli from domiciliary (100 strains) and hospital (100 strains) urinary tract infections to Mecillinam fig.1 and Ampicillin fig. 2.

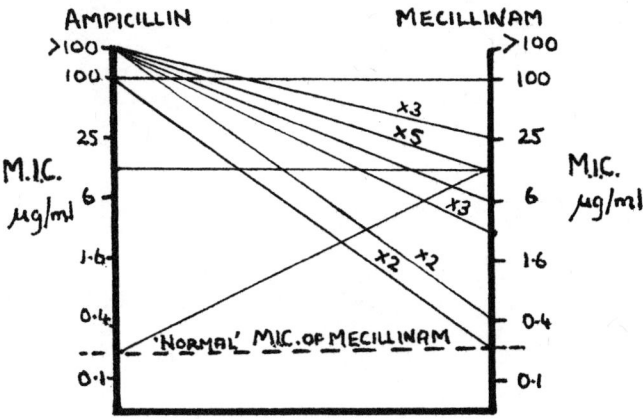

Fig. 3 Cross resistance patterns to Mecillinam and Ampicillin of 19 strains of Escherichia coli.
Cross Resistance

CROSS RESISTANCE

The cross resistance patterns of 10 Escherichia coli strains chosen for their Ampicillin resistance and 9 chosen for their increased resistance to Mecillinam are shown in figure 3. 16 out of 19 (84%) strains showed a degree of cross resistance. However, the degree of resistance to Mecillinam seen is still well within the theoretical treatment range in urinary tract infections as the minimum inhibitory concentrations were still well below the normal levels of Mecillinam achieved in the urine.

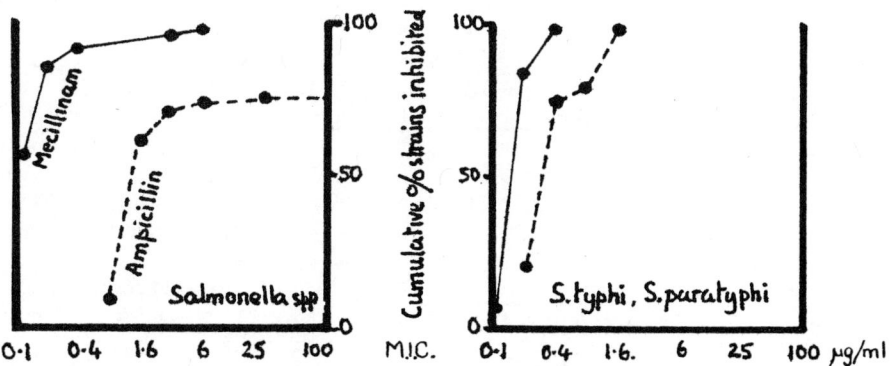

Sensitivity of Salmonella species to Ampicillin and Mecillinam
fig. 4 (a) Salmonella spp. (100 strains) fig. 4 (b) Salmonella typhi and paratyphi (25 strains).

Synergy testing of these same organisms showed only three with a fourfold on greater decrease in the M.I.C. of Mecillinam when an equal amount of Ampicillin was present in the agar. Of these two organisms had M.I.C.'s. to Mecillinam of greater than 100 μg/ml.

SENSITIVITY OF SALMONELLA SPECIES

The high degree of sensitivity of 100 salmonella strains to Mecillinam is seen in figure 4. When compared with Ampicillin not only is Mecillinam more effective on individual strains but it is also effective against a much larger proportion of strains.

The sensitivity of strains of S. typhi and S. paratyphi shown in fig. 4b shows a similar high degree of activity of Mecillinam. Ampicillin is effective against there particular strains though to a lesser degree than Mecillinam. The use of Mecillinam and Ampicillin in equal amounts with S. typhi and S. paratyphi strains showed no evidence of synergy.

CLINICAL RESULTS

In a pilot study 11 of 20 patient were treated successfully for urinary tract infection. Side effects were vomiting, anorexia and eosinophilia each inone patient. Several of the patients were elderly.

DISCUSSION

The high activity of Mecillinam against Escherichia coli make it's use in the treatment of urinary tract infection a possibility. However, although over 75% of domiciliary infections are caused by this organism, less the 50% of hospital infections are and although many strains of Proteus mirabilis may in theory be treatable results have been disappointing with this organism and in vitro studies suggest that it is difficult to achieve a bacterial effect in urine with this organism. The efficacy of Mecillinam in treatment of micrococcal urinary infection remains to be seen. The use of Mecillinam on patients with enteric fever or who are chronic carriers of Salmonella spp. seems to be a realistic prospect. The organisms are very sensitive and Mecillinam is excreted in bile with high and persistant levels being achieved. (Sales, Wilson and Rimmer, 1975).

Cases of enteric fever have been treated with Mecillinam and initial clinical improvement, and the time taken for the temperature to return to normal were found to be comparable with Chloramphenicol, Ampicillin or Hetacillin therapy, furthermore the Mecillinam dose of 300 mg. 6 hourly is one sixth of the effective dose of Ampicillin or Heticillin (Limson 1973, Jonsson 1974, Schiraldi 1974). This would make the use of Mecillinam in enteric fever during pregnancy a possibility.

CONCLUSION

Mecillinam shows great activity against Escherichia coli and Salmonella species including S. typhi and S. paratyphi. Its potential use in urinary tract infection caused by Escherichia coli and in Enteric fever and chronic Salmonella carriage seem to warrant further clinical trials.

REFERENCES

Jonsson M. (1974) Is Chloramphenicol the Drug of Choice for the Treatment of Enteric Fever? Infection 2 1974 Nr. 3.

Limson B.M. (1973) FL 1039, A new semisynthetic penicillin. Preliminary report on its use in Enteric Fever. Philippine Journal of Internal Medicine. Vol 11 No. 1

Sales J. L. Wilson A. Rimmer D. 1975. 9th International Congress of Chemotherapy.

Schiraldi. O. 1974 Comments on a Clinical Trial with FL 1039, unpublished.

A CLINICAL INVESTIGATION OF PIVMECILLINAM, A NOVEL β-LACTAM
ANTIBIOTIC, IN THE TREATMENT OF URINARY TRACT INFECTIONS

R. Wise,* D.S. Reeves, J.M. Symonds, and P.J. Wilkinson

Department of Medical Microbiology

Southmead Hospital, Bristol

SUMMARY

Pivmecillinam (FL1039) is the pivaloyloxymethyl ester of mecillinam (FL1060) which has considerable in vitro activity against Enterobacteriacae.

Thirty eight hospital inpatients who had proven urinary tract infections were treated with 400 mgs of pivmecillinam 4 times daily for 5 - 7 days. The MIC of mecillinam to the infecting organisms was determined as were the serum and urinary concentrations of the antibiotic.

The patients were followed up for 4 - 6 weeks after the end of treatment. Three patients were lost to follow up. Of the 35 patients who were adequately followed up, 29 (83%) were classified as cured and there were 6 failures. Reported side effects were of a minor nature.

INTRODUCTION

Lund & Tybring (1972) described a new group of β-lactam antibiotics, the 6 beta-amidinopenicillanic acids, the most active of which is mecillinam, which has been shown to be active against a wide range of urinary tract pathogens, with the exception of Gram positive organisms. Mecillinam is poorly absorbed by the oral route, but the hydrochloride of its pivaloyloxymethyl ester, pivmecillinam, is well absorbed being rapidly hydrolysed enzymatically and resulting in satisfactory levels of mecillinam (Roholt et al., 1975). This investigation was designed to study the clinical efficacy of the drug in treating urinary tract infections, and to study its clinical pharmacology.

MATERIALS AND METHODS

Thirty eight hospital inpatients with proven urinary tract infections (at least 100,000 organisms/ml of the same bacterial species in two consecutive specimens of urine) were treated with 400 mgs of pivmecillinam given orally every 6 hours. In 22 patients, the serum levels of mecillinam were determined, samples being taken at 0, 1, 2, 4 and 6 hours following the first dose. The urine levels of mecillinam were measured on four 6 - hourly specimens from most patients, 10 ml aliquots of the urine being frozen on the wards prior to transport to the laboratory in order to minimise loss of activity. Two days after the end of 5 - 7 days treatment and 4 - 6 weeks later, specimens of urine were examined for the presence of pathogens. A cure was defined as the inability to re-isolate the original infecting organism from either specimen.

On all patients a full blood count, alkaline phosphatase, S.G.O.T., S.G.P.T., serum bilirubin and blood urea were determined before and after treatment. The patients were questioned for possible gastrointestinal side effects and signs of penicillin allergy.

Antibiotic assays were performed by a standard microbiological plate diffusion method, using Esch. coli (NCTC 10418) as indicator organism. The antibiotic levels were expressed as mg/litre of mecillinam (anhydrous). For serum estimations standards were prepared in pooled human serum. Urine was assayed using standards in phosphate buffered physiological saline (pH 7.2), and the urine was diluted using the same buffer. The media used was 'Oxoid Diagnostic Sensitivity Test' agar. The majority of specimens were assayed the day they were taken, but if not they were stored at -20°C and assayed the following day. The 95% confidence limits of the assay were $\pm$ 14%.

The minimum inhibitory concentration (MIC) of mecillinam to the infecting organism was determined by a routine plate dilution method in the same media, using a light inoculum of $10^3 - 10^4$ organisms/ml.

RESULTS

Pharmacology

Serum mecillinam assays were performed on 22 patients and the mean 1, 2, 4 and 6 hour concentrations were 3.93, 3.48, 1.3 and

0.74 mg/litre respectively. As can be seen from Table I, the range of values obtained was considerable. It was noted that a raised blood urea was associated with a diminished excretion of mecillinam and hence a raised 6 hour serum concentration, in one case to 2.3 mg/litre. There were too few cases with impaired renal function to quantify or confirm this observation. The serum half-life of the drug, in patients with normal renal function was 1.5 - 2 hours. Urine was assayed from 6 hour samples from 33 patients. As is usually the case, the levels obtained were very variable, the mean concentration being 187 mg/litre (range 37 - 787 mg/litre). It was not possible to assess the effect of impairment of renal function upon the urinary excretion of the drug, as there were very few patients with any considerable degree of renal failure. The highest blood urea noted was 86 mgs per 100 ml (14.3 mmol/litre) and this patient had an average concentration of 133 mg/litre of mecillinam in four 6 hourly collections.

Clinical

Thirty eight patients were admitted to the trial and of these 1 died on the 3rd day of treatment of an unrelated cause (acute leukaemia) and 2 patients could not be followed up. Of the remaining 35 patients, 29 (83%) were considered to be cured and there were 6 failures. These 6 patients are summarised in Table II. In cases 1 & 16 the infecting organism at the beginning and end of treatment was the same serotype in each case. Diene's testing of the isolates from case 27 showed the organism to be of the same type. The Esch. coli isolates from cases 15 & 37 could not be serotyped with available sera. From Table III it can be seen that the majority of clinical isolates were Esch. coli with an MIC to mecillinam of 0.25 mg/litre. In those cases where treatment was considered to have failed, the susceptibility of the post-treatment isolates to mecillinam was found to be the same as, or one dilution either side of, the pre-treatment MIC.

TABLE I. Serum level mg/litre (range)
Time after dose, hours

1	2	4	6
3.93 (6.4 - 1.3)	3.48 (7.6 - 0.9)	1.3 (5.8 - 0.3)	0.74 (2.3 - 0)

Serum levels of mecillinam (anhydrous) following oral administration of 400 mg of pivmecillinam.

TABLE II. Summary of patients who failed to respond to treatment

Case No.	Infecting organism	Pathological condition present in urogenital tract
1	E. coli	Prostatic hypertrophy. Retention & overflow
15	E. coli	Nil
16	E. coli	Multiple myeloma - immunosuppressive therapy
27	Proteus mirabilis	Carcinoma prostate - indwelling catheter
33	Proteus morganii	Chronic urinary tract infection ? aetiology
37	E. coli	Prostatic hypertrophy - indwelling catheter

TABLE III. Infecting organisms MIC mg/litre) of mecillinam

	0.25	0.5	1	2	4	8	16	32	64	>64
E. coli	22		2				1			
Proteus mirabilis		1					1	3	1	
Proteus sp.							1			
Klebsiella sp.								2		
Citrobacter	1									

There were no significant differences in any of the haematological parameters measured. Two patients, who had S.G.O.T. and S.G.P.T. levels within the normal range before treatment had levels of these enzymes slightly higher than normal at the end of treatment. No explanation for this could be found. Another patient complained of diarrhoea and had oral candidiasis from the last day of treatment.

DISCUSSION

Mecillinam has a high degree of activity, in vitro, against a wide range of Gram negative organisms (Reeves et al., 1975). A typical MIC to an Esch. coli being 0.25 mg/litre, Klebsiella sp., Proteus mirabilis and the indole positive Proteus sp. have a more variable susceptibility, with the MICs in range 0.25 - 64 mg/litre. There is very little activity against the Gram positive organisms.

In this study we have demonstrated that the levels attained in the urine should be sufficient to treat susceptible pathogens even in patients with moderate degrees of renal impairment. A cure rate of 83% compares favourably with commonly used oral antibiotics which are effective against urinary tract pathogens isolated from hospital inpatients. Davies et al., (1971) showed that cephalexin and ampicillin had a cure rate of about 60% in hospital patients with urinary tract infections. The cure rate amongst similar patients treated with co-trimoxazole was 67% (Reeves, Faiers, Parsell & Brumfitt, 1969). Amongst those 6 patients in whom treatment failed it was interesting to note that 4 had pathological conditions present in their urogenital tract, and therefore treatment failure was not unexpected.

The possibility of the emergence of resistant variants after treatment with pivmecillinam has been raised by Greenwood et al., (1974). We paid particular attention to this possibility in our study. In those patients where pivmecillinam failed to eradicate the infecting organism, the sensitivity of pre and post treatment bacterial isolates were similar, indicating that in this trial at least, the emergence of resistant variants was not a clinical problem. Christoffersen et al., (1974) and Verrier-Jones and Asscher (1975) have also noted that there was no development of resistance to mecillinam during clinical usage. The combined experience of these three studies would seem to indicate that the in vitro findings are not repeated in the clinical situation and the likelihood of resistance emerging from clinical usage of pivmecillinam would therefore seem to be no greater than that of any other β-lactam antibiotic.

ACKNOWLEDGEMENTS

We should like to thank Mrs. H. Bennett for her technical assistance, and Dr. B. Marsh and Mr. P. Menday of Leo Laboratories for supplying the antibiotic and their helpful advice.

* Present address: Department of Medical Microbiology, Dudley Road Hospital, Birmingham.

REFERENCES

Christoffersen, J.C., Iversen, H.G., Jacobsen, J., Korner, B., Petersen, H.K., Rasmussen, F. & Tybring, L. FL1039 in bacteriuria following prostatectomy. Scandinavian Journal of Urology & Nephrology. (In Press).

Davies, J.A., Strangeways, J.E.M., Mitchell, R.G., Beilia, L.J., Ledingham, J.G.C., & Holt, J.M. Comparative double blind trial of cephalexin and ampicillin in treatment of urinary tract infections. British Medical Journal 3: 215-217 (1971).

Greenwood, D., Brooks, L.H., Gargan, R., & O'Grady, F. Activity of FL1060 a new β-lactam antibiotic, against urinary tract pathogens. Journal of Clinical Pathology 27: 192-197, (1974).

Lund, F., & Tybring, H., 6 β-amidinopenicillanic acids - a new group of antibiotics. Nature, New Biology 236: 135-137, (1972).

Reeves, D.S., Faiers, M.C., Pursell, R.E., & Brumfitt, W. Trimethoprim-Sulphamethoxazole: Comparative study in urinary tract infections in hospital. British Medical Journal 1: 541-544, (1969).

Reeves, D.S., Wise, R., & Bywater, M.J. A laboratory evaluation of a novel β-lactam antibiotic mecillinam; a treatment for bacterial infection. (To be published).

Roholt, K., Nielsen, B., & Kristensen, E. Pharmacokinetic studies with mecillinam and pivmecillinam. (In Press).

Verrier-Jones, E.R., & Asscher, A.W., Treatment of recurrent bacteriuria with pivmecillinam (FL1039). The Journal of Antimicrobial Chemotherapy. 1: 193-196, (1975).

ANTIBACTERIAL ACTIVITY OF EIGHT CEPHALOSPORINS (CEFAMAN-
DOLE INCLUDED) ON TWO COMMON RESPIRATORY PATHOGENS (HAE-
MOPHILUS INFLUENZAE AND DIPLOCOCCUS PNEUMONIAE)

E. YOURASSOWSKY, E. SCHOUTENS and
M.P.VANDERLINDEN
Hôpital Universitaire Brugmann
Service de Biologie Clinique
1020 - Bruxelles. Belgium

ABSTRACT

Two hundred recent clinical isolates of Haemophilus and Pneumococcus were tested in vitro against eight
cephalosporins by means of disc diffusion and agar dilution tests.
Cefamandole was the most active cephalosporin
against Haemophilus, 97% of the strains being inhibited by 0,78 mcg per ml of this drug. In order of decreasing bacteriostatic effectiveness, the other drugs
were classified as follows: cephapirin, cephalothin,
cefoxitin, cephaloridine, cefazolin, cephradine and
cephalexin. This, study suggest that prediction of
the susceptibility of Haemophilus strains to cephalosporins, on the basis of one drug of this group testing
alone, is likely to be hazardous.
The most active cephalosporins against D. pneumoniae were cephaloridine, cephapirine, cefazolin, cefamandole and cephalothin which inhibited 90% of the
strains at 0,19 mcg per ml. Cefoxitin, cephradine and
cephalexin were clearly less active, requiring 3,12mcg
per ml to exhibit the same antibacterial activity.
Nevertheless, none of the strains were clearly resistant to these drugs.

INTRODUCTION

Although changing prevalence of pathogenic bacteria in several infections is a widely accepted notion

(2) by far, the commonest bacterial pathogens in chronic bronchitis still remain H. influenzae and D. pneumoniae (4).

Until recently, the remarkable sensitivity pattern of these two bacteria (5,8) was considered sufficiently constant to justify blind chemotherapy with ampicillin in the routine management of chronic bronchitis. Unfortunately, ampicillin resistant Haemophilus are now encountered (6) which makes this therapeutic option hazardous. Moreover, this drug cannot be used in patients hypersensitive to penicillin.

As cephalosporins could be an alternative choice in such cases, the present study was undertaken to compare the in-vitro activity of several substances of this group of antibiotics, against recent clinical isolates of D. pneumoniae and Haemophilus.

MATERIALS and METHODS

The strains were mostly isolated from transtracheal aspirations, sputum and throat swabs. They were preserved in liquid nitrogen until sensitivity testing. Included in the survey were 100 strains of D. pneumoniae and 100 strains of Haemophilus (28 H. influenzae, 24 H. parainfluenzae, 8 H. haemolyticus, 34 H. parahaemolyticus and 6 H. paraphraphilus).
Antibiotics were furnished as follows: cefamandole, cephalexin, cephaloridine and cephalothin, Lilly; cefazolin, Bristol; cefoxitin, Merck, Sharp and Dohme ; cephapirin, Mead-Johnson and cephradine, Squibb.
Minimal inhibitory concentrations (MIC) were determined by an agar plate dilution method using trypticase soy agar supplemented with 2% Fildes enrichment for Haemophilus strains, and Mueller Hinton agar supplemented with 5% horse blood for Pneumococcus strains. Overnight broth cultures in Mueller Hinton broth supplemented with 5% Fildes enrichment were diluted to contain 10^5 organisms per ml. The plates were inoculated with an automatic multipoint inocular (Dynatech, Billingshurst, Sussex, GB).
Results were read after 18 hr incubation in an atmosphere of 10% CO_2. The MIC was determined as the lowest concentration yielding no growth.
Antibiotic sensitivity testing was also performed by the filter-paper-disc method using 30 mcg discs and the same media as in MIC determinations. Diameters of the inhibition zones were measured with a caliper after overnight incubation in a CO_2 enriched atmosphere.

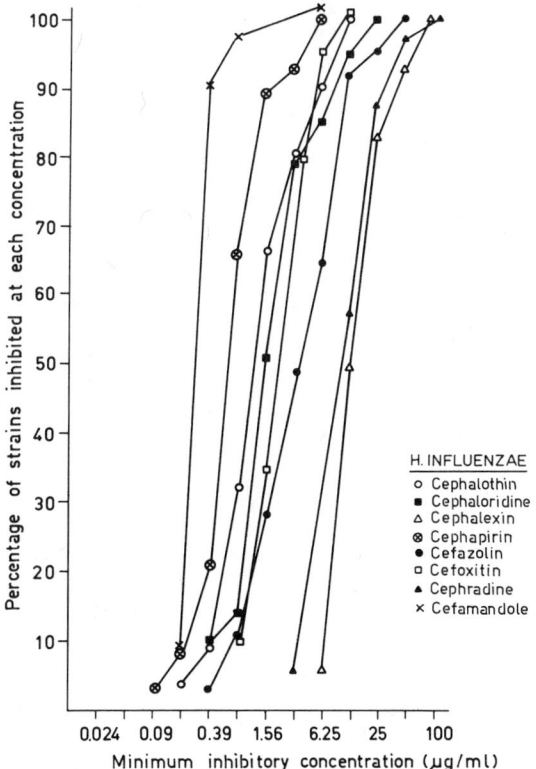

Fig. 1 : Activity of eight cephalosporins against 100 strains of Haemophilus.

RESULTS

MIC values of the Haemophilus strains are summarized in fig. 1.
Of the eight cephalosporins tested, cefamandole is the most active with 97% of the strains inhibited by 0,78 mcg per ml. In order of decreasing bacteriostatic effectiveness, the other drugs can be classified as follows: cephapirin, cephalothin, cefoxitin, cephaloridine, cefazolin, cephradine and cephalexin. Mean values and standard deviations of the zone diameters obtained with the Haemophilus strains are: cephalothin : 29,73 (± 5,77)mm, cephapirin : 29,38 (± 5,60)mm, cefoxitin: 28,16 (± 5,40)mm, cephaloridine: 27,39 (± 5,18)mm, cefamandole: 25,91 (± 3,63)mm, cefazolin: 25,35 (± 5,42)mm, cephradine: 23,49 (± 3,86)mm, cephalexin: 23,16 (± 4,85)mm. Cephalexin and cephradine are the least effective drugs with many resistant strains

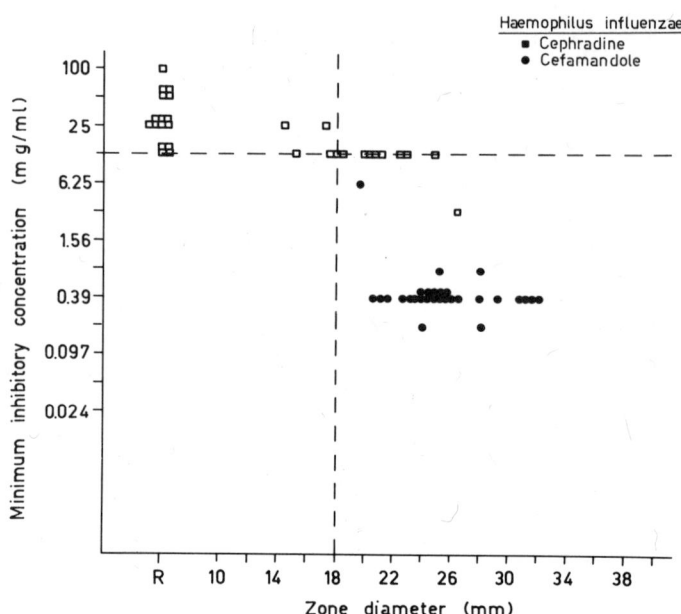

Fig. 2 : Comparison of agar dilution with disk diffusion susceptibility tests for 100 Haemophilus strains against cephradine and cefamandole.

(MIC $>$ 25 mcg/ml, zone diameter $<$ 14mm).
The relationship between MIC values and zone sizes is generally good; as examples, results obtained with cefamandole and cephradine are shown in Fig. 2.

MIC values of the Pneumococcus strains are summarized in Fig. 3.
The cephalosporins can be grouped in two categories: included in the most active are cephaloridine, cephaloridine, cephapirin, cefamandole, cefazolin and cephalothin with 90% of strains being susceptible to 0,19 mcg per ml. In contrast, cefoxitin, cephradine and cephalexin require 3,12 mcg per ml for comparative inhibitory power. However all strains are inhibited by 12,5mcg per ml of these drugs.

The relationship between MIC values and zone sizes for cephaloridin and cephalexin are shown in Fig. 4.

Mean values and standard deviations of the zone diamters obtained with the Pneumococcus strains are: cefamandole: 45,83 ($\pm$ 5,13)mm, cephalothin: 42,62 ($\pm$ 6,28)mm, cephaloridine: 42,48 ($\pm$ 3,37)mm, cefazolin:

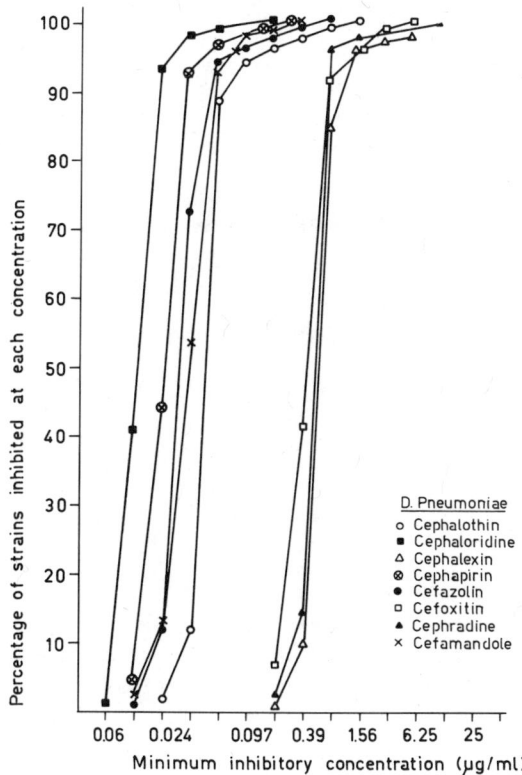

Fig. 3 : Activity of eight cephalosporins against 100 strains of D. pneumoniae.

41,45 (± 3,30)mm, cephapirin: 41,19 (± 6,35)mm, cefoxitin: 34,77 (± 4,70)mm, cephradine: 33,51 (± 5,13)mm, cephalexin: 25,33 (± 3,63)mm.
No strain has a zone size < 14mm.

DISCUSSION and CONCLUSIONS

Striking differences in in-vitro effectiveness are demonstrated among cephalosporins against two common respiratory pathogens: in the case of Pneumococcus, these drugs can be divided into two categories, the least effective including cefoxitin, cephradine and cephalexin.
However, no resistant strains are encountered.
In the case of Haemophilus, the most active drug (cefamandole) is one hundred times as active as the least

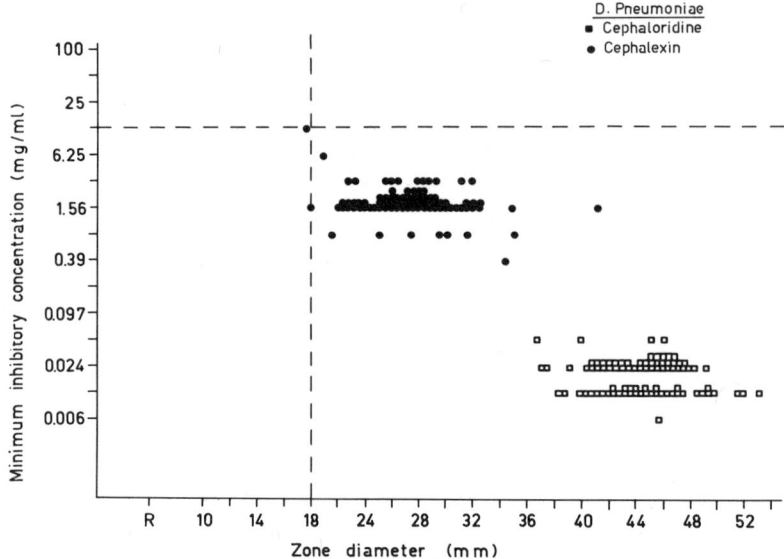

Fig. 4 : Comparison of agar dilution with disk diffusion susceptibility tests for 100 D. pneumoniae strains against cephaloridine and cephalexin.

effective one (cephalexin), the other antibiotics of this group being evenly distributed between these two extremes. Many strains are resistant to cephradine and cephalexin.
These data correlate well with those previously published by Williams et al (7).

Clinical laboratories most often use the disk agar diffusion method (1) as routine technique for susceptibility testing.
The present study suggests that prediction of the sensitivity of Pneumococcus strains to all cephalosporins on the basis of one drug of this group being tested alone (generally cephalothin) is a suitable procedure as each strain exhibits comparable sensitivities to the different antibiotics of this group. This is not rue for Haemophilus, strains being encountered which are resistant to cephradine and cephalexin, although sensitive to cephalothin.

It is difficult to extrapolate from laboratory results to clinical indications for therapy and it is not the purpose of the present paper. Cases in which cephalosporins would be the oustanding drugs of choice are still to be define (3). The eventual role of these antibiotics in the chemotherapy of pulmonary tract infections will likely depend on further comparative trials of efficacy, toxicity and cost.

   Acknowledgments. The technical assistance of J. SCHOONJANS and her colleagues is gratefully acknowledged.

REFERENCES

1. BAUER A.W., KIRBY W.M.M., SHERRIS J.C. and TURCK M. :
Antibiotic susceptibility testing by a standardized single disk method.
   Amer.J.Clin.Pathol.45: 493-496 (1966).

2. FINLAND M. :
Changing ecology of bacterial infections as related to antibacterial therapy.
   J.Infect.Dis.122: 419-431 (1970).

3. HAMILTON-MILLER J.M.T., BRUMFITT W. :
Whither the cephalosporins ?
   J.Infect.Dis.130: 81-83 (1974).

4. MAY J.R. :
The chemotherapy of chronic bronchitis and allied disorders.
   The English Universities Press Ltd, 1968.

5. SABATH L.D., STUMPF L.L., WALLACE S.J. and FINLAND M. :
Susceptibility of Diplococcus pneumoniae, Haemophilus influenzae, and Neisseria meningitidis to 23 antibiotics.
   Antimicr.Ag.Chemother.1970: 53-56.

6. SCHIFFER M.S., MaC LOWRY J., SCHNEERSON R., ROBBINS J.B. :
Clinical, bacteriological and Immunological characterisation of ampicillin-resistant Haemophilus influenzae type B.
   Lancet, ii, 257-259 (1974).

7. WILLIAMS J.D., ANDREWS J. :
Sensitivity of Haemophilus influenzae to antibiotics.
   Br.Med.J. 1: 134-137 (1974).

8. YOURASSOWSKY E., SCHOUTENS E., VANDERLINDEN M.P., PRUDHOMME M.R. :
   Susceptibility of Haemophilus to antibiotics : present status.
   Infection 3: 15-18 (1975).

RELATIONSHIP BETWEEN LYTIC AND INHIBITORY CONCENTRATIONS OF CEPHALOSPORINS

J.M.T. Hamilton-Miller

The Royal Free Hospital

Pond Street, Hampstead, London NW3 2QG

The β-lactam antibiotics owe their bactericidal activity to their lytic action on the bacterial cell wall. This property sets them apart from other bactericidal antibiotics, such as the aminoglycosides. Shortly after the introduction of benzylpenicillin some 30 years ago much attention was paid to the lysis phenomenon, especially in relation to the "zone effect" (Eagle & Musselman 1948). However, interest in this aspect waned. The recent increase in the number of semisynthetic β-lactam antibiotics has caused a renewed interest in lytic activity, which has been lead by O'Grady and his colleagues (e.g. Greenwood & O'Grady 1973, 1975). An intriguing finding by these workers is that cephalexin is "lytic-deficient", in that filamentation rather than lysis is the bacterial response over a wide range of antibiotic concentrations (Greenwood & O'Grady 1973). As cephalexin was unique among the β-lactam compounds which they tested, in that it has a 3-methyl sidechain, it seemed possible that there was some simple relationship between chemical structure and lytic ability among cephalosporins. The present study was designed to investigate this possibility.

MATERIALS AND METHODS

Bacterial Strains

Two standard laboratory strains were used, Staphylococcus aureus NCTC 6571 (Oxford strain), and Escherichia coli K12. Both were sensitive to a wide range of antimicrobial compounds. This specimen of E.coli K12 produces a β-lactamase at a low level (Hamilton-Miller, Smith & Knox 1965); despite this, it is fully sensitive to all the cephalosporins tested.

Cephalosporins

Eleven compounds were tested; they are listed, together with the nature of their 3- and 7- substituents, in Table 1. We gratefully acknowledge the generous gifts of their products by the following manufacturers: Glaxo Research Laboratories (cephaloridine, cephalexin, cephalosporin C and 87/312); Lilly Research Laboratories (cephalothin and its deacetyl and deacetoxy analogues); Merck, Sharp & Dohme (cefoxitin); E.R. Squibb (cephradine); Fujisawa Pharmaceuticals (cefazolin); CIBA-Geigy (cephacetrile). Compound 87/312 was tested against S.aureus only and the deacetyl and deacetoxy analogues of cephalothin against E.coli only; the other cephalosporins were tested against both species.

Compound	3-sidechain	7-sidechain
Cephalosporin C	acetoxy	α-aminoadipoyl
Cephalothin	acetoxy	2-thienylmethyl
Cephacetrile	acetoxy	cyanomethyl
Cephalexin	methyl	α-aminobenzyl
Cephradine	methyl	α-aminocyclohexadienyl
Deacetoxycephalothin	methyl	2-thienylmethyl
Deacetylcephalothin	hydroxymethyl	2-thienylmethyl
Cefazolin	thiadiazolyl	tetrazolylmethyl
Cefoxitin	carbamoyl	2-thienylmethyl
Cephaloridine	pyridinium	2-thienylmethyl
87/312	2,4-dinitrostyryl	2-thienylmethyl

Table 1. Structures of cephalosporins tested

Microbiological Procedures

Growth curves were followed thus: organisms were cultured in 10 ml. volumes of Hartley's digest broth (Southern Group Laboratories) statically overnight. Such cultures contained about 500 million staphylococci/ml. or about 1,000 million E.coli/ml. 5 ml. of culture was added to 95 ml. brain heart infusion broth (BHI; Oxoid), which has an osmolality of 387 mOsm./Kg. 8 ml. amounts were pipetted into each of 10 T-tubes, which were plugged and swung (60 cycles/min) in a waterbath at 37C. Growth was followed using a Spekker Absorptiometer. Full details of this system have been published elsewhere (Hamilton-Miller 1974). Under these conditions, the mean generation times of S.aureus and E.coli were found to be 22 and 19 min., respectively. When E had reached 0.5 - 0.6 (after about 120 - 150 min.), 2 ml. of BHI broth, containing serial doubling concentrations of a cephalosporin, was added to each tube. The final concentrations of antibiotic in the tubes extended over a wide range on either side of the MIC. One tube acted as control. Monitoring of each tube on the Spekker continued.

MIC were estimated by the conventional agar serial dilution technique. A large inoculum (1 drop of overnight culture) was used in order to simulate as closely as possible the conditions of the growth curve. Antibiotic dilutions were made in molten BHI agar which was dispensed in 2 ml. volumes into separate divisions of compartmented plastics plates (10 cm. square; Dyos Plastics). Complete inhibition of growth after overnight incubation was taken as endpoint.

A more accurate measure than MIC is given by the determination of "critical concentrations", the parameter M' of Cooper (1963). Hamilton-Miller (1971) referred to this as MNIC - maximal non-inhibitory concentration. 5 ml. amounts of overnight culture were added to 95 ml. molten BHI agar, and 11 ml. were then poured into each 8 cm. plastics plate, giving an agar depth of 2 mm. Four wells (8 mm. diameter) were cut from every plate, and each was filled with an appropriate concentration of a cephalosporin, one drug per plate. Plates were prepared in duplicate. Zone diameters were read after overnight incubation, and plotted against log. dose. The regression lines thus obtained were produced back to determine that concentration which would give a "zone size" of 8 mm.; this concentration is M'.

RESULTS AND DISCUSSION

Relation of MIC to M'

The ratio of MIC to M' was greater for S.aureus than for E.coli, mean values being 2.98 and 1.63, respectively. Cooper found this ratio to be between 2 and 4.

Relation of Inhibitory to Lytic Concentrations

S.aureus required relatively lower concentrations of all cephalosporins tested to bring about lysis; thus, mean values for the 9 compounds tested were 0.74 X MIC or 1.56 X M'. No one compound was outstanding either for its ability or inability to cause lysis. In particular, both the 3-methyl cephalosporins tested, cephalexin and cephradine, were lytic at 0.5 X MIC.

Against E.coli, taking mean values for the 10 compounds, 3.73 X MIC or 5 X M' were required for lysis. Cephradine and cephalexin were lytic-deficient, 16 X and 8 X of respective MIC being needed to initiate lysis. In contrast, the other 3-methyl cephalosporin tested, deacetoxycephalothin, was not lytic-deficient, only 2 X MIC causing lysis. The closely related compound deacetylcephalothin was also not lytic-deficient. It can therefore be concluded that lytic ability against S.aureus is independent of gross chemical structure, and that the lytic deficiency of cephalexin and cephradine against E.coli cannot be explained solely in terms of of there being 3-methyl cephalosporins.

Morphological Effects

Greenwood & O'Grady (1973) reported that filamentation of E.coli in response to cephalexin could be observed microscopically at concentrations below the MIC. We have now also observed this phenomenon for cephradine. At higher concentrations (2 - 4 X MIC), filamentation was so marked that tubes exhibited "flow birefringence", which was strikingly obvious to the naked eye. This effect was not seen when cephalexin or cephradine acted upon staphylococci (where a lytic response was observed), nor when the deacetoxy or deacetyl analogues of cephalothin acted on E.coli. Thus morphological and lytic events appeared to be correlated.

REFERENCES

Cooper, K.E. in Analytical Microbiology (ed. Kavanagh, F.) p. 1 Academic Press, New York, 1963.
Eagle, H. & Musselman, A.D. 1948 J.exp.Med., 88, 99.
Greenwood, D. & O'Grady, F. 1973 J.inf.Dis., 128, 211.
Greenwood, D. & O'Grady, F. 1975 J.med.Microbiol., 8, 205.
Hamilton-Miller, J.M.T. 1971 J.med.Microbiol., 4, 227.
Hamilton-Miller, J.M.T. 1974 Lab.Practice, 23, 569.
Hamilton-Miller, J.M.T., Smith, J.T. & Knox, R. 1965 Nature, 208, 235.

CEPHACETRILE : PLASMA CONCENTRATIONS DURING AND AFTER CONSTANT INFUSION

K.G. Naber, H.G. Meyer-Brunot and I. Reitz

Department of Urology, University of Marburg, Germany
Research Department, Pharmaceuticals Division
CIBA-GEIGY Ltd., Basle, Switzerland

Since in case of severe infection antibiotics are frequently administered by intravenous infusion in order to achieve high and effective plasma concentrations over a long period of time, we determined the plasma concentrations of cephacetrile during and after constant infusion using various dosage regimens.

MATERIALS AND METHODS

Twenty-five infusion experiments were performed in five male and two female volunteers (age: 24-33 years, weight: 50-87 kg, height 160-186 cm, body surface: 1.50-2.15 m^2). Five different dosage regimens were used (2 g of cephacetrile was infused during 1 hour, 2 g during 2 hours, 4 g during 0.5 hours, 4 g during 1 hour and 4 g during 2 hours). The amount of cephacetrile was dissolved in 500 ml of 0.9% NaCl and administered intravenously into the cubital vein using an infusion pump (Infusomat, Braun, Melsungen). Heparinized blood samples were drawn from the contralateral cubital vein at intervals during infusion and up to three hours after the end of infusion.

Cepahacetrile was bioassayed by an agar well test (1) on NUNC-BIO assay plates No. 1015 using B. subtilis (Difco) as test organism. All standard curves were made up by diluting the antibiotic with blank plasma of each volunteer resulting in concentrations of 100, 50, 25, 12.5 and 6.25 mcg/ml. If necessary, plasma was diluted with blank plasma by two folds.

RESULTS AND DISCUSSION

Four of the twenty-five experiments hat to be rejected from further calculations because of technical defects during infusion.

Figure 1 shows the plasma concentrations in the five different groups. In all groups peak concentrations were reached at the end of infusion indicating that in none of the dosage regimens steady state conditions were achieved during time of infusion. It is remarkable that three hours after start of infusion the three groups 4 g/0.5 hours, 4 g/1 hour and 2 g/2 hours show approximately the same plasma concentration of 20 mcg/ml. Higher plasma concentrations at this time were achieved only in group 4 g/2 hours. This may lead to the conclusion that a constant infusion during a period of 2 hours is preferable to that during a period of 1 or 0.5 hours., if the same total amount of antibiotic is administered. It is unlikely that for example the mean peak concentration of 129 mcg/ml in the group 4 g/0.5 hours is of a much greater value than that of 98 mcg/ml in the group 4 g/2 hours.

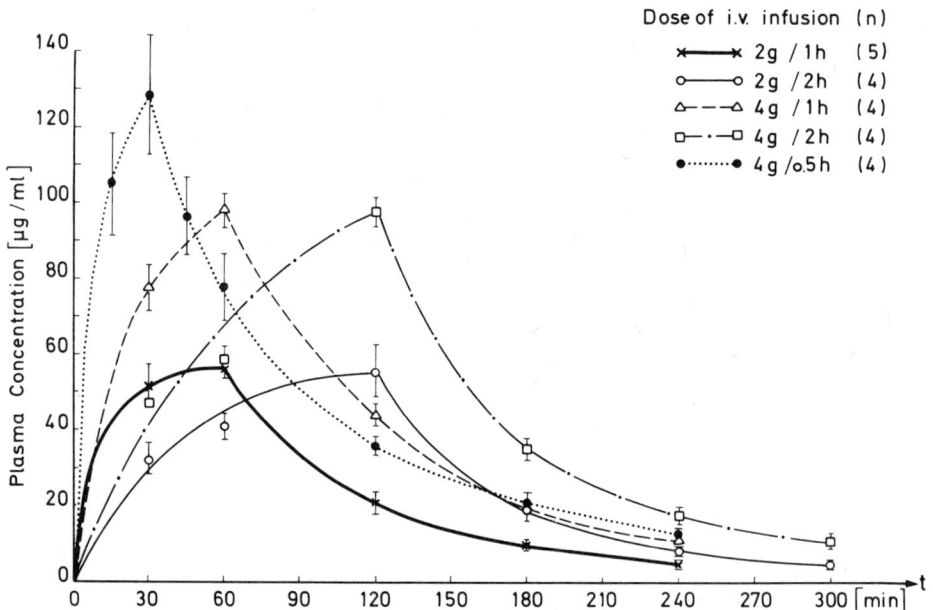

Figure 1: Plasma concentrations during and after constant intravenous infusion of cephacetrile in human volunteers with five different dosage regimens. Mean ± SE, (n) number of experiments.

Dose of infusion	No. of experiments	c_τ Plasma conc. at end of infusion [mg/l]	$t_{50\%}$ Plasma half life [h]	k_e Elimination rate constant [h^{-1}]	V Apparent volume of distribution [l]	C_p Total virtual plasma clearance [ml/min]
2g/1h	5	56.2 ± 5.7	0.96 ± 0.19	.743 ± .125	25.3 ± 2.5	313 ± 53
2g/2h	4	56.1 ± 14.6	1.02 ± 0.09	.965 ± .056	20.8 ± 6.7	232 ± 58
4g/0.5h	4	128.5 ± 31.3	1.15 ± 0.22	.622 ± .130	28.0 ± 6.6	294 ± 119
4g/1h	4	98.0 ± 9.1	1.04 ± 0.15	.675 ± .097	30.0 ± 3.9	333 ± 7
4g/2h	4	97.9 ± 7.7	1.19 ± 0.27	.605 ± .128	23.9 ± 2.4	238 ± 37

Table 1: Pharmacokinetic data in the five different groups of cephacetrile infusion. Mean ± SE.

From the curve of plasma concentration we calculated the half-life, the elimination rate constant, the apparent volume of distribution and the total virtual plasma clearance (2) for all five groups (Table 1).

A relatively wide range of the apparent volume of distribution was found (4). There was some correlation to the rate of infusion. There was a significant difference ($p < 0.05$) between group 4 g/1 hour and 4 g/2 hours in volume of distribution and plasma clearance. The mean half-lives ranged from 0.96 to 1.19 hours with no significant differences between the various groups.

The areas under the curve (Figure 2) showed a good correlation to the total amount of antibiotic administered indicating that the kinetics of elimination are not different between the various groups.

In Table 2 the pharmacokinetic data of cephacetrile are compared to those of five different cephalosporins as reported by KIRBY and REGAMEY (3). These authors also used the constant infusion technique. The half-life of cephacetrile is in the range of that of cephaloridine and cephalexin, shorter than that of cefazolin and cephanone and longer than that of cephalothin. In addition to a convenient half-life, cephacetrile displays a low protein binding.

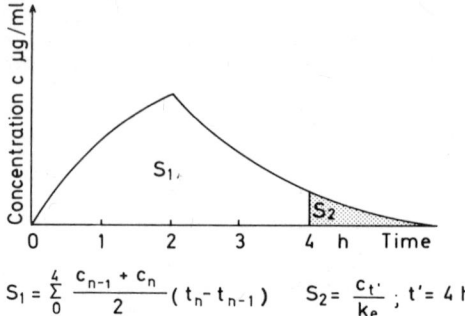

$$S_1 = \sum_{0}^{4} \frac{c_{n-1} + c_n}{2} (t_n - t_{n-1}) \qquad S_2 = \frac{c_{t'}}{k_e} ; \; t' = 4 \, h$$

Experiment	S_1 $\left[\frac{\mu g \cdot h}{ml}\right]$	S_2 $\left[\frac{\mu g \cdot h}{ml}\right]$	$S_1 + S_2$ $\left[\frac{\mu g \cdot h}{ml}\right]$
2g / 1h	101	6	107
2g / 2h	126	12	138
4g/0.5h	195	20	215
4g / 1h	182	17	199
4g / 2h	209	29	238

Figure 2: Areas under the curve in the five different groups of cephacetrile infusion

Parameter	Cephacetrile (range)	Cefazolin*	Cephanone*	Cephaloridine*	Cephalexin*	Cephalothin*
Total virtual plasma clearance C_p [ml/min/1.73 m^2]	218 ± 24 – 336 ± 33	62 ± 6	56 ± 2	167 ± 20	248 ± 11	472 ± 59
Plasma half life $t_{50\%}$ [h]	0.96±0.19 – 1.19±0.27	1.8±0.2	2.5±0.1	1.12 ± 0.07	0.9 ±0.02	0.47 ± 0.13
Apparent volume of distribution V [l/1.73 m^2]	19.4±3.5 – 30.1± 2.2	10±0.4	12±0.4	16 ± 2.7	16 ±1.3	18 ± 4.0
Protein binding [%]	19 – 24	86	88	20	15	65

Mean ± SE.   *KIRBY and REGAMEY, 1973

Table 2: Pharmacokinetic data of cephacetrile as compared to those of five different cephalosporins.

PLASMA CONCENTRATIONS OF CEPHACETRILE

SUMMARY

Cephacetrile was administered to human volunteers using constant intravenous infusion technique. Five different dosage regimens were used: 2 g cephacetrile were infused during 1 hour, 2 g during 2 hours, 4 g during 0.5 hours, 4 g during 1 hour and 4 g during 2 hours. The mean plasma concentrations at the end of infusion of each group were 56 mcg/ml, 56 mcg/ml, 129 mcg/ml, 98 mcg/ml and 98 mcg/ml. Three hours after the start of infusion the three groups 2 g/2 hours, 4 g/0.5 hours and 4 g/1 hour showed almost identical concentrations of 20 mcg/ml. It was concluded that a 2 hours infusion may be preferable to a 1 or 0.5 hour infusion if the same total amount of antibiotic is administered. The plasma half-life was in the range of 0.96 to 1.19 hours, the apparent volume of distribution of 19.4 to 30.1 l/1.73 m^2 and the plasma clearance of 218 to 336 ml/min./1.73 m^2. The pharmacokinetic data were compared with those of five different cephalosporins.

REFERENCES

1. Bauer, K., Hiltmann, R., Schmid, J., Anhagen, E.:
   Neue kristallisierte Penicillinsalze und ihre Prüfung auf Depotwirkung am Kaninchen.
   Med. und Chemie 5, 25, 1956

2. Gladtke, E., von Hattingberg, H.M.
   Pharmakokinetik. Springer, Berlin, 1973 p. 20

3. Kirby, W.M.M., Regamey, C.
   Pharmacokinetics of cefazolin compared with four other cephalosporins
   J. Inf. Dis. 128 Suppl. 341, 1973

4. Maurice, P.N., Riess, W., Welke, A., Amson, K.
   Celospor (C 36 278-Ba), ein neues Antibiotikum aus der Cephalosporinreihe: Pharmakokinetik und klinische Prüfung
   Schw. Med. Wschr. 103, 718, 1973

CLINICAL EVALUATION OF CEFOXITIN

G.K. Daikos, H. Giamarellou, K. Kanellakopoulou, and G. Piperakis

1st Department of Propedeutic Medicine
Athens University School of Medicine
King Paul's Hospital, Athens

This study reports the results of a clinical trial with Cefoxitin. Of the 28 patients treated, there were 9 urinary tract infections, 4 cases of chronic bronchitis in exacerbation, 2 cases of pneumonia, 2 cases of chest empyema, 3 cases of postoperative fistulas, 2 cases of salmonellosis, 2 cases of chronic vaginitis and one of the following: soft tissue infection, acute cholocystitis, chronic osteomyelitis and septicemia.

Causative organisms were mainly Klebsiella, E.Coli and Proteus Ind. (+), as well as Staph aureus and few anaerobic bacteria

Cefoxitin was given as a 2gm infusion over 30 min q^{8h}. The peak serum levels ranged between 150-200 µg/ml, but the trough levels were less than 1µg/ml. Urinary levels ranged between 160µg/ml-6000µg/ml.

The drug proved very effective both clinically and bacteriologically.

Except for a patient with drug allergy, Cefoxitin was well tolerated.

Cefoxitin is a semisynthetic cephamycin, (1,2,3,), which is much less easily destroyed by b-lactamases produced by the enterobacteriaceae than the other cephalosporins (4). Previous in vitro sensitivity studies in this laboratory with Cefoxitin. (Fig.1), using 25 strains of each different species, indicated that about 70% of freshly isolated Klebsiella sp., E.Coli and Proteus ind (+) have MICs of 16 µg/ml or

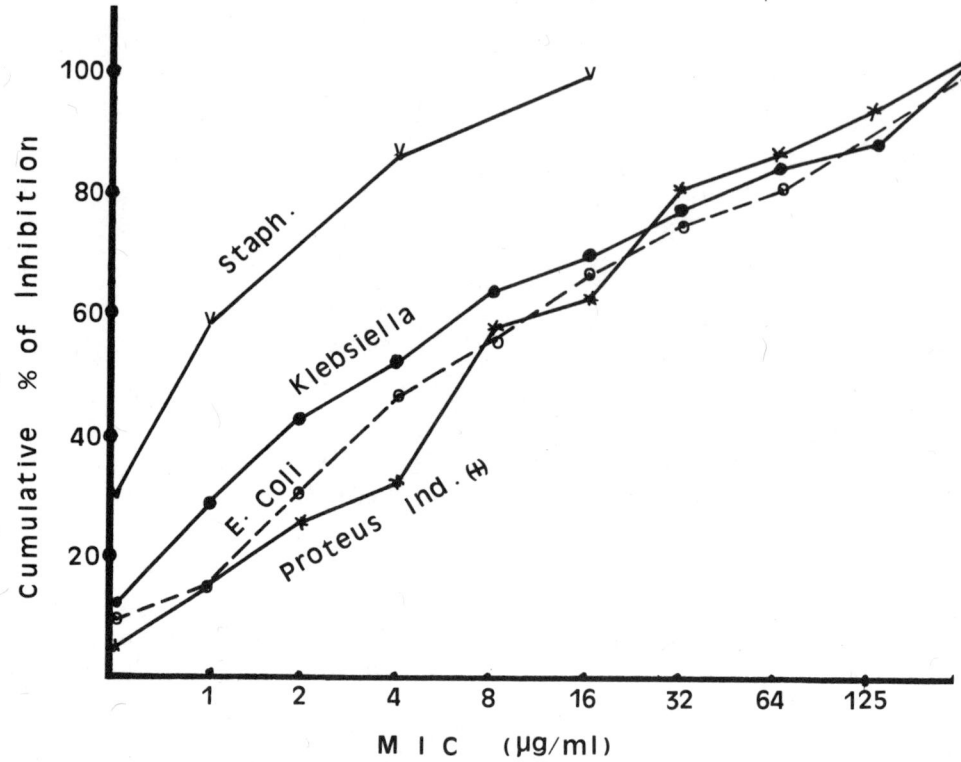

FIG.1.The in vitro susceptibility of different genera of bacteria to Cefoxitin.

less. All strains of Pseudomonas aeruginosa were resistant to 250 µg/ml, while from the Gram (+) bacteria, 85% of Staphylococci were inhibited by 4 µg/ml or less. It is noteworthy that most of the above bacteria had higher MICs, or were resistant to Cephalothin in comparison with Cefoxitin. The MBCs for about 70% of Klebsiella sp., E. coli, and Proteus Ind (+) were 32 µg/ml or less. In some Staph. strains the phenomenon of persistence was observed. We have therefore studied both the clinical efficacy and the pharmacological properties of the new drug.

PATIENTS AND METHODS

Sensitivities were done by the Kirby-Bauer method using 30 µg discs. Minimal inhibitory concentrations were determined by the microtiter technique using tryptose phosphate broth as the basic medium with a standard bacterial inoculum of 10^6 bacteria per ml. Minimal bactericídal concentrations was designated as the concentration of Cefoxitin that produced a reduction in viable organisms of at least 99.9%.

The antibiotic levels in serum and urine were estimated by the agar well diffusion method using a special strain of staph aureus (MB-27 86) and Cefoxitin standard two-fold dilutions of 128 µg/ml to 1µg/ml.

A total of 28 patients varying in age from 19 to 69 y were treated with Cefoxitin. These included 12 males and 16 females. Distribution of infections is shown in table I.

The daily dose of Cefoxitin was 2gm I.V. q^{8h} with each dose infused over a period of 30 min, for 10-15 days.

Toxicity studies were done on all patients.

RESULTS

The MICs of the bacteria isolated from the patients ranged between 0.25-8mg/ml while the MBCs between 0.5-16µg/ml. A zone size of 22mm or more by the Kirby-Bauer method could reliably be considered as indication of sensitivity. There was a rather good correlation between the two methods.

Analysis of the patients treated with Cefoxitin is shown in table II. The overal clinical effect was very good in 25 out of 28 cases (89%) including 15 cured and 10 improved cases, while there was elimination of the pathogens in 18 cases. All 4 cases of chronic bronchitis were in critical condition. During treatment with Cefoxitin, there was much improvement with clearance of sputum to mucoid and volume reduction. Although pathogens persisted in 3 patients, they were in small numbers, with the same sensitivity pattern.

The 2 cases of anaerobic chest empyema are of particular interest because the anaerobic bacteria (Bacteroides species and anaerobic cocci) were in adittion isolated from blood. Both improved initially, but because surgical assistance and prolonged treatment were needed, Cefoxitin was shifted to other antibiotics.

TABLE I

Distribution of Infections Treated with Cefoxitin	
Respiratory	8
Urinary	9
Miscellaneous	11
Total	28

TABLE II. Clinical and Bacteriologic Effects of Cefoxitin on Various Infections

Infection	No of cases	Clinical Cured	Improved	Failure	Bacteriologic Elimination	Failure
Respiratory tract:						
Chronic bronchitis in exacerbation	4		4		1	3
Lobar Pneumonia	2	1	1		1	1
Empyema of chest	2		2		not	done
Urinary tract	9	7	1	1	8	1
Miscellaneous:						
Postoperative fistula	3	2		1	2	1
Soft tissue	1	1			1	
Chronic vaginitis	2	2			2	
Acute cholocystitis	1		1		not	done
Osteomyelitis	1		1		1	
Septicemia	1			1		1
Salmonellosis	2	2			2	
Totals:	28	15	10	3	18	7

Of the 9 patients with urinary tract infections, only one with transplanted kidney failed to respond, while a second one with obstructive uropathy, relapsed during the follow-up period. The remaining 7 patients remained free from infection for at least 8 weeks after completion or treatment.

11 patients suffering from miscellaneous infections were treated with Cefoxitin. 7 were cured, 2 improved and 2 failed. Among the improved patients, a case of chronic posttraumatic osteomylitis due to staph aureus was completely cleared, while all previous schedules with various antistaphylococcal drugs, to which the pathogen was sensitive in vitro, have failed. The 2 patients who did not respond to Cefoxitin were suffering, the first from a postoperative fistula due to E. coli, and the second patient being also leukopenic because of A.M.L. from Staph aureus septicemia.

Concerning the different pathogens (Table III), E. coli was easily eradicated. Of the 6 Klebsiella strains, 1 was eliminated, but the remaining 5 strains persisted in small numbers with the same sensitivities. 4 species were isolated from patients with chronic bronchitis. Of the 4 Proteus Ind(+) strains, 3 (2 vulgaris and 1 morgani) were eradicated, while 1 Proteus rettgeri persisted.

Cefoxitin serum levels were done in 4 patients. After 1/2h infusion

TABLE III. Bacteriologic and Clinical Effects of Cefoxitin on Various Pathogens

Species	Clinical				Bacteriologic	
	Number	Cured	Improved	Failure	Elimination	Failure
E.Coli	11	10	1		11	
Klebsiella	6		5	1	1	5
Proteus Ind.(+)	4	3		1	3	1
Salmonella (non group D)	2	2			2	
Bacteroides:						
melaninogenicus	1		1		not done	
fragilis	1		1			
Staph aureus	1	1			1	
Peptostreptococcus	1		1		not done	
Peptococcus	1		1		not done	

of 2gm of Cefoxitin the peak serum level ranged between 150-200 µg/ml. 6h post infusion the drug levels were about 5µg/ml, but the trough level was almost 0 before the next infusion. The obtained serum levels were above the patients' MBCs for at least 4 hrs. The urinary excretion of Cefoxitin was between 80-90% of the dose given, ranging between 160-6000 µg/ml of urine.

No side effects were observed. Only one patient not included in the present study, with a history of food and drug allergy but not to penicillins, suffering from pyometra due to E. coli and B. fragilis, became hypotensive with diffuse maculopapular erythema, immediately after starting the infusion. Toxicity studies were in the normal limits. No pain or phlebitis was noted at the site of infusion.

COMMENTS

Cefoxitin is an effective new antibiotic. Although more clinical trials are needed, the following factors, make Cefoxitin a promising new drug:
1) Cefoxitin is very active against most Gram negative bacteria, especially against indole (+) Proteus species, which are usually resistant to the commonly used cephalosporins. Although Staph aureus species appear as less sensitive to Cefoxitin, the obtained MICs are within the attainable blood levels.
2) The lack of toxicity with the possible limitation of previous allergy to penicillins.
3) Although blood levels were very high (5,6) they were not long sustained with the above schedule. Most of the treatment failures, can be attributed to the above drowback, which can be overcome by intramuscular administration of Cefoxitin and shorter intervals between doses.

The extremely high urinary levels, even as trough levels, are very important in the treatment of urinary tract infections.
4) The favorable clinical results in our patients even for infections which have been unsuccessfully treated in the past with other antibiotics. All the above factors justify the need for further clinical evaluation of Cefoxitin.

REFERENCES

1. Nagarajan,R.,Boeck,L.D.,Gorman,M.,Hamill,R.L.,Higgens,C.E., Hoehn, M.M.,Stark,W.M. and Whitney,J.G. (1971) J.Amer.Chem.Soc. 93 2308-2310
2. Stapley,E.O.,Jackson,M.,Hernandez,S.,Zimmerman,S.B., Currie,S.A., Mochales,S.,Mata,J.M.,Woodruff,H.B.,and Hendlin,D.(1972) Antimicrob.Ag.Chemother. 2.122-131 .
3. Karady,S.,et al (1972) J.Amer.Chem.Coc., 95 , 1410.
4. Daoust,D.R.,Onishi,H.R.,Wallick,H.,Hendlin,D., and Stapley,E.O. (1973) Antimicrob.Ag.Chemother. 3. 254-261 .
5. Kosmidis,J.,Hamilton-Miller,J.M.T.,Gilchrist,J.N.G.,Kerry,D.W.and Brumfitt,W.(1973).Cefoxitin, a New Semisynthetic Cephamycin: An in-vitro and in-vivo comparison with Cephalothin.B.M.J., 3, 653-655 .
6. Kosmidis,J.,Hamilton-Miller,J.M.T.,Gilchrist,J.N.G.,Kerry,D.W. and Brumfitt,W.Comparative Clinical Pharmacology of Cefoxitin and Cephalothin in Humans,Progress in Chemotherapy,Proceedings of the 8th International Congress of Chemotherapy,Athens 1974, 1, 592 - 597

SYNERGISTIC INTERACTION OF CEPHALOSPORINS AND HUMAN SERUM ON

GRAM-NEGATIVE BACTERIA

P. Orsolini, M.R. Milani

Laboratori Glaxo S.p.A. - Research Division

Verona, Italy

SUMMARY

Different kinds of interaction have been observed when certain antibiotics were added to serum. Chloramphenicol and demethyl-chlortetracycline showed a negative interaction while streptomycin did not significantly change the activity of guinea pig serum against E.coli. Cephalexin and cephaloridine showed synergistic interactions with guinea pig and human serum against E.coli. Heat inactivation, ultrafiltration, bentonite-absorption of serum did not abolish the synergistic effect with cephaloridine.

INTRODUCTION

Several possible interactions between antibiotics and serum factors in killing bacteria are known. A direct negative effect on serum bactericidal factors (specific immunoglobulins, complement components, calcium and magnesium ions, lysozyme) has been attributed to several antibiotics, such as chloramphenicol, bacitracin, polymyxin B, tetracyclines (Zschiesche and Augusten, 1968; Forsgren and Gnarpe, 1973). Different mechanisms are involved such as protein synthesis inhibition and calcium and magnesium chelation. On the other hand an enhancement of immune response of mice treated with cyclacillin due to the release of larger amounts of immunogenic components of bacteria has been reported (Friedman et al., 1974). A direct effect of serum on an antibiotic may decrease the effectiveness of the antibiotic because of its binding to serum proteins; however, in some cases non-bactericidal proteins of human serum seem to increase antibiotic activity via unknown mechanisms (Adam, 1973). Apart from direct interactions, antibiotic and humoral factors may each modify the structure or metabolism of bacteria and consequently their sensitivity to the action of either the humoral factors or the antibiotic (Warren and Gray, 1965; Traub and Sherris, 1970). Finally, a joint independent action of serum and antibiotics has been described (Treffers and Muschel, 1954).

Little data are available about the interaction of cephalosporins with serum (Toshioka et al., 1971; Adam, 1975) and the present study was undertaken to obtain additional information.

MATERIALS AND METHODS

E.coli O20, E.coli O25, S.typhimurium 804E, were maintained on slanted nutrient agar and transferred monthly. Chloramphenicol and 6-demethyl-7-chlortetracycline were obtained from Gianni, Milan, and streptomycin, cephalexin (sodium salt) and cephaloridine from Glaxo, Verona. Sera were obtained from the blood of normal and C4-deficient guinea pigs and from human volunteers. In some experiments serum was incubated at 56°C. for 30 minutes for inactivation, or absorbed with bentonite to deplete lysozyme and β-lysin. Ultrafiltration of human serum was performed with a PSED membrane (nominal molecular weight limit of 25,000), using a Millipore micro-ultrafiltration chamber. Lysozyme and bactericidal activity were absent in the ultrafiltrate.

For the determination of the bactericidal activity, serum, antibiotics or their combinations were serially diluted in phosphate buffer M/150 in saline pH 7 to a final volume of 1 ml and each tube was inoculated with 0.2 ml of a suspension of the micro-organism standardized at 1×10^5 cells/ml. After inoculation the tubes were incubated for 1 hour at 37°C and a plate count was performed on each tube. The phosphate buffer control was similarly treated.

RESULTS

Activity of Antibiotics and Guinea Pig Serum against E.coli O20.

Chloramphenicol (10-25-50 µg/ml), demethylchlortetracycline (2.5-10-25-50 µg/ml), streptomycin (10-25-50 µg/ml) and fresh guinea pig serum (1:10) were tested together and separately against E.coli O20. Serum alone was bactericidal and the reduction of viable count depended on the dilution of serum. Chloramphenicol and streptomycin did not reduce the viable count at the concentrations tested while with demethylchlortetracycline at 50 and 25 µg/ml, 56% and 73% of the inoculum survived. When the antibiotics were added to guinea pig serum (1:10) and then serially diluted, an antagonistic effect, i.e. a partial neutralization of the reduction of viable count brought about by the serum alone, was observed for chloramphenicol and demethylchlortetracycline. Such effect is dose dependent and the highest negative effect

observed for chloramphenicol was at 50 µg/ml (Fig.1A) while the
antagonistic effect of demethylchlortetracycline was maximum at
25 µg/ml, probably because at the highest concentration of antibiotic
the antagonistic effect is partially compensated by its killing
activity. An addition of 25 µg/ml of streptomycin did not appreciably
change the bactericidal activity of serum (Fig.1A).

Sodium cephalexin at 50 and 25 µg/ml reduced the viable count
by 31% and 21%, respectively. When sodium cephalexin at 50 µg/ml
was added to guinea pig serum (1:15), the combination was more
effective than antibiotic or serum alone in killing bacteria (Fig.1B).

Cephaloridine at 15 and 7.5 µg/ml reduced the viable count by
60% and 50%, respectively. The addition of 15 µg/ml of cephaloridine
to guinea pig serum (1:15), followed by serial dilution, greatly
enhanced the reduction of viable count in comparison with that
brought about by the serum or antibiotic alone (Fig.1B). Experiments
were then performed with serum depleted of some non-specific
bactericidal factors. The synergistic effect of cephaloridine
combined with heat inactivated guinea pig serum was exactly the same
as with normal serum (Fig.1B). C4-deficient or bentonite-absorbed
guinea pig serum also gave the same kind of synergism.

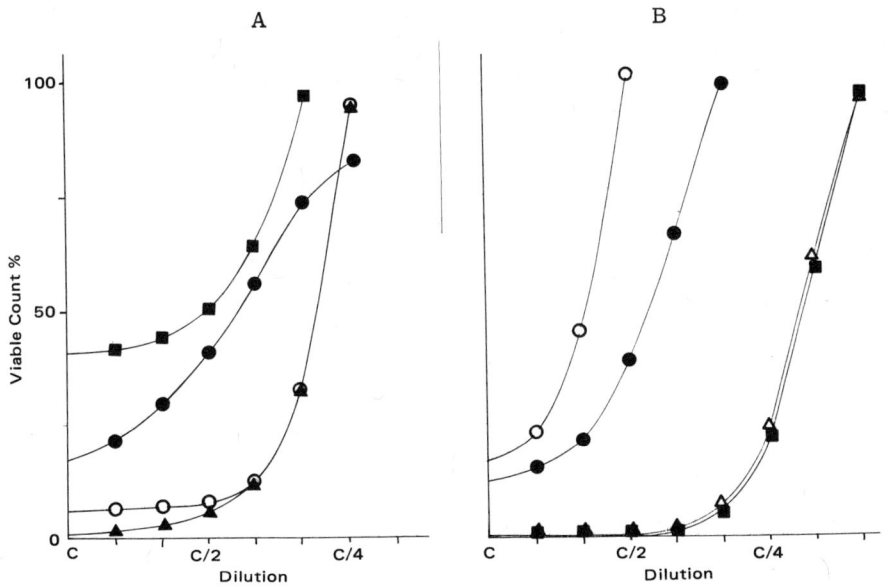

Fig.1 - Antibiotics and Guinea Pig Serum against E.coli 020.
A) ○ Serum c = 1:10, ● Serum + Demethylchlortetracycline c =
25 µg/ml, ■ Serum + Chloramphenicol c = 50 µg/ml, ▲ Serum +
Streptomycin c = 25 µg/ml;
B) ○ Serum c = 1:15, ● Serum + Cephalexin c = 50 µg/ml, ■ Serum +
Cephaloridine c = 15 µg/ml, △ Heat-inactivated serum +
Cephaloridine c = 15 µg/ml.

Activity of Cephalosporins and Human Serum against E.coli O20.

The addition of 50 ug/ml of sodium cephalexin to human serum (1:125) resulted in increased killing (Fig.2). Expected results on the hypothesis of joint, independent actions of serum and antibiotic were calculated for each dilution from the equation (Treffers and Muschel, 1954):

$$P = P_1 + P_2 (1-P_1)$$

in which P is the total mortality and P_1 and P_2 are the mortalities resulting from serum and antibiotic applied separately. Observed reduction of viable count was 10-20% higher than that expected, leading to the conclusion that the results were due to a synergistic interaction between human serum and sodium cephalexin.

Cephaloridine at 15 µg/ml added to human serum (1:125) gave a clear synergistic effect similar to that observed with guinea pig serum (Fig.2). Experiments were then performed with serum depleted of bactericidal factors by ultrafiltration (molecular weight limit of 25,000) or by bentonite absorption. Ultrafiltered or bentonite-absorbed human serum was serially diluted to 1:4096 and one ED_{50} of cephaloridine was added to each dilution, resulting in an increased killing of above 95% up to a dilution of 1:500 (Fig.3). The mixture of normal human serum and cephaloridine gave the same results while with serum alone, killing above 95% was found at dilutions of 1:100 or less.

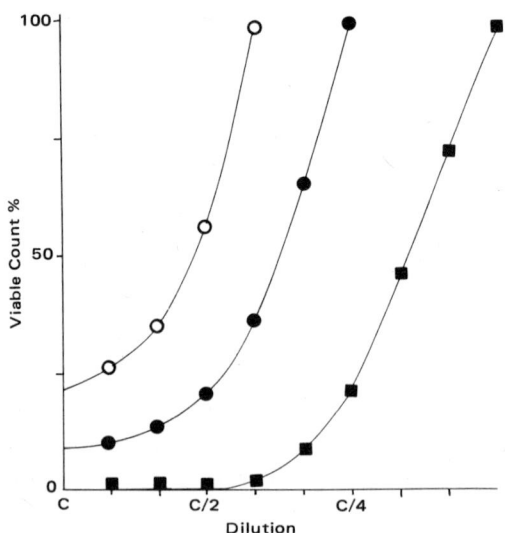

Fig.2 - Cephalosporins and Normal Human Serum against E.coli O20.
○ Serum c = 1:125; ● Serum + Cephalexin c = 50 µg/ml, ■ Serum + Cephaloridine c = 15 µg/ml.

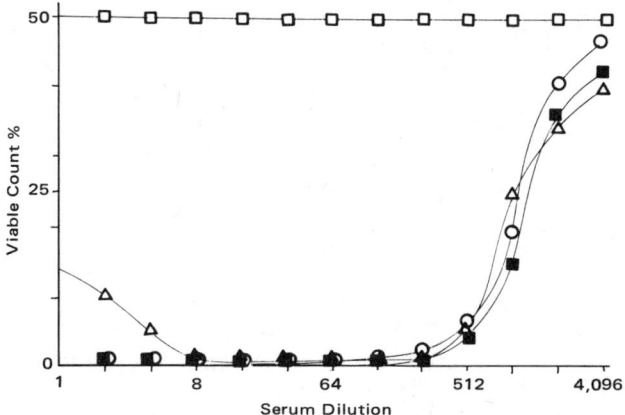

Fig.3 - Cephaloridine and Depleted Human Serum against E.coli O20.
□ Cephaloridine 7.5 µg/ml, ■ Normal serum + Cephaloridine 7.5 µg/ml,
○ Bentonite-absorbed serum + Cephaloridine 7.5 µg/ml,
△ Ultrafiltered serum + Cephaloridine 7.5 µg/ml.

Studies with other Gram-negative Bacteria

A synergistic effect of the mixture of cephaloridine and inactivated guinea pig and human serum was also found against E.coli O25 which is partially resistant to the killing activity of the serum alone. Against Salmonella typhimurium 804E the synergistic effect was less marked than that observed with the two E.coli strains.

DISCUSSION

Different kinds of interaction have been observed when antibiotics are added to serum. Chloramphenicol and demethyl-chlortetracycline showed a negative interaction, determining a reduction of the bactericidal activity of guinea pig serum, in accordance with data published by other Authors (Forsgren and Gnarpe, 1973; Weisbren and Brown, 1964). The addition of streptomycin did not appreciably change the activity of guinea pig serum. The absence of a clear additive effect is probably due to the resistance of the bacterial strain to streptomycin.

Cephalosporins showed synergistic interactions with guinea pig and human serum. The effect observed with sodium cephalexin was related to the bactericidal activity of the serum and the total mortality was higher than expected, when calculated on the hypothesis of joint independent actions of serum and antibiotic. A different synergistic interaction was observed for cephaloridine, being also evident when serum was diluted much beyond the range of activity or when it was heat inactivated. These results suggest that the complement system is not involved as confirmed by the experiment where C4-deficient guinea pig serum was used. Serum depleted of lysozyme and β-lysin by bentonite absorption, gave the same synergistic effect with cephaloridine thus excluding a rôle of these factors. The synergistic effect was also found when human serum ultrafiltrate (molecular weight limit of 25,000) was used, thus suggesting that immunoglobulins are not involved. Complement, lysozyme, β-lysin and immunoglobulins seem not to be involved in the determination of the synergistic effect observed with cephaloridine, indicating that other non-bactericidal serum factors may interact directly or indirectly with the antibiotic.

In conclusion, if the results found in vitro were to be confirmed in vivo the particular advantage of synergistic interactions between cephalosporins and host factors is relevant, particularly in the treatment of Gram-negative infections in immunologically deficient patients.

REFERENCES

Adam, D., (1973), in: "Non-Specific" Factors Influencing Host Resistance, eds. W.Braun and J.Ungar (Karger, Basel), p. 452.

Adam, D., (1975), Infection, 3, 44.

Forsgren, A., Gnarpe, H., (1973), Nature New Biol., 244, 82.

Friedman, H. et al., (1974), in: Progress in Chemotherapy (Hellenic Soc.Chemotherapy, Athens), Vol.II, p.119.

Toshioka, T. et al., (1971), Nippon Univ.J.Med., 13, 155.

Traub, W.H., Sherris, J.C., (1970), Chemotherapy, 15, 70.

Treffers, H.P., Muschel, L.H., (1954), J.Exp.Med., 99, 155.

Warren, G.H., Gray, J., (1965), Proc.Soc.Exp.Biol.Med., 120, 504.

Weisbren, B.A., Brown, I., (1964), Amer.J.Med.Sci., 248, 56.

Zschiesche, W., Augusten, K., (1968), Chemotherapy, 13, 257.

A COMPARATIVE STUDY OF CEFTEZOL (DEMETHYL-CEFAZOLIN) AND CEFAZOLIN: ABSORPTION, DISTRIBUTION AND METABOLISM

S. Ishiyama, I. Nakayama, H. Iwamoto, S. Iwai,
I. Sakata, I. Murata, H. Mizuashi
Department of Surgery
Nihon University School of Medicine
8, 1-chome, Kandasurugadai, Chiyoda-ku, Tokyo, Japan

Ceftezol is a new synthetic cephalosporin antibiotic, recently developed as a cefazolin analogue.

The chemical structure is characterized by an absence of methyl-radical in thiadiazol of the side chain of cefazolin, therefore it may be also called a demethyl-cefazolin. (Fig.1)

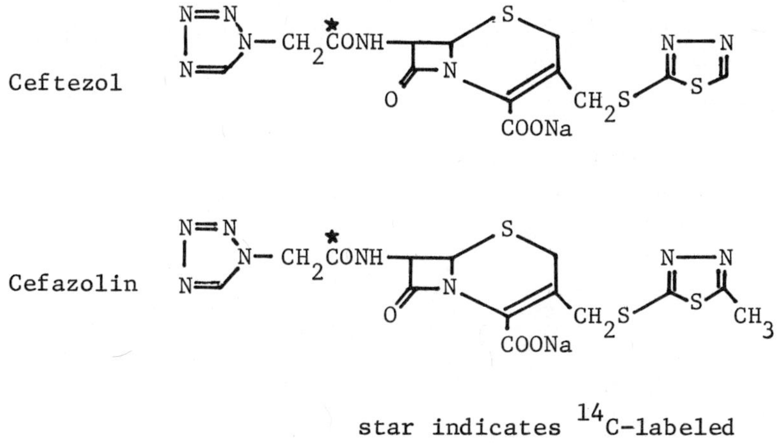

star indicates ^{14}C-labeled

Fig. 1. The Chemical Structure of Ceftezol and Cefazolin

The antibacterial spectrum of ceftezol and its sensitivity distribution for clinical isolates (Staph. aur., E. coli, Klebsiella, Proteus.) are similar to those of cefazolin. (Table 1)

	≤0.1	0.2	0.4	0.8	1.56	3.13	6.25	12.5	25	50	100	>100
Staph.aur. (54)												
Ceftezol		16	18	13	7							
Cefazolin		10	23	10	11							
E. coli (54)												
Ceftezol				13	26	6			2	1	2	4
Cefazolin				2	27	7	4	4	3		3	4
Klebsiella (27)												
Ceftezol				1	8	6	2	2	2	4		2
Cefazolin				1	3	10	3	2	1	4	1	2
Proteus mir. (27)												
Ceftezol						1	6	8	8	1		3
Cefazolin						1	1	13	7	2		3

MIC (µg/ml)

Table 1.   Sensitivity Distribution of Clinical Isolates to Ceftezol and Cefazolin

The serum levels in three healthy adult volunteers after a single intramuscular administration were determined by use of the cylinder plate method with Bacillus subtilis ATCC6633 as a test organism. When a single dose of ceftezol 500 mg was given, average serum concentrations of it were respectively 25.1, 20.8, 11.0, 3.1 and 1.9 µg/ml at each half, 1, 2, 4 and 6 hours after injection. The peak level reached at 30 minutes. These results were lower than those of cefazolin. (Table 2)

	1/2	1	2	4	6	hrs.
K.N. (6.7mg/kg)	31.0	23.0	9.6	4.8	2.5	µg/ml
I.N. (6.0mg/kg)	26.0	23.8	11.5	1.7	1.4	µg/ml
H.K. (5.6mg/kg)	18.3	15.5	12.0	2.7	1.8	µg/ml
Average (6.1mg/kg)	25.1	20.8	11.0	3.1	1.9	µg/ml

500 mg i.m.

Table 2.   Serum Levels of Ceftezol

	1/2	1	2	4	6	hrs.
M.T. (9.3mg/kg)	29.0	38.4	19.6	11.1	6.5	µg/ml
T.M. (7.6mg/kg)	25.6	37.5	15.2	10.8	5.0	µg/ml
S.N. (7.7mg/kg)	22.0	26.4	20.5	14.2	7.0	µg/ml
Average (8.2mg/kg)	25.5	34.1	18.4	12.0	6.2	µg/ml

500 mg i.m.

Table 3. Serum Levels of Cefazolin

The urinary concentrations were estimated by a paper disc method using Bacillus subtilis ATCC 6633 as a test organism. When a single dose of 500 mg of ceftezol and cefazolin was given to 3 healthy adult volunteers; Ceftezol and cefazolin were excreted with high concentration. Average concentrations of ceftezol were respectively 250, 1,457, 977, 441 and 71 µg/ml at each half, 1, 2, 4 and 6 hours after injection. Urinary concentrations of cefazolin were respectively 1,291, 4,000, 2,450 787 and 207 µg/ml at each half, 1, 2, 4 and 6 hours after injection. The maximum excretions of ceftezol and cefazolin were found in 1 hour urine. Of these doses given, 66.5% of ceftezol and 62.6% of cefazolin was recovered from 6 hour urine spamples. Urinary elimination of ceftezol are more rapid than those of cefazolin. (Table 4)

	1/2	1	2	4	6	hrs.	recovery
K.N. (6.7mg/kg)	175 210 16.8	1000 114 114.0	430 168 72.2	223 294 65.6	34 580 19.8	µg/ml ml mg	361.3mg 71.3 %
I.N. (6.0mg/kg)	310 220 68.2	2100 34 61.4	1280 90 111.5	370 222 82.3	54 84 4.5	µg/ml ml mg	327.9mg 65.6 %
H.K. (5.6mg/kg)	265 120 31.8	1270 48 61.0	1220 102 124.4	730 170 124.1	125 160 20.0	µg/ml ml mg	308.3mg 61.7 %
Average (6.1mg/kg)	250 45.6	1457 78.8	977 102.7	441 90.7	71 14.7	µg/ml mg	332.5mg 66.5 %

500 mg i.m.

Table 4. Urinary Excretions of Ceftezol

A Sprague-Dawley strain rat, in groups of three, each 6 to 7 weeks old and weighing 180-200g received 20mg/kg (1.7 μCi/rat) of ^{14}C-labelled ceftezol (containing 0.51 μCi/mg which has 94.4 per cent in radioactivity) intramuscularly, and sacrificed after complete withdrawal of blood.
At each 1/4, 1/2, 1 and 2 hours administration, and serum, brain, heart, lungs, liver and kidneys were removed.

These samples, after homogenization, were subjected to both radiochemical and biological assay, the former by use of a liquid scinitillation counter and the latter by the disc method with Bacillus subtilis ATCC 6633 as the test organism.
The tissue concentrations were high in the range of kidneys, serum, lungs, liver and spleen in that order. These were same distribution pattern in both biological and radiochemical assays.

The same method was performed for ^{14}C-labeled cefazolin (Containing 4.70 μCi/mg). The results of both assays were similar in the various tissues examined. The concentrations in tissues were in the descending order of serum, kidneys, liver, lungs, heart and spleen. The concentration in the brain was lower than that in the spleen, and detectable by the radiochemical assay but not biologically. (Table 5)

Time (hrs.)		Tissue concentration (μg/g)							Serum (μg/ml)
		Brain	Heart	Liver	Kidney	Lung	Spleen	Muscle	
1/2	Radio.	1.0	9.0	33.0	175.0	50.0	39.0	97.5	54.6
	Bio.	trace	18.0	28.2	204.0	28.2	13.5	6.9	67.0
1	Radio.	10.0	10.0	13.0	190.0	31.8	11.8	24.8	50.2
	Bio.	trace	7.8	23.4	144.0	11.4	20.4	22.2	44.0
2	Radio.	0.8	6.0	8.0	95.0	7.8	2.5	11.4	18.7
	Bio.	trace	3.5	9.0	54.0	3.5	1.7	1.3	17.5
4	Radio.	n.d.	0.5	1.0	12.6	1.5	0.8	9.0	2.9
	Bio.	n.d.	trace	1.8	3.1	trace	trace	trace	1.7

Radio. = Radioassay
Bio. = Bioassay

Table 5. Tissue Concentrations of ^{14}C-Ceftezol

Six hours of rat urine, which was received 5.0 μCi as radioactive ceftezol, was studied through a thin-layer chromatograph and radio scanning. There was only one peak was reached at Rf 0.6 in the active zone of radioautogram. It suggested that there was only one radioative substance corresponding to ceftezol itself and no metabolite.

On the otherhand, after injection of 500mg of ceftezol, a bioautogram was taken of human urine samples spanning 0 to 6 hours. It was positively determined that there was no metabolite formation within the urine. A bioautogram of human urine and bile which was given 500mg cefazolin also showed clearly sure there was no metablolite formation.

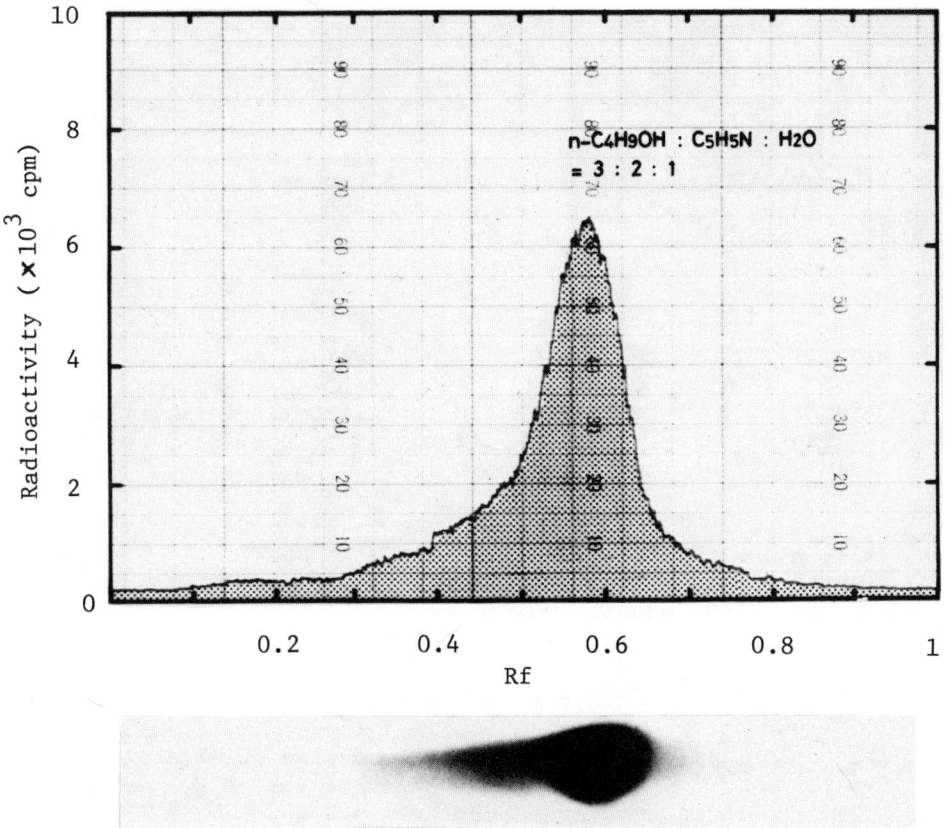

Fig. 2. Radio Scanning and Radioautogram in Rat's Urine

Summary

Ceftezol is a new cephalosporin antibiotic which is a demethyl analogue of cefazolin. Antibacterial spectrum and activities in the clinical isolates are similar to those of cefazolin.

Absorption and urinary elimination are more rapid than those of cefazolin. The tissue concentration of ceftezol turned out higher in the order of kidney, serum, lung, liver and spleen, and those of cefazolin were high in the range of kidney, serum, liver, heart and spleen.

There was no metabolite of ceftezol in human urine.

Literature

1) Ishiyama, S., I. Kawakami, and I. Nakayama.
   Laboratory and clinical results of cephaloridine in surgical infections.
   Postgrad. Med.J.43:148-151. 1967

2) Nishida, M., T. Matsubara, T. Murakawa, Y. Mine, Y. Yokota, S. Goto, and S. Kuwahara.
   Cefazolin. a new semisynthetic cephalosporin antibiotic.
   Absorption, excretion and tissue distribution in parenteral administration. J. Antibiot. (Tokyo) 23:184-194. 1967.

3) Okui, M., K. Hattori, and M. Nishida.
   Studies on the metabolism of cephalosporins. J. Antibiot. (Tokyo) 20:287-293. 1967.

4) Ishiyama, S., I. Nakayama, H. Iwamoto, S. Iwai, M. Okui and T. Matsubara
   Absorption, Tissue Concentration, and Organ Distribution of Cefazolin
   Antimicrobial Agents and Chemotherapy 476-470. 1970

IN VITRO AND IN VIVO EVALUATION OF TWO NEW ORALLY ACTIVE

CEPHALOSPORIN DERIVATIVES

O. Zak, C. Schenk, W.A. Vischer

Research Department, Pharmaceuticals Division

CIBA-GEIGY Limited, Basle, Switzerland

CGP 81 and CGP 3940 (7-phenylglycyl derivatives of 3-H-and 3-methoxy-cephem) are semisynthetic, orally active cephalosporin antibiotics. Their synthesis and their physicochemical characteristics have already been described (1-3). This paper is concerned with their experimental evaluation in vitro and in vivo in comparison with cephalexin.

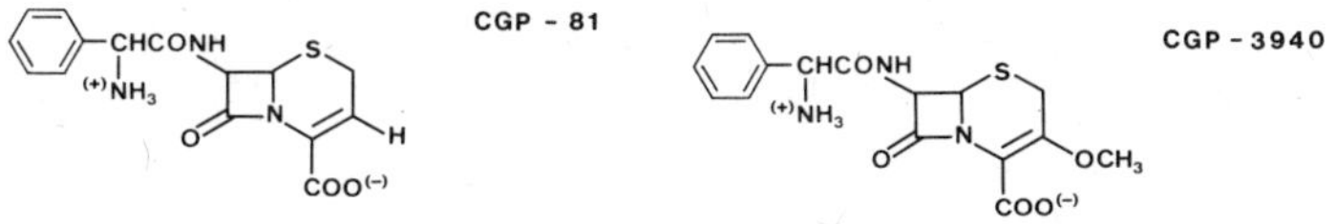

Fig. 1

MATERIALS AND METHODS

In vitro studies: The experiments were performed with both laboratory strains and fresh clinical isolates. The minimum inhibitory concentrations (MIC) were determined by the gradient-plate technique (4) in Brain-Heart Infusion Agar (Difco); the plates were incubated at 37°C over a period of 20 hours. The bactericidal effect of the compounds was tested on proliferating cells in Brain-Heart Infusion Broth; the number of viable organisms was determined by the pour-plate method at various times after the addition of the antibiotic. For the determination of the binding to human serum proteins equilibrium dialysis was used. The concentrations of the antibiotics in the blood of mice and in the plasma of human subjects were measured by the agar-well diffusion technique, Sarcina lutea ATCC 9341 being used as test organism. In vivo studies: MF2 mice were infected by intraperitoneal injection of standardized bacterial suspensions and treated orally with the antibiotics, as indicated in the tables. The dose affording protection in 50 % of the animals (ED_{50}) was calculated by probit transformation from the survival rates recorded on the 5th day after infection. Bilateral pyelonephritis was induced in Wistar rats by instillation of a suspension of E.coli through the urethra into the bladder and the renal pelvis. The antibiotics were administered daily in 2 doses for 3 days starting 1 day p.inf. Bacteriological examination of kidneys and urine was performed 6 days after infection.

The acute systemic toxicity was assessed in mice, rats and dogs after an observation period of 10 days.

RESULTS

CGP 81, the 3-unsubstituted cephem, was found to be approximately as active in vitro at pH 6.5 against gram-positive and gram-negative micro-organisms as cephalexin. Only against penicillin-resistant staphylococci did it prove slightly less effective. At pH 7.4, however, at which it is less stable, CGP 81 was several times less active than both cephalexin and CGP 3940. In the mouse this instability did not become manifest and the results obtained with CGP 81 were roughly comparable with those produced by cephalexin (Table 1).

The 3-methoxy cephem, CGP 3940, proved active in vitro against a broad spectrum of gram-positive and gram-negative bacteria. The MIC's were similar to those of cephalexin (Fig. 2). Both these cephalosporins proved inactive against Pseudomonas and indole-positive strains of

STRAIN	pH OF MEDIUM	MIC (mcg/ml)			NUMBER OF DOSES	ED_{50} (mg/kg)		
		CGP 81 (H)	CGP 3940 (OCH_3)	CEPHALEXIN (CH_3)		CGP 81 (H)	CGP 3940 (OCH_3)	CEPHALEXIN (CH_3)
Staph.aureus 10 B	6.5 / 7.4	2.5 / 20	1.5 / 1	1.5 / 1.5	1*	2.7	6	5.5
Staph.aureus 2999 i⁺p⁺	6.5 / 7.4	25 / 50	20 / 30	3.5 / 9.4	1	200	210	95
E.coli 205	6.5 / 7.4	3.5 / 30	3.5 / 3	4 / 7.5	2**	20	30	60
Salm.typhimurium 277	6.5 / 7.4	3 / 10	3 / 2	4.7 / 3.3	2	50	65	145
Klebs.pneumoniae 327	6.5 / 7.4	2.5 / 20	3 / 1.5	3.3 / 1.8	2	85	120	125

<u>Table 1</u> Activity in vitro at different pH and chemotherapeutic activity against systemic infections in mice
* Single dose administered simultaneously with infection
** Two doses; the first administered simultaneously with infection, the second 3 hours later

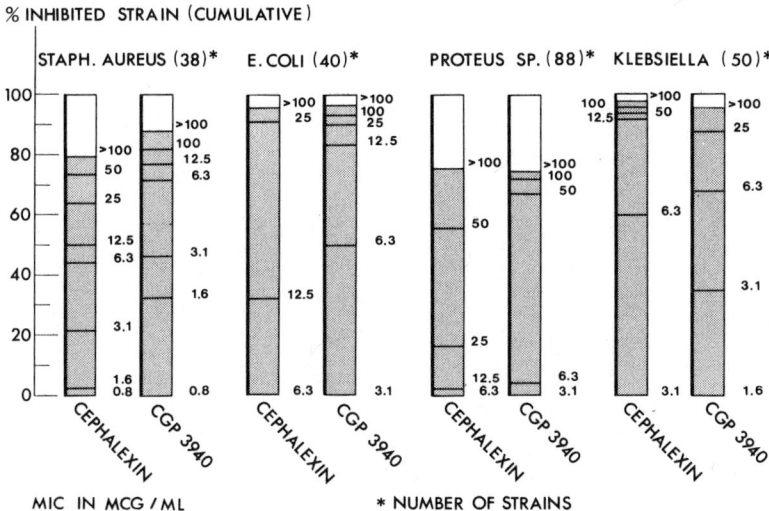

Fig. 2 Susceptibility of various pathogenic bacteria (clinical isolates) to CGP 3940 and cephalexin

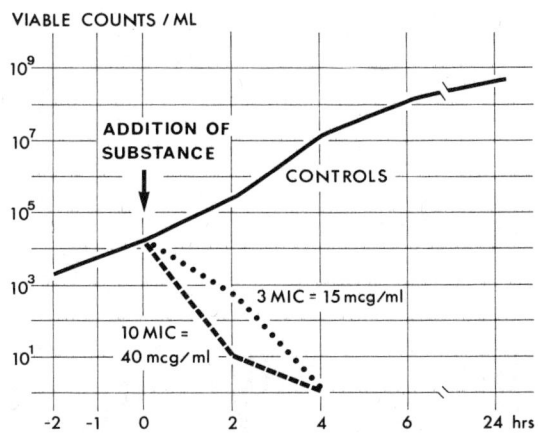

Fig. 3 Bactericidal effect of CGP 3940 on proliferating cells of E.coli (strain 1097)

Proteus, and they had only a weak effect on Enterococcus. CGP 3940 exerted a bactericidal action at concentrations very close to the MIC's (Fig. 3). Less than 10 % of CGP 3940 was bound to proteins, which is apporximately the same as the figure quoted in the literature for cephalexin.

When administered by mouth, CGP 3940 proved to be as active as cephalexin against infections due to gram-positive bacteria and E.coli, including strains producing β-lactamase. CGP 3940, however, was more

INFECTION (i.p.)	NUMBER OF DOSES	ED$_{50}$ (mg/kg)	
		CGP 3940	CEPHALEXIN
Staph.aureus Smith	1	6	8
Staph.aureus 102 #	1	100	110
Str.pyogenes Aronson	2	2.5	8
Dipl.pneumoniae III/84	2	16	55
E.coli 2018	2	13	13
E.coli 2018 R$^+$TEM ⊙	2	38	50
E.coli 205 R$^+$TEM ⊙	2	48	34
E.coli 5 ⊙	2	13	28
E.coli 16 ⊙	2	56	25
Salm.thyphimurium 273	2	60	170
Shigella flexneri 11836	2	25	95
Klebs.pneumoniae 329 ⊙	2	40	90
Proteus vulgaris 1076 ⊙	2	25	50
Proteus rettgeri	2	14	50
Proteus mirabilis 774	2	54	130
Proteus mirabilis 564	2	27	60
Proteus morganii 2359 ⊙	2	>300	>300
Enterob.cloacae P 99 ⊙	2	>300	>300
Ps.aeruginosa 799 ⊙	2	>300	>300

Table 2 Activity in systemic bacterial infections in mice

⊙ Ampicillin-resistant strains   # Methicillin-resistant strain

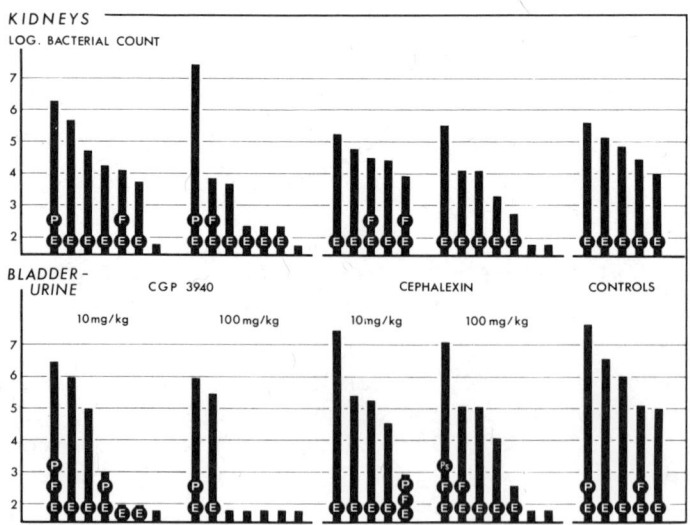

Fig. 4 Effect of CGP 3940 and cephalexin on acute E.coli-induced Pyelonephritis in rats

EVALUATION OF TWO NEW CEPHALOSPORIN DERIVATIVES

effective against infections due to Salmonella, Shigella, Klebsiella and various Proteus sp. (Table 2). On the other hand, both cephalosporins turned out to be inactive in infections with Enterobacter cloacae, some indole-positive Proteus and Pseudomonas aeruginosa. This is in accordance with the findings of Preston and Wick (5). CGP 3940 was also active against pyelonephritis induced with E.coli in the rat. It caused a greater reduction in the bacterial count, especially in the urine, than cephalexin (Fig. 4).
As can be seen from Table 3, the toxicity of CGP 3940 is very favourable.

SPECIES	ROUTE OF ADMINISTRATION	NUMBER OF ANIMALS	LD_{50} (mg/kg)
Mouse	p.o.	20	>6000
	i.p.	80	3800 ± 290
Rat	p.o.	8	>5000
Dog	p.o.	2	>300

<u>Table 3</u> Acute toxicity of CGP 3940

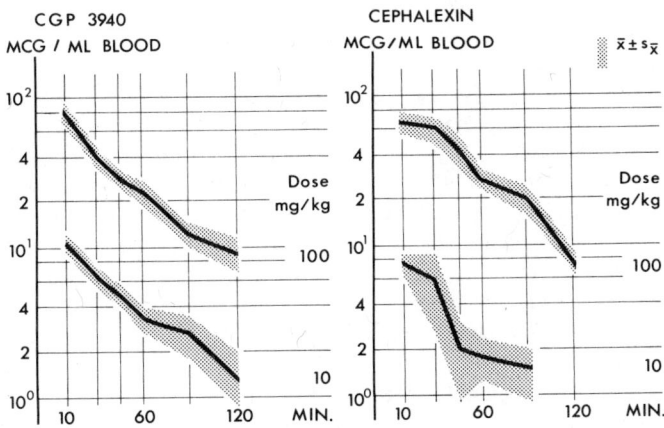

<u>Fig. 5</u> Antibiotic concentration in blood after oral administration to MF2 female mice (n = 20)

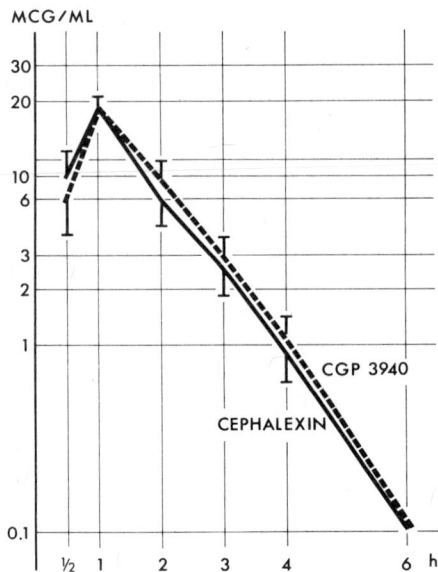

Fig. 6 Antibiotic concentrations in plasma after a single oral dose of 500 mg in healthy volunteers

CGP 3940 was readily absorbed after oral administration. The maximum concentrations in the blood of the mouse were already attained within ten minutes. The compound remained demonstrable in the blood for approximately the same length of time as cephalexin (Fig. 5). The absorption of CGP 3940 after the administration of an oral dose of 500 mg. was also compared with that of cephalexin in a cross-over study in three volunteers. The plasma concentrations of the two drugs follow an almost identical course (Fig. 6). On the average, 91 % of the dose of CGP 3940 and 84 % of that of cephalexin were excreted in the urine in active form within 24 hours of administration.

To sum up: CGP 81 and CGP 3940 are orally active cephalosporins. In their activity in vitro they resemble cephalexin, with the exception that CGP 81 is less stable at pH 7.4. In several experimental infections in the mouse and the rat, CGP 3940 proved more effective than cephalexin. After oral administration, CGP 3940 is very readily absorbed, in man as well as in animals, and in addition it has certain advantages from the toxicological point of view.

References: 1. Scartazzini R., Bickel H.: 1972, Helv.chim.Acta 55, 423; 2. Peter H., Bickel H.: 1974, ibidem 57, 2044; 3. Scartazzini R., Bickel H.: 1974, ibidem 57, 1919; 4. Bryson V., Szybalski W.: 1952, Science 116, 45; 5. Preston D.A., Wick W.E.: Abstracts 14th ICAAC, 1974, 426.

A NEW PARENTERAL CEPHALOSPORIN. SK&F 59962: SERUM LEVELS AND URINARY RECOVERY IN MAN

Paul Actor, Donald H. Pitkin, George Lucyszyn and Jerry A. Weisbach

Smith Kline & French Laboratories, Philadelphia Pennsylvania USA

José L. Bran

Hospital General San Juan de Dios, Guatemala City Guatemala   C.A.

SUMMARY

The pharmacokinetic profile of SK&F 59962, a new parenteral cephalosporin, was found to be similar to that of cephalothin after intravenous or intramuscular administration to human volunteers. SK&F 59962 was well-tolerated when administered parenterally. No overt pain was observed in 15 of 17 subjects after intramuscular administration of SK&F 59962 in contrast to cephalothin where pain was observed in all of the subjects following intramuscular administration.

INTRODUCTION

SK&F 59962 [7-Trifluoromethyl-thioacetamido-3-(1-methyl-1H-tetrazol-5-ylthiomethyl)-3-cephem-4-carboxylic acid, sodium salt] is a new parenteral cephalosporin first synthesized in the Smith Kline & French Laboratories (DeMarinis et al. 1975). In laboratory studies reported by Actor et al. 1975, SK&F 59962 was found to have a high order of in vitro and in vivo antibacterial activity against a broad spectrum of clinical isolates. In in vitro trials employing gram-negative organisms, SK&F 59962 was consistently more active than cefazolin and far superior to cephalothin. Against gram-positive bacteria, SK&F 59962 showed activity equal to cephalothin. In mouse infection-protection studies using bacterial pathogens, SK&F 59962 had protective activity of the order of that of cefazolin and superior to that of cephalothin. The serum antibiotic levels in laboratory animals were similar to that of cephalothin. The study to be reported here describes the safety and comparative serum levels and urinary recovery of SK&F 59962 and cephalothin after parenteral administration to human volunteers using a crossover designed study.

MATERIALS AND METHODS

SK&F 59962 was prepared in one gram vials and reconstituted with sterile water for parenteral administration. A commercial one gram formulation of cephalothin (Keflin®, Eli Lilly & Co.) was prepared in the same manner. Normal adult male volunteers were selected on the basis of: (1) a complete medical history to exclude those having a history of hematologic, hepatic or renal disease or a history of allergic sensitivity to penicillins or cephalosporins, (2) a complete physical examination and (c) laboratory studies which included CBC, serum bilirubin, SGOT, alkaline phosphatase, serum glucose, BUN and urinalysis. The physical examination and laboratory tests were repeated 24 hours after cephalosporin administration. SK&F 59962 or cephalothin were administered in one gram doses either intramuscularly or intravenously to two groups of subjects and periodic blood and urine samples were obtained for antibiotic analysis. After one week, those subjects having received SK&F 59962 were dosed with cephalothin and those who previously received cephalothin were dosed with SK&F 59962. Blood and urine samples were collected in the same manner and at the same time intervals as in the first phase of the study. Antibiotic serum and urine levels were determined by disc-diffusion assay using a previously reported method (Fare et al. 1974).

RESULTS AND DISCUSSION

Intramuscular Crossover Study

Table 1 shows the average antibiotic serum concentrations obtained for 17 subjects after intramuscular administration of one gram of SK&F 59962 or cephalothin in a crossover design. Gross examination of these data reveal a similarity in antibiotic serum levels with both antibiotics at almost every time interval examined. There was, however, statistically higher antibiotic serum levels obtained with SK&F 59962 at 30, 60 and 120 minutes after administration ($p = < 0.01$). No measurable serum levels were obtained with either antibiotic at four hours post-administration. The serum profile observed for cephalothin was found to be similar to our previously reported data for this antibiotic (Cahn et al. 1974).

	Average Serum Concentration in mcg/ml				
Antibiotic	10 Min.	20 Min.	30 Min.	60 Min.	120 Min.
SK&F 59962	31.5	38.9	35.1	23.1	7.1
S.E. ±	4.1	3.9	2.3	1.0	0.4
Cephalothin	33.9	31.7	28.9	16.8	5.2
S.E. ±	3.3	2.6	1.7	1.0	0.6

Table 1. Antibiotic Serum Concentrations Obtained in 17 Subjects After Intramuscular Administration of 1 Gram of SK&F 59962 or Cephalothin - Crossover Study

Table 2 presents a summary of the intramuscular crossover study. The estimated peak serum concentration, calculated from a computer model, for SK&F 59962 was 41.6 mcg/ml as opposed to 36.1 mcg/ml for cephalothin. The calculated peak serum time for SK&F 59962 was somewhat longer than that of cephalothin and there was a greater area under the serum antibiotic curve for SK&F 59962. The average urinary recovery for the first six hours after administration was similar for the two antibiotics. Although there was a wide range of urinary recovery in individual subjects, the greater percentage of both antibiotics were excreted in the urine within the first two hours after drug administration. The average urinary recovery of SK&F 59962 was found to be 76.0 percent of the administered dose at six hours post-administration as compared with cephalothin which was 66.0 percent. No separate estimate was made for the desacetyl metabolite of cephalothin. There were no significant differences between the two cephalosporins with respect to the urinalysis, hematology or blood chemistry values. Neither drug gave significant values outside the pre-dosing range for these laboratory tests. Pain at the site of injection was the only adverse effect observed with either drug. All of the subjects receiving cephalothin reported pain lasting from 15 minutes to one hour following intramuscular administration, whereas, only 2 of 17 subjects reported pain with SK&F 59962.

	SK&F 59962	Cephalothin
Peak Serum Concentration (mcg/ml)	41.6 ± 3.9	36.1 ± 3.3
Peak Time (Minutes)	25.4	18.1
Area Under Serum Curve	2601 ± 95	2123 ± 78
Percent Urinary Recovery (0-6 Hr)	76.0 ± 5.1	65.6 ± 3.8

Table 2. Summary of Crossover Study in 17 Subjects Receiving 1 Gram SK&F 59962 and 1 Gram Cephalothin Intramuscularly

	Average Serum Concentration in mcg/ml				
Antibiotic	5 Min.	15 Min.	30 Min.	60 Min.	120 Min.
SK&F 59962	367.7	84.5	38.6	13.2	2.6
S.E. ±	55.3	21.5	4.0	1.3	0.3
Cephalothin	221.7	57.2	23.3	6.6	1.5
S.E. ±	27.6	4.7	2.0	0.6	0.2

Table 3. Antibiotic Serum Concentrations Obtained in 16 Subjects After Intravenous Administration of 1 Gram of SK&F 59962 or Cephalothin - Crossover Study

Intravenous Crossover Study

Table 3 shows the average antibiotic serum concentrations for 16 subjects after intravenous administration of one gram of SK&F 59962 or cephalothin. Measurable serum values were obtained with both antibiotics for up to 120 minutes after intravenous administration. No significant serum levels were observed at 240 minutes after administration. In general, the serum antibiotic levels obtained with SK&F 59962 were higher than those observed with cephalothin. The average serum antibiotic levels of SK&F 59962 were statistically higher than those of cephalothin from 15-20 minutes after intravenous administration ($p = < 0.01$). A summary of the intravenous study with the calculated pharmacokinetic parameters is shown in Table 4. The average peak serum concentration was 367.7 mcg/ml for SK&F 59962 as compared to cephalothin which was 221.7 mcg/ml. The peak time for both antibiotics was five minutes after administration, the earliest time sampled. The area under the serum curve for SK&F 59962 was significantly greater than that of cephalothin, however, the half-lives were similar with

	SK&F 59962	Cephalothin
Peak Serum Concentration (mcg/ml)	367.7 ± 55.3	221.7 ± 27.6
Peak Time (Minutes)	5	5
Area Under Serum Curve	5265 ± 413	3329 ± 261
Average Serum Half-Life (Hr)	0.436	0.468
Apparent Volume of Distribution (l)	2.59	4.45
Percent Urinary Recovery (0-6 Hr)	68.2 ± 7.3	54.4 ± 7.9

Table 4. Summary of Crossover Study in 16 Subjects Receiving 1 Gram SK&F 59962 and 1 Gram Cephalothin Intravenously

no statistical difference observed. The apparent volume of distribution using a two-compartment model as the basis for the calculation (Rattie and Ravin 1975) was 4.45 liters for cephalothin and 2.59 liters for SK&F 59962. The average urinary recovery at 6 hours was found to be 68 percent for SK&F 59962 and 54 percent for cephalothin. As was found in the intramuscular study, there were no significant abnormalities in the values observed with either antibiotic with respect to the blood chemistry, hematology or urinalysis determination. No side effects were observed after intravenous administration of either antibiotic.

REFERENCES

Actor, P. A., Uri, J. V., Guarini, J. R., Zajac, I., Phillips, L., Sachs, C. S., DeMarinis, R. M., Hoover, J. R. E. and Weisbach, J. A. (1975), J. Antibiotics, 28, 471.

Cahn, M. H., Levy, E. J., Actor, P. and Pauls, J. F. (1974), J. Clin. Pharmacol., 14, 61.

DeMarinis, R. M., Hoover, J. R. E., Dunn, G. L., Actor, P., Uri, J. V. and Weisbach, J. A. (1975), J. Antibiotics, 28, 463.

Fare, L. R., Actor, P., Sachs, C. S., Phillips, L., Joloza, M., Pauls, J. F. and Weisbach, J. A. (1974), Antimicr. Agents Chemother., 6, 150.

Rattie, E. S. and Ravin, L. J. (1975), Antimicr. Agents Chemother., 7, 606.

PHARMACOKINETICS OF CEPHRADINE

E. BERGOGNE, N. LAMBERT & J. L. ROUVILLOIS

BICHAT HOSPITAL

170 Boulevard Ney, 78877 PARIS CEDEX 18, France

The main features of Cephradine, a new semi-synthetic cephalosporin antibiotic, are its broad spectrum of activity and its facility of use, since it can be administered both orally and parenterally. The purpose of the present investigation was to test Cephradine for its diffusion into various body fluids. To this end, we have determined by microbial assays the concentrations of the drug in sera and biles of adults, sera and cerebrospinal fluids of children and sera and amniotic fluids of pregnant women near delivery. As regards the pregnant women, determinations of the concentrations achieved simultaneously in maternal blood, blood of umbilical cord and amniotic fluid allowed the transplacental passage of the drug to be checked.

I. STUDY PROTOCOL

1) Serum, bile and amniotic fluid samples were frozen at -20°C immediately after drawing and stored until assayed. Serum and cerebrospinal fluid samples from children with purulent meningitis were sent to us in frozen storage from Dakar hospital. Samples were used pure or diluted in pH6 buffer (bile samples).

2) Serum quantitative determinations were carried out after intravenous administration of Cephradine.

3) The material investigated came from 3 very different categories of subjects including : 2 healthy adult male volunteers for serum and bile samples; 10 children with purulent meningitis caused by various organisms for serum and cerebrospinal fluid; 7 pregnant women awaiting delivery in a department of obstetrics for blood of umbilical vein and artery, and amniotic fluid.

4) Quantitative determination method (according to the GROVE & RANDALL technique) : Culture medium : Difco pH 6.6 Antibio Medium No.2; test organism : strain IP 5832 of Bacillus subtilis (suspension titrated at 5.10^7 spores/ml); diffusion originated from stainless steel cylinders at 5 mm; serial dilutions : from 0.15 to 20 mcg/ml.

II. INTERPRETATION OF RESULTS

In Vitro Results

1) <u>Serum Concentrations</u>. a) In general, significant levels were achieved for about 3 hours, sometimes more. After 4 hours, the levels became barely assayable. b) In adults, peak serum concentrations were achieved rapidly. Although early measurements were few, a peak level of 18.5 mcg/ml was reached in 10 minutes in 1 case. At 45 minutes, the level was 6 mcg/ml. Between 1 1/2 and 3 hours, levels ranged from 1.75 to 5 mcg/ml. In fact, serum concentrations reached various levels often superior to the MIC of Cephradine against susceptible organisms. c) Half-life in serum : The mean concentrations achieved at various times served to plot the concentration curve of Cephradine against time on semi-logarithmic paper. Hence the half-life of Cephradine was estimated to be 65 minutes; this value compares favourably with the half-lives of other cephalosporin derivatives such as Cephacetrile (BLACK), Cephalothin (DUVAL & MORA) and Cephaloridin.

2) <u>Cerebrospinal Fluid Concentrations</u>. In 2 cases, the ratio of cerebrospinal fluid to serum concentration was very high at 1 hour after intravenous administration of 75 mg/kg of Cephradine (1.1 mcg/1.4 mcg and 1.5 mcg/5 mcg respectively). In 3 cases, no detectable amount of drug passed into the cerebrospinal fluid in spite of a serum concentration as high as 10 mcg/ml in one instance. In the other 2 cases, serum levels were very low (0.2 mcg/ml) or nil. In 5 cases, even though the concentration ratios were not quite as high, they were nevertheless valid. Therefore, responses varied greatly. In the 2 children who died, cerebrospinal fluid concentrations were either nil or practically inexistent. Thus, on the whole, Cephradine was found to pass irregularly through the blood brain barrier when infection is present.

3) <u>Bile Concentrations</u>. All the assays yielded high bile concentrations; a level of 20 mcg/ml was reached at 1 hour in a subject. Very significant levels were still present at 2 1/2 hours in the samples from both subjects tested (3.4 and 7.2 mcg/ml respectively). Bile concentrations were always higher than corresponding serum concentrations.

4) <u>Passage through the Placenta</u>. a) Sampling was no doubt carried out too late to enable us to measure peak concentrations in venous blood from pregnant women, since the first determinations were performed on samples collected 45 minutes after administration.

The venous blood levels achieved averaged 6 and 3 mcg/ml 45 minutes and 2 hours after administration, respectively. b) The ratio between the maternal serum concentrations and umbilical cord concentrations of Cephradine was worthwhile; it was high and seemed to increase in the course of time. c) A similar increase was observed with respect to amniotic fluid concentrations which can become higher than corresponding serum concentrations. d) A number of isolated determinations were carried out on samples of amniotic fluid taken from pregnant women who had received 1 g of Cephradine daily for 3 days orally. Sampling was effected on the 3rd day 2 to 3 hours after oral ingestion. The amniotic fluid levels achieved by this route of administration were similar to those obtained intravenously, averaging 3 mcg/ml at the 3rd hour.

COMMENTS AND CONCLUSIONS

Peak concentration levels were achieved rapidly, as is usual after intravenous administration. In comparison with results reported in the literature, the highest concentrations assayed in this study may seem to be low. But only few determinations were carried out on samples collected soon enough after administration; most samples were probably taken after the occurrence of the peak.

Diffusion of Cephradine into the cerebrospinal fluid was not very important in most cases, as currently encountered with other cephalosporins such as Cephalexin and Cephacetrile.

As far as passage into the bile was concerned, it was very satisfactory. Drug concentrations were higher in the bile than in the serum and they largely exceeded the MIC of Cephradine against sensitive organisms.

The passage of Cephradine through the placenta was excellent. High amniotic fluid levels were achieved. BARR & GRAHAM have given evidence of the passage of Cephaloridin through the placenta after intramuscular injection of 1 g. of this antibiotic. Relying on the pharmacokinetic data reported by these authors, ROUVILLOIS & Al. treated until delivery 150 women, whose birth membranes had prematurely ruptured, with 2 g. of Cephaloridin daily for periods ranging from 1 to 32 days. At birth, samples of blood (for hemocultural purposes) and of gastric, cerebrospinal and lacrymal fluids were drawn from every newborn child. A prenatal infection was suspected clinically in only 11 cases and bacteriologically confirmed in 9. Of them, only 1 had an unfavourable issue. Accordingly, it would seem that Cephradine might also be of definite interest in this type of patient.

Cephradine, a broad spectrum cephalosporin antibiotic allows high drug levels to be obtained in the serum. It passes through the blood brain barrier in small amounts, but its excretion in bile is considerable,in normal adults, at least. Cephradine also passes through the placenta in significant amounts, and the levels measured in samples from amniotic fluid and umbilical cord blood substantiate its indication in obstetrics for the treatment of a number of particular cases.

STUDIES ON THE DIFFUSION OF CEPHRADINE AND CEPHALOTHIN INTO HUMAN TISSUE

D. Adam, A.G. Hofstetter, W. Jacoby, and B. Reichardt

Children's Hospital, University of Munich
Munich, West Germany, Lindwurmstrasse 4

The clinical effectiveness of antibiotics and chemotherapeutic agents depends on various factors as serum half-lives, elimination rates, renal excretion, protein binding, minimal inhibition concentrations, pH and enzyme stability. The capability of antibiotics to diffuse into the infected tissue is one of the most important factors for their therapeutic effect. The tissue level of a drug is certainly better correlated to its effectiveness than the level in blood serum. The absolut values of tissue and serum levels as well as their numerical relation are important characteristics of a drug. These were the reasons for investigating the tissue concentrations of cephradine and cephalothin, two derivatives of ß-lactam group antibiotics which are widely used in hospitals.

Material and Methods:

The studies were carried out with three different human tissues: 1. heart muscle, 2. prostatic tissue, 3. brain tissue. The serum and tissue levels of these antibiotics were determined by biological assay with the Kirby-Bauer Agar-diffusion method using Bacillus subtilis ATCC 6633 as test organism. Serum diluted standard curves were made with activity standardised samples of cephradine and cephalothin. All assays were performed in triplicate. The tissue material was homogenized in a buffered solution with the Colworth Stomacher No.80. Zone diameters of serum and tissue samples were measured to the nearest 0.05 cm with the help of an overhead projection device and plotted in a logarithmic system for determining of serum and tissue standard curves.

Heart muscle samples were collected from children with Fallot's disease exactly 60 minutes after application of 100 mg/kg of cephalothin and cephradine respectively. Heart muscle was removed after an ischemia of 5 minutes so that the blood portion in the tissue was very low. Before homogenizing the tissue samples were washed free from blood three times in saline. Serum samples were collected before the application of the antibiotic as control and exactly at the time of tissue removing.

Prostatic tissue was removed from patients with prostatic adenoma. From all patients 10 ml of venous blood were collected before beginning of the operation as controls and thereafter 2 grams of cephalothin and cephradine respectively were injected by the intravenous route. Approximately 30 minutes later adenoma tissue was removed and washed with saline so that macroscopically no blood was visible at the tissue sample. At the time of removal the second blood sample for determining the antibiotic concentration was drawn. Serum and tissue samples were frozen at $-20^\circ C$ and transported to the bacteriological laboratory.

Brain tissue was removed from patients with cerebral tumors. The material was collected when making a channel during operation necessary for access to the tumor in depth of the brain or from other healthy parts in case resection of brain lobe was necessary. All materials were freed from visible blood by washing in buffered saline. All patients received 2 or 4 grams of cephalothin and cephradine respectively at the intravenous route in a 20 or 40 minutes infusion period. Blood samples were collected before injection of the antibiotics and at the time of tissue resection, i.e. 60, 70 and 80 minutes after beginning of the infusion.

Results

1. Heart Muscle and Serum Studies

8 children each with Fallot's disease and an average age of 8 1/2 years (ranging from 3 1/2 to 16) were included in this investigation.
Before cephalothin or cephradine were given, no serum sample had detectable antimicrobial activity. After application of 100 mg/kg cephradine the serum concentration ranged 60 minutes from 53.7 mcg/ml to 157.5 mcg/

ml with an average of 92 mcg (see figure 1). The cephradine concentrations in heart muscle tissue ranged 60 minutes after administration of the drug from 11.5 mcg/g to 21.4 mcg/g with an average value of 15.4. The cephalothin serum values varied between 27.5 mcg/ml and 87.5 mcg/ml with an average of 51 and in the heart tissue from 0.7 mcg/g to 2.0 mcg/g with an average of 1.4 mcg/g. Under identical dosing the mean serum concentrations of cephradine were 2 times higher and the mean tissue concentrations of cephradine were 10 times higher than the corresponding concentrations of cephalothin.
(Figure 1)

2. Prostatic Tissue and Serum Studies

9 patients with prostatic adenoma and an average age of 70 years (ranging from 60 to 81) were included in the study with cephradine and 7 patients with an average age of 74 years (ranging from 65 to 80) in the study with cephalothin.
After 2 grams of cephradine the serum concentrations at the time of tissue removing ranged from 22 to 125 mcg/ml with an average value of 77. The tissue levels ranged at corresponding points of time from 6.7 to 89.5 mcg/g with an average value of 27 whereas the mean values of cephalothin were 33.3 in serum and 8 mcg/g in prostatic tissue. Therefore the levels of cephradine were two times higher in the patients serum and 3.4 times higher in the prostatic tissue than the corresponding concentrations of cephalothin.
(Figure 2)

3. Brain Tissue, Cerebro-Spinal Fluid and Serum Studies

14 patients with an average age of 43 years (ranging from 13 to 65) were included in the study with cephradine and 4 patients with an average age of 40 years (ranging from 28 to 55) in that with cephalothin.
One group of patients received two grams of the drug and a second received 4 grams. In every case blood was collected 60 minutes after beginning of the infusion. At the same time the first tissue material was removed. As shown in figure 3 the mean serum concentration value 60 minutes after infusion of 2 grams of cephradine was 35.7 mcg/ml and 136.5 mcg/ml after a dosage of 4 grams i.v. The serum concentration of cephalothin after the latter dose was 4 times lower with a mean value of 34 mcg/ml.
(Figure 3)

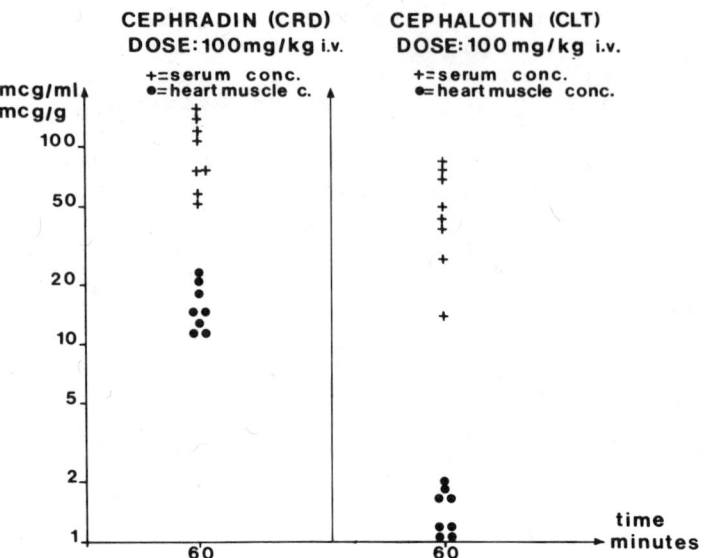

Fig. 1. Heart muscle and serum studies.

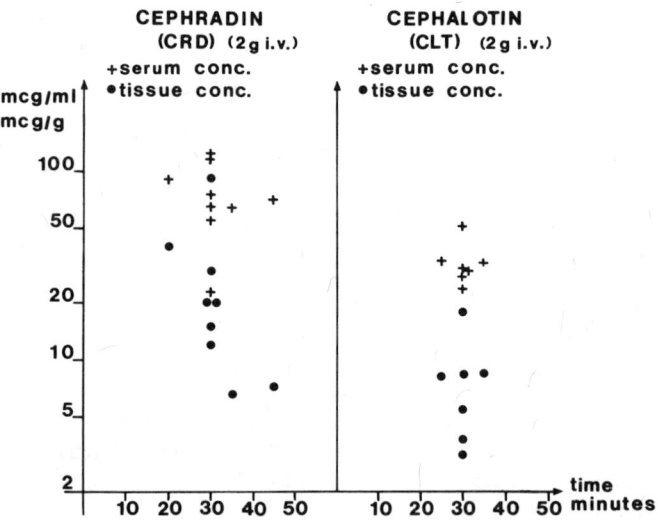

Fig. 2. Prostatic tissue and serum studies.

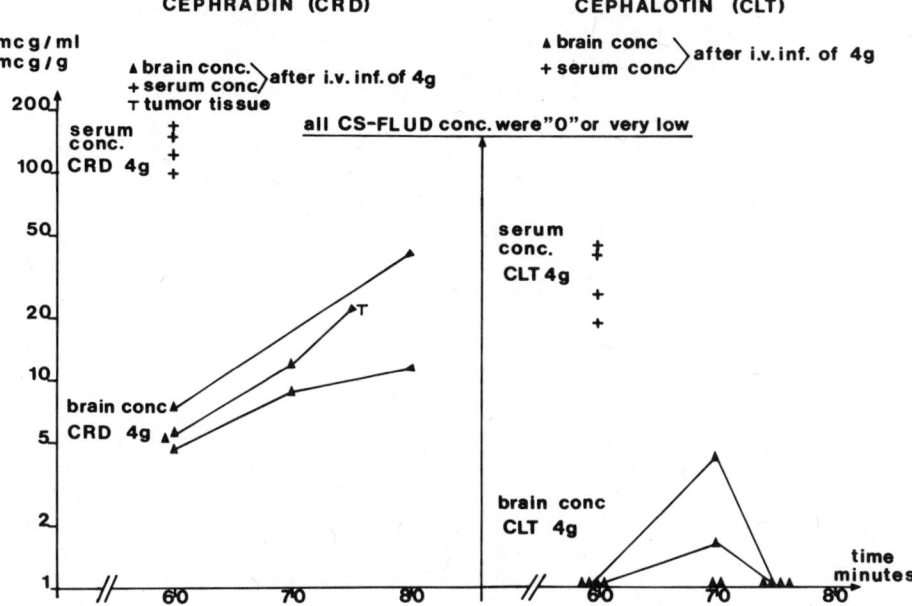

Fig. 3. Brain tissue CS-fluid and serum studies.

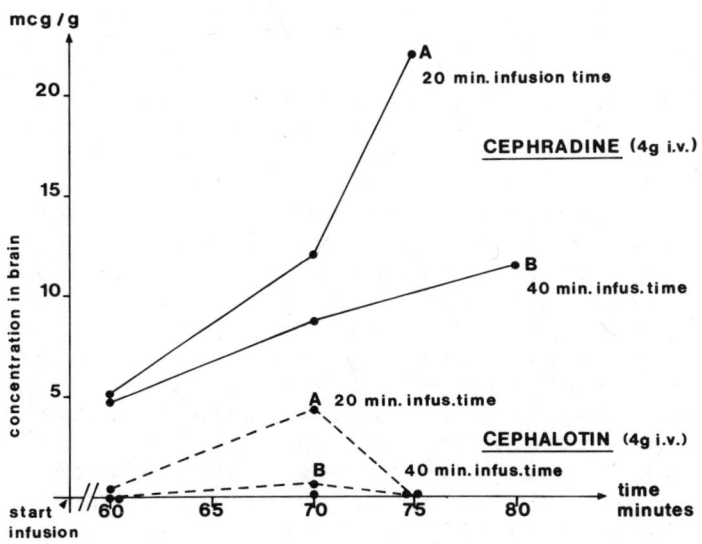

Fig. 4. Brain tissue studies.

After application of 2 grams of cephalothin no measurable values of this drug were detectable in brain tissue. Also the patients who received 2 grams of cephradine had relatively low concentrations of this drug in brain tissue with a mean value of 1.75 mcg/g ranging from 0 to 3.8 respectively to 5.2 in the tissue of a brain tumor. After a 4 gram dosage of cephradine the mean tissue concentration rose up to 12.75 mcg/g ranging from 4.2 to 41.5 whereas 4 grams cephalothin gave a mean value of only 1 mcg/g. There were no or very low concentrations of both substances in the cerebrospinal fluid after application of 2 or 4 grams of the drugs. The highest values were 1.2 respectively 1.5 mcg of cephradine per ml.

Figure 4 demonstrates clearly that the highest concentrations of cephradine in brain tissue were obtained when giving the i.v. infusion within 20 minutes. Also the rise after a time of 5 or 10 minutes was higher with a 20 minutes infusion time than with a 40-minutes infusion time. After a dosage of 4 grams of cephalothin the tissue levels were very low and fell down to 0 already after 15 minutes compared with cephradine which still rose up at this point of time.
(Figure 4)

Discussion of Results

Our relatively low serum levels of cephalothin compared with cephradine are in line with the data of the literature. The explanation for this fact may lie in the short half life of cephalothin, the metabolisation and inactivation of 32 to 40% of the substance. If one considers the protein-binding which is low for cephradine and relatively high for cephalothin (60 - 65%) the discrepancy is still more pronounced. The fact that the brain tissue levels of cephradine are higher can again be explained by its minimal protein-binding since only the free (not protein-bound) levels of the drugs in the blood and in the tissues tend to reach a balance. Our investigations show that also the speed of infusion plays its part. Infusing 4 grams in 20 minutes the brain tissue levels are higher than after a 40 minutes infusion period. This may be explained by delayed entrance of lower concentrations of the substance in the tissue because of the blood brain barrier. In addition, in the case of the 40 minutes infusion period because of the excretion of the substance the offer over the time interval to the brain tissue may be relatively low compared with the amount which is available after a 20 minutes

infusion period.
The high tissue levels of cephradine shown in this study fulfill an important condition for the antibacterial chemotherapy of infections.

Summary:

The penetration of cephradine and cephalothin into human heart muscle, prostatic tissue, brain tissue, and the CSF was studied each in two patient groups. The serum levels of cephalothin were 2 times lower than those of cephradine. The mean tissue concentrations of cephradine in heart muscle were 10 times higher and in prostatic tissue 3.4 times higher than those of cephalothin. Brain tissue values of cephalothin were not detectable after application of 2 grams of the drug whereas the mean values of cephradine were 1.75 mcg/g. After a dosage of 4 grams the values rose to 12.75 mcg/g in the case of cephradine and only to 1 mcg/g after cephalothin application. In the CSF were no or very low concentrations of both substances. The findings will be explained with the metabolisation rate of cephalothin with 32-40% whereas cephradine is not metabolized. The difference of protein binding of both substances was not regarded when comparing the serum levels, but it may play an important role for the ability of each drug to reach the tissues. The high tissue levels of cephradine fulfill an important condition for the antibacterial chemotherapy of infections.

DOSAGE SCHEDULE OF ANTIMICROBIAL AGENTS

Yoshihito Ban, Yasuo Shimizu, Yukimichi Kawada, and Tsuneo Nishiura

Department of Urology
Gifu University School of Medicine
40, Tsukasa, Gifu, Japan

In general, dosage schedule of antimicrobial agents have to be established theoretically in relation to the serum concentration and minimal inhibitory concentration against infecting organisms. But, in practice, those theoretical schedule was not always kept. Nevertheless, excellent therapeutic effects have been often obtained. According to those facts, basic experiments were employed in order to reexamine about the dosage schedule of antimicrobial agents.

METHODS AND RESULTS

Standard strain of E.coli(JC-2) was inoculated into 10 ml volumes of trypticase soy broth which contained cephalotin(CET) or ampicillin(ABPC) in various concentrations. The inoculum size was set finally at about 10^6 cells/ml. The turbidity produced by bacterial growth was observed with biophotometer(BIO LOG-II) continuously (Fig.1). Drug concentrations illustrated on these figures were based on minimal inhibitory concentrations of those drugs against E.coli(JC-2). The curves on these figures show the bacterial growth. In the medium containing lower than 1/2 MIC of CET or ABPC the bacteria was able to grow. But, in the medium containing more than 1 MIC of both drugs, no bacterial growth was observed within 24 hours.

In the next, it was tested when E.coli(JC-2) was exposed for only 3 hours. Namely, CET in the medium was inactivated by addition of cephalosporinase after 3 hours incubation. In the medium containing from 1/8 to 1 MIC of CET, all the growth curves began to rise at nearly the same time(Fig.2). In the cases of higher concentrations a similar tendency was observed. These facts suggest that if the exposure time was limited to a specific short time, i.e. 3 hours, bacterial growth inhibition time was not so affected with antibiotic concentrations.

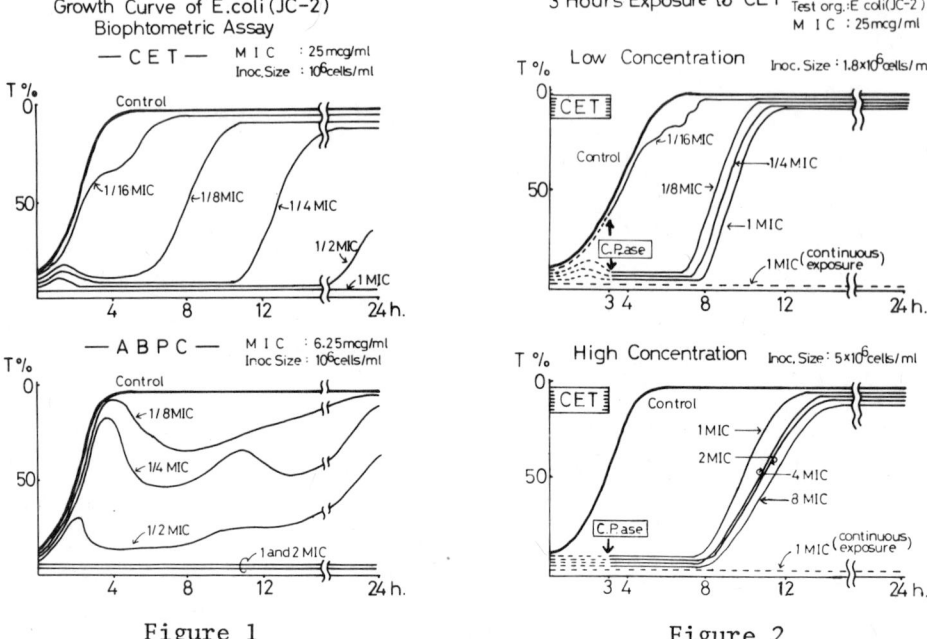

Figure 1   Figure 2

Figure 3 shows the case when sulbenicillin(SBPC) was used. In spite of exposure at such a low concentration as 1/8 MIC, its growth inhibition time was revealed to be similar to that of 1 MIC. On the other hand, viable cells were counted simultaneously in order to observe the relationship between biophotogram and viable cell counts. Biophotogram had good correlations with viable cell counts (Fig.3). In the case of higher concentrations of more than 1 MIC of SBPC showed nearly the same growth inhibition time as that of 1 MIC. ABPC was also tested similarly and it was found that with from 1/4 to 4 MIC of ABPC, nearly the same growth inhibition times were seen(Fig.4). In summary, these tendencies were observed in all those drugs CET, SBPC and ABPC.

The exposure time was varied from 1 hour to 6 hours in a constant concentration of 4 MIC of SBPC in this case(Fig.5). It was found that in spite of exposure to such a high concentration as 4 MIC for as long as 6 hours, the bacteria was able to grow after inactivation of SBPC. Namely, within these conditions, growth inhibition time after inactivation seemed to be constant whether exposure time was long or short. The lower figure in figure 5 shows the cases of large inoculum size of E.coli in logarythmic phase to carbenicillin(CBPC) for 3 hours. The bacteria began to grow in spite of the exposure at such a high concentration as 32 times of MIC. That is, when the exposure time was within 6 hours, it was considered that bacteria could not be always killed even if a considerablly highly concentrated drug was used against E.coli. Thus, it seemed important to lengthen the growth inhibition time

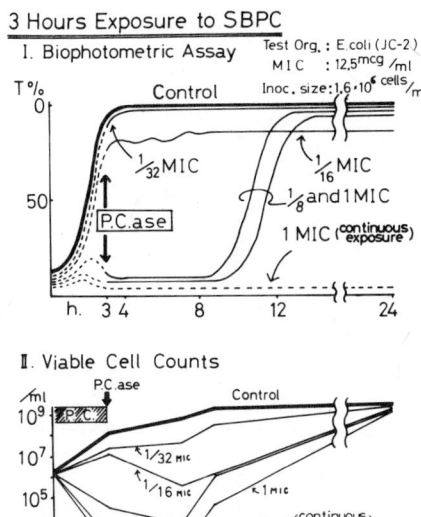

Figure 3

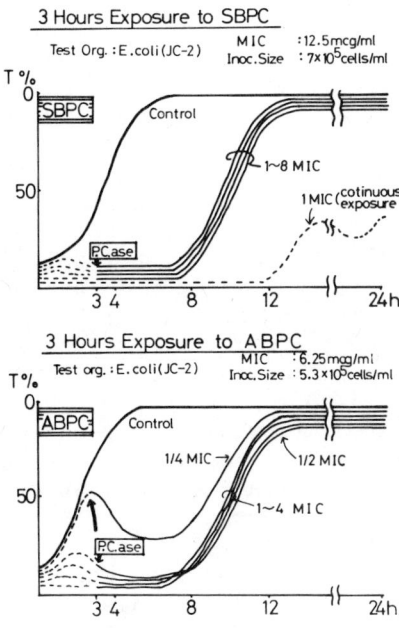

Figure 4

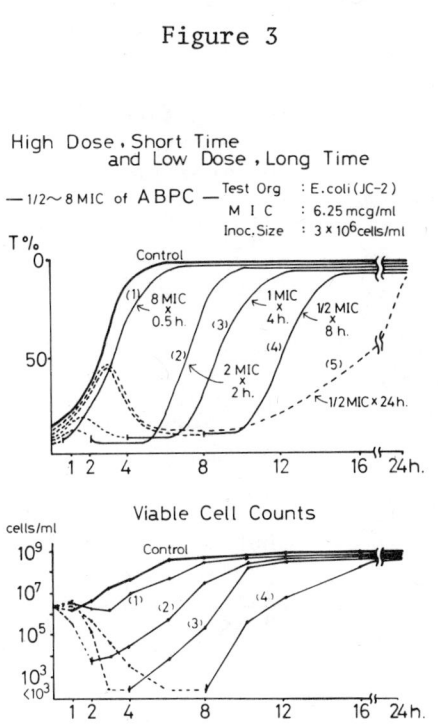

Figure 5

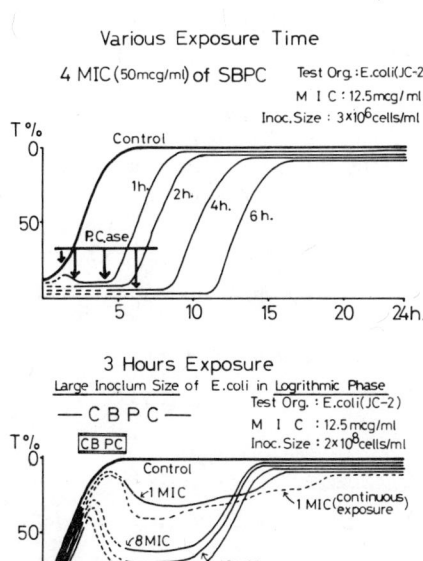

Figure 6

of bacteria.

What manner is better to use drugs in high concentration for short time or in low concentration for long time? For this question we conducted this experiment as shown in figure 6. The arranged concentrations were from 1/2 MIC of ABPC and exposure time were varied from 8 to 1/2 hours. Namely, the product of concentration by exposure time was arranged at constant 4. As a result, the longest growth inhibition time was obtained when exposed to 1/2 MIC for 8 hours. The study about viable cell counts revealed the same result (Fig.6). Then, it seemed more effective to expose for longer time in lower concentration than to expose to higher concentration for shorter time. The comparison was made with double exposure in low concentration and a single one in high concentration. E.coli was exposed to 1/2 MIC of ABPC for two hours and the same exposure was repeated after six hours. In order to confirm the growth curve on the biophotogram, viable cells after 12 hours incubation were counted as shown in figure 7. It seemed better to expose twice to low concentration than to expose once to high concentration. Clinically isolated E.coli(4897) was also used. The tendencies concerning growth inhibition time was found to be almost the same time as those of standerd strain of E.coli(JC-2).

Then, experimental treatment of mouse infections were carried out in order to compare the curative effects with two different dosage schedules. Figure 8 shows the antibiotic concentrations of mouse after intramuscular injection of ABPC. The mice used in these experiments were male SHIZUOKA albino mice weighting from 18 to 20 g. As you can see in figure 8, in these mice, peak serum levels happened to be almost equivalent to the injected dosages. So, when the equivalent dosage of 1 MIC of ABPC was injected in mouse, the blood concentration 15 minutes after injection was considered to be 1 MIC level. Groupes of ten mice were infected intraperitoneally with E.coli and treated with intramuscular injection of ABPC. One group was injected ABPC only one time 1 hour after intraperitoneal inoculation and another group was injected two times, 1 and 5 hours after inoculation (Fig.9). In the case of single injection, median effective dose (ED_{50}) was 8 MIC per gram of mouse or more, but in the case of double injection it was revealed to be 2.48 MIC per gram of mouse. The curative effects obtained by double injections of one half volume twice was superior than by single injection of

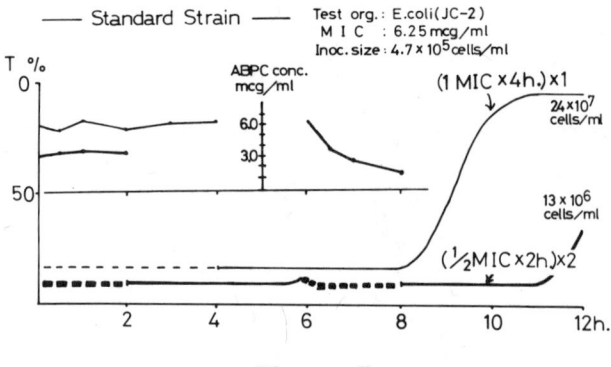

Figure 7

total volume. Figure 10 shows the case that total dosage was divided into fifths. When each equivalent dosage of ABPC was injected 5 times, the ED_{50} was 3.8 MIC per gram of mouse, which was somewhat higher than that obtained by double injections. But, when one half of total dosage was injected at the first injection and followed with 4 injections of 1/8 respectively, that was the smallest dosage of all these different dosage schedules. Furthermore, we conducted similar experiments with clinically isolated Proteus morganii(0237) against which the MIC of ABPC was as high as 250 mcg/ml. The curative effect was superior when whole dosage was divided into two parts than whole dosage was injected at one time.

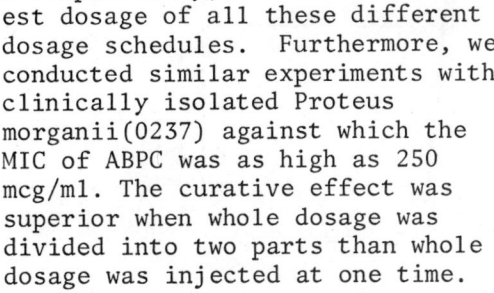

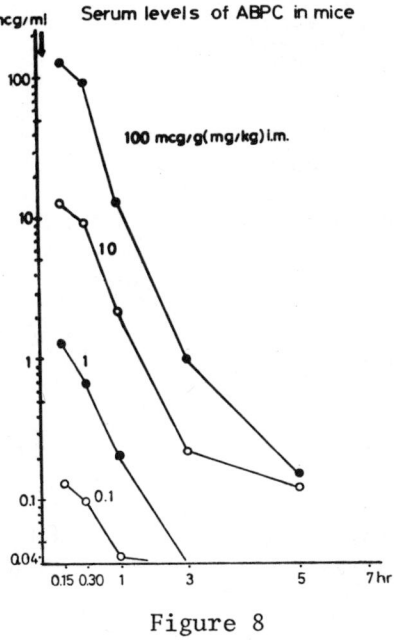

Figure 8

DISCUSSION

In regard to administration schedule of antimicrobial agents we can see some papers, some of which were reported by Eagle et al. in the 1950's. They carried out a lot of fundamental experiments both in vitro and in vivo concerning administration schedule of penicillin and reported that "penicillin time" was important. Since the time to today, many antimicrobial agents have been discovered and in general, dosage administration schedule have been established in relation to the serum concentration and minimal inhibitory concentration against infecting organisms. But, in practice, those theoretical schedule were not always kept. Nevertheless, excellent therapeutic effects have been often obtained. On the other hand, it became popular in these days to use large doses of penicillin and cephalosporin in serious infections and good curative effects have been obtained clin-

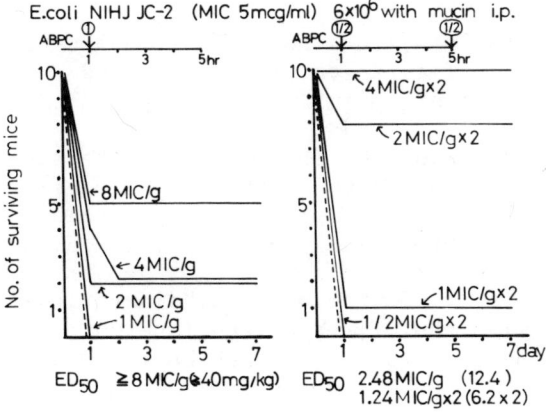

Figure 9

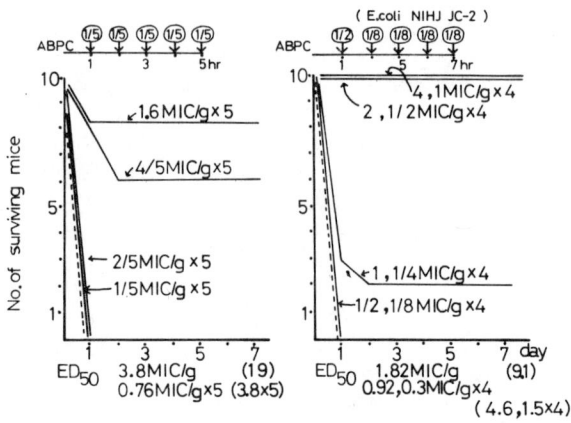

Figure 10

ically. But, it seemed that laboratory and fundamental experiments about massive dose therapy were not sufficiently performed. According to those facts, basic examinations were carried out in order to reexamine about the dosage schedule of antimicrobial agents. Biophotometer(BIO LOG-II) was used mainly and in order to stop the bactericidal action of drugs, inactivating enzymes were used. In the animal experiments, the total dosage was fixed in a definite volume and injected singly or multiply.

Results are summarized as follows.
In the cases drug exposure terms were limited within a specific short time, i.e. 6 hours, the growth curves began to rise at nearly the same time even if the bacteria was exposed to low concentration or high concentration. Then it seemed important to lengthen the growth inhibition time. The longer inhibition time was obtained when exposed for longer time even if to low concentration and when exposed multiply. According to animal experiments, multiple injections revealed superior to single injection of whole volume. Namely, using penicillin and cephalosporin in these experiments, it is suggested that continuous exposure at low concentration is superior to transient exposure of high concentration.

REFERENCES

1) Eagle,H.,Fleischman,R.and Musselman,A.D. The bactericidal action of penicillin in vivo: the participation of the host and the slow recovery of the surviving organisms. Ann.Int.Med.,33:544-571,1950
2) Eagle,H.,Fleischman,R.and Musselman,A.D. The effect of the schedule of administration on the therapeutic efficacy of penicillin: the importance of the aggregate time for which penicillin remains at effectively bactericidal levels. Am.J.Med.,9: 280-299,1950
3) Eagle,H.,Fleischman,R.and Levy,M. "Continuous" vs."discontinuous" therapy with penicillin: the effect of the interval between injections on therapeutic efficacy. New Engl.J.Med., 248:481-488,1953

SCHEDULE OF INTERMITTENT CEPHALOTHIN THERAPY

Kaoru Shimada and Hiroshi Kato

Tokyo Metropolitan Geriatric Hospital, Tokyo and

Shionogi Research Laboratories, Osaka, Japan

In eighteen patients (nine with septicemia and nine with respiratory tract infections) who had not responded to 6 grams or less of cephalothin daily given for 3 to 10 days, the total daily dose was increased to 8 grams or more.

The individual dose of cephalothin was administered by intravenous drip infusion in 500 ml of saline or 5% dextrose solution over a 2-hour period.

Out of the eighteen, ten responded satisfactorily when the total daily dose was increased.

The total daily dose was increased in three different ways.

In two patients, the individual dose was increased without increasing the number of doses. One patient out of the two responded.

In ten patients, the number of doses was increased by shortening the interval between individual doses but without increasing the individual dose. Six patients out of the ten showed a satisfactory response.

In six patients, both the individual dose and the number of doses were increased. Three patients out of the six responded satisfactorily.

These results suggest that not only the individual dose, but also the interval between drip infusions are playing an important role in determining the therapeutic outcome.

We conducted a study concerning the number of surviving E. coli exposed to cephalothin and attempted to apply the result of the study to the clinical use of cephalothin.

Six strains of E. coli in a final suspension of 10^6 organisms per ml during the logarithmic phase of growth were exposed at 37°C to various concentration of cephalothin in Antibiotic Medium for 1 or 3 hours.

After 1 or 3 hour exposure, the suspension was centrifuged at 15,000 g for 20 minutes, and bacterial sediment was immediately resuspended in a broth free of antibiotics and was incubated at 37°C.

Throughout the whole process, the number of viable organisms in the suspension was periodically determined by colony counting on the plate.

Fig. 1 shows the number of viable E. coli when it was exposed to various concentrations of cephalothin for 1 hour.

Fig. 2 shows similar data when E. coli was exposed to cephalothin for 3 hours. Exposure of growing E. coli to one MIC or higher of cephalothin for one or three hours resulted in a sharp decrease in the number of viable cells. When the organisms were removed from a medium containing cephalothin to an antibiotic-free medium, the decrease in the number of surviving organisms continued for some time after which they resumed multiplication. The recovery rate varied, depending on bacterial strains, concentration of cephalothin in which the bacteria had been exposed and the duration of the exposure.

The average time required to kill 99% of E. coli was 104 minutes with 1 MIC, 80 minutes with 2 MIC's and 55 minutes with 4 MIC's, respectively.

As is shown in the table, the average time required for the number of the organisms to recover to 1% of the inoculum after the termination of exposure to cephalothin. Exposure to 1 MIC of cephalothin for 1 hour failed to reduce the number of viable E. coli to 1% of the inoculum. In other condition listed in the table, the time required for the number of E. coli to recover to 1% of the inoculum ranged from 2.1 to 8.7 hours. These results were obtained in vitro and, therefore, can be compared in vivo to a situation in which there is no host defense.

Eagle[1] reported that in vivo the recovery time of penicillin-damaged gram-positive cocci was usually longer than that observed in vitro. His data show that the recovery time in vivo is prolonged by 3 to 5 hours from that in vitro. This can be regarded as the effect of host defense mechanism.

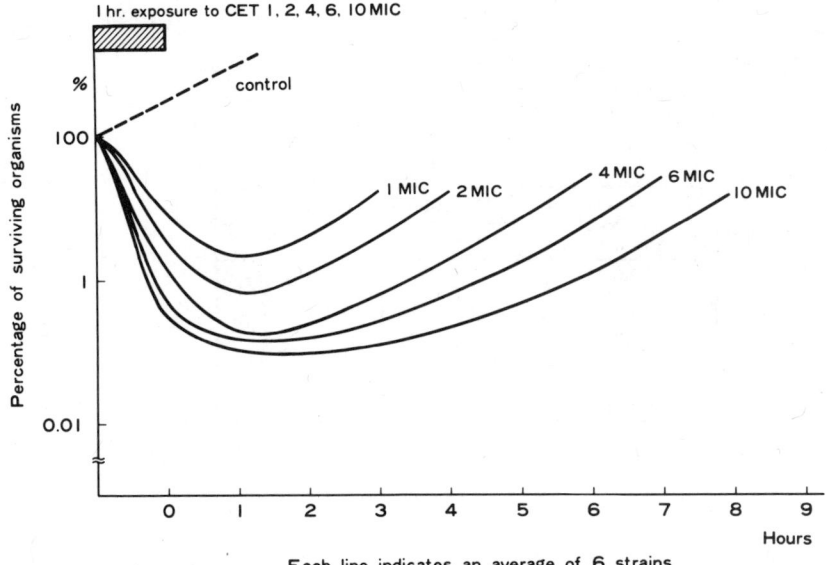

Fig. 1. The recovery of cephalothin-treated E. coli in vitro (Medium: ABM 3).

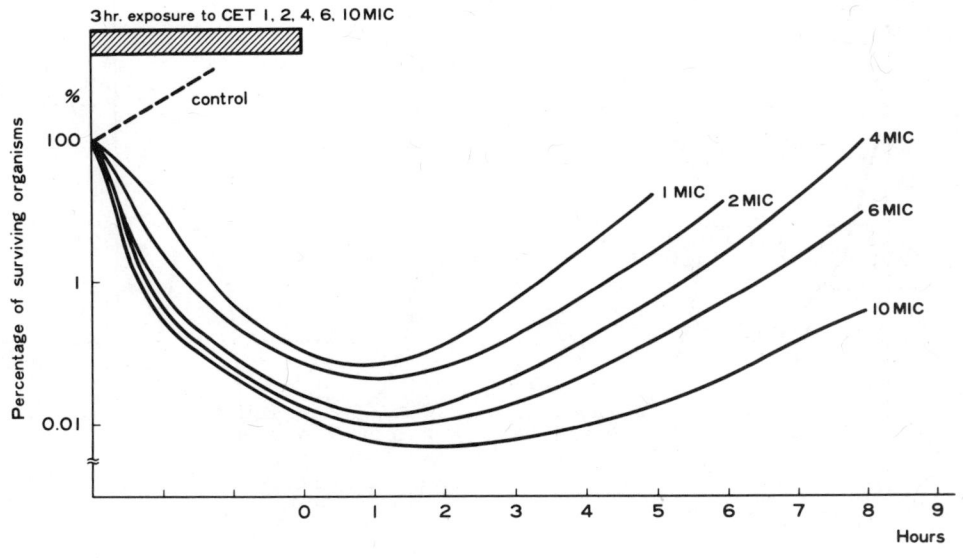

Fig. 2. The recovery of cephalothin-treated E. coli in vitro (Medium: ABM 3).

Table 1. Time required to recover to 1% the inoculum after termination to exposure to cephalothin (average of 6 strains)

Concentration	Duration of exposure	
	1 hr	3 hr
1 MIC	—	3.5 (hr)
2 MIC	2.1 (hr)	4.3
4 MIC	3.6	5.4
6 MIC	4.3	6.6
10 MIC	5.5	8.7

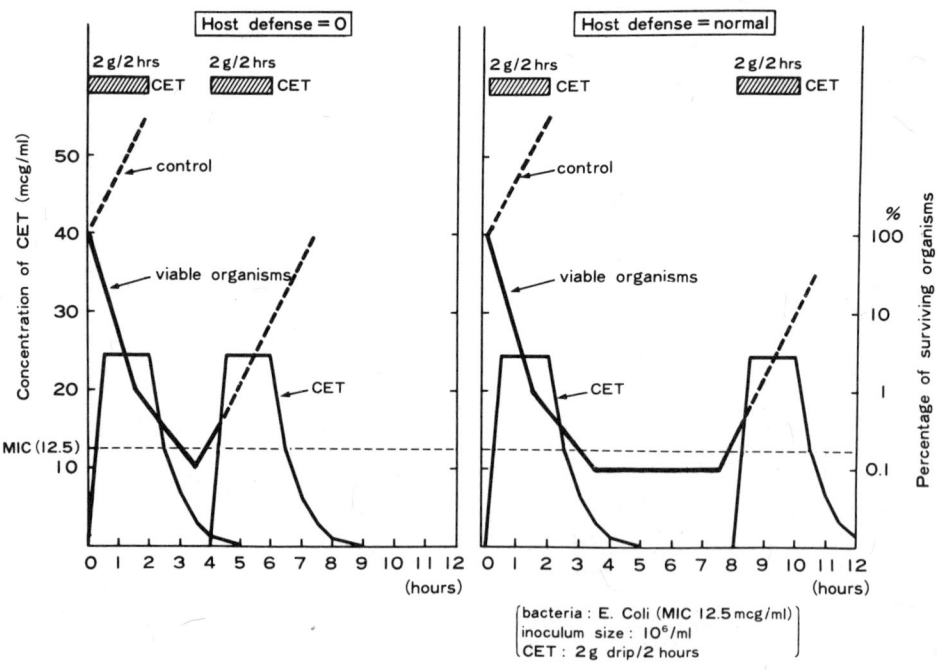

Fig. 3. Relationship between concentration of CET and number of viable organisms.

An attempt has been made to apply the data so far discussed to the clinical situation in which cephalothin is given by drip infusion in a patient with E. coli infection.

First, we have to know the concentration of cephalothin in contact with the organisms at the site of infection. This is the tissue concentration. Because the tissue concentration is not necessarily easy to determine, we use the blood levels instead. Mashimo and Fukaya[2] determined the blood levels of cephalothin in the constant drip infusion to patients and noted that a fairly uniform peak serum concentration was obtained 30 minutes after starting the drip infusion. This peak level was maintained until the end of the drip infusion after which the concentration decreased at a half time of 30 minutes. Based on the result, they proposed a formula to calculate the peak concentration.

Based on the result, the cephalothin concentration in serum which results from a drip infusion of 2 grams of cephalothin over a 2-hour period can be depicted as the trapezoids in Fig. 3. If we assume that the MIC of E. coli which causes the infection is 12.5 µg per ml, the peak cephalothin level attained is about 2 MIC's. Based on the data already discussed, the number of viable organisms is expected to be reduced to 1% or less of the original one in approximately one and a half hours after the start of the drip infusion. In vitro study data also suggest that, without the host defense, it will take approximately 3 hours after the cessation of the drip infusion before the number of the viable organisms recovers over 1% of the original. Therefore, if the next dose of cephalothin is started within 3 hours after the cessation of the previous dose, effective eradication of the organisms could be expected.

By extrapolating Eagle's observation with penicillin-damaged gram-positive cocci to cephalothin-damaged E. coli, we assume that the recovery time for E. coli in vivo with normal host defense will be prolonged by 3 to 5 hours. Therefore, if the next dose of cephalothin is started within 6 hours after the cessation of the previous dose (or if the cephalothin administration is given once every 8 hours or less), effective eradication of the organisms could be expected.

Of course, the actual tissue concentration differs from the serum concentration described in Fig. 3. This is especially true, for example, in the central nervous system infections.

Therefore, what is described in Fig. 3 should be interpreted as a means of emphasizing the importance of selecting proper dose and timing so that an adequate concentration of cephalothin should be maintained for an appropriate period of time and repeated at an appropriate interval.

However, by refining this kind of analysis, we would be able to decide dose and timing of antibiotic administration on much more rational basis than what is conventionally employed.

BIBLIOGRAPHY
1. Eagle. H. et al.: The Bactericidal Action of PC in Vivo. Ann. Intern. Med. 33:544-571, 1950.
2. Mashimo, H. et al.: Absorption, Excretion and Distribution in High Dose of Cephalothin-Summarized Results of Blood Levels in Many Institutions, Saishin-Igaku 29(5):845-849, 1974.

ABSORPTION AND EXCRETION STUDIES OF CEPHALOSPORINS IN HUMAN SUBJECTS

A. G. Paradelis

Department of Experimental Pharmacology, Medical Faculty
Aristotelian University of Thessaloniki
Thessaloniki, Greece

Brotzu (1948) showed that filtrates of the fungus Cephalosporium acremonium had strong antibiotic activity against many gram-negative and gram-positive bacteria. Further investigation revealed that this fungus contained three distinct antibiotics. One of these was labeled cephalosporin C and was of special interest because of its action on penicillin-resistant staphylococci and gram-negative organisms.

With the isolation of the nucleus of cephalosporin C,7-aminoce-phalosporanic acid, and with the addition of side chains, it became possible to produce semisynthetic compounds with antibacterial activity much greater than the parent substance. Among these semisynthetic compounds are cephaloridine, cephradine and cephazolin. The molecular structures of the above semisynthetic compounds are shown in figure 1.

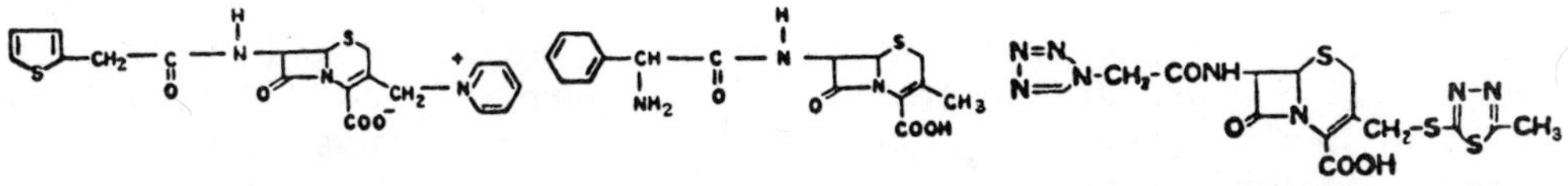

Cephaloridine Cephradine Cephazolin

Fig.1. Molecular structures of cephaloridin, cephradine and cephazolin.

Cephradine is almost completely absorbed from the upper small intestine, while cephaloridine and cephazolin are poorly absorbed from the gastrointestinal tract. These cephalosporins are excreted almost unchanged in the urine, partly by glomerular filtration and partly by tubular secretion (Gadebusch et al.1972, Gower et al.1973,Nishida et al.1969).

The following pharmacological experiment consists of a comparison of blood serum concentrations and urinary excretions after intramuscular or intravenous injection of a single dose of cephaloridine, cephradine and cephazolin in healthy male volunteers.

MATERIALS AND METHODS

Serum and urine concentrations of cephaloridine, cephradine and cephazolin were determined in young male volunteers, weighing approximately 60 Kg each.

The volunteers were divided in six groups of fifteen each. An intramuscular or intravenous injection of 0.5 g of cephaloridine, cephradine and cephazolin was given in every group.

Blood samples were taken by venepuncture at 1/4,1/2,3/4,1,1 1/2,2,3,4,5 and 6 hours after the intramuscular or intravenous injection of the above antibiotics. All blood samples were allowed to clot, and after centrifugation the serum was stored at $-20^\circ C$.

Urine specimens were collected during the following periods of time 0 - 2, 2 - 4, 4 - 6, 6 - 12 and 12 - 24 hours after administration of cephalosporins, total volumes were measured and aliquots frozen for assay.

The cephalosporins were assayed in serum and urine by the large plate agar diffusion method against Sarcina lutea (Logaras and Paradelis,1973,O'Callaghan et al.1971). A spore suspension of Sarcina lutea ATCC 9341 was inoculated at 0.01% into agar made up as follows: 0.5% peptone (Oxoid),0.3% Lab.Lemo,1.0% sodium citrate and 1.5% agar (Oxoid) at pH 7.

Standard solutions of cephalosporins were prepared at 0.5 mg/ml in 0.2 M phosphate buffer at pH 6 and stored at $4^\circ C$ for upto 4 days. Working standards at required concentrations were freshly prepared each day by dilution into pooled human serum and urine.

A logarithmic equation was fitted to the data according to the theory of least squares in order to measure the elimination of the drug from the blood as a function of time after the top serum value (concentration) had been reached.

The mean half-lives were estimated by cumulative distribution of the mean serum concentrations.

Protein binding. The degree of binding of cephaloridine, cephradine and cephazolin to serum proteins was measured by ultrafiltration through Viskin tubing (size 8/32). The cephalosporins present in the protein-free ultrafiltrates were assayed by large plate agar diffusion method against Sarcina lutea (Nishida et al. 1969, Logaras and Paradelis, 1973).

RESULTS

The mean serum concentrations of cephaloridine, cephradine and cephazolin, after administration of 0.5 g intramuscularly, are illustrated in table 1 and shown in figure 2.

All cephalosporins reach peak serum levels half an hour after intramuscular injection. The maximal level in serum is 15.38 ± 2.63 µg/ml for cephaloridine, 16.74 ± 2.41 µg/ml for cephradine and 14.47 ± 2.38 µg/ml for cephazolin. The mean serum concentrations of cephradine are slightly superior to those of cephaloridine and cephazolin (table 1).

The mean serum half-lives (t 1/2) are 1.07 hours for cephaloridine, 1.18 hours for cephradine and 1.22 hours for cephazolin.

The mean serum concentrations, after intravenous injection of 0.5g of the above cephalosporins, are illustrated in table 2 and shown in figure 3.

Table 1. Mean serum concentrations of cephaloridine, cephradine and cephazolin after administration of 0.5g intramuscularly.

Time after injection (hours)	Number of subjects	Mean serum concetrations $\pm$ SD (µ/ml)		
		Cephaloridine	Cephradine	Cephazolin
1/4	15	4.37 ± 1.30	5.00 ± 1.51	4.24 ± 1.35
1/2	15	15.38 ± 2.63	16.74 ± 2.41	14.47 ± 2.38
3/4	15	15.04 ± 2.38	16.44 ± 2.33	14.30 ± 2.19
1	15	13.03 ± 1.99	14.17 ± 2.36	12.74 ± 2.20
1 1/2	15	9.10 ± 1.30	10.34 ± 1.39	9.11 ± 1.40
2	15	6.83 ± 1.19	7.40 ± 0.91	6.68 ± 1.15
3	15	4.18 ± 1.19	4.26 ± 0.96	4.22 ± 1.22
4	15	2.73 ± 0.83	3.38 ± 0.98	2.22 ± 0.73
5	15	1.98 ± 0.66	2.31 ± 0.87	1.90 ± 0.66
6	15	2.05 ± 0.83	2.20 ± 0.84	2.03 ± 0.81

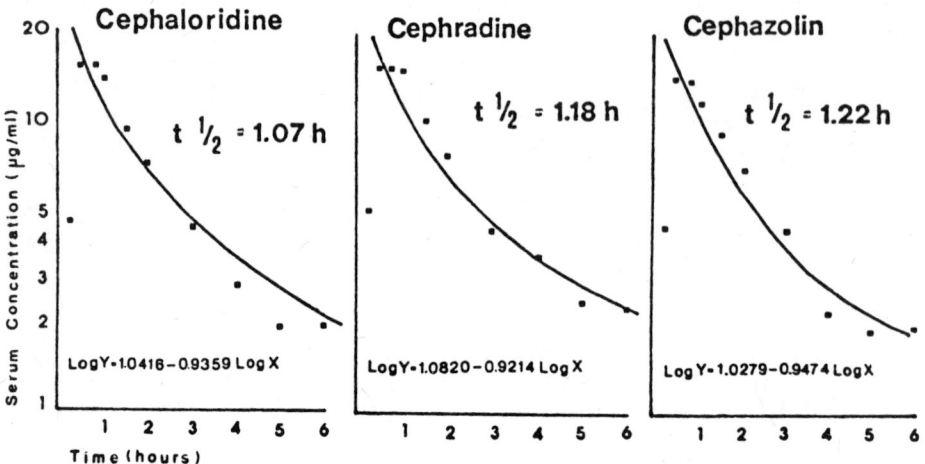

Fig. 2. Fitted regression curves on the mean serum concentrations of cephaloridine, cephradine and cephazolin after intramuscular administration of 0.5 g. t 1/2 = the mean serum half-life.

Table 2. Mean serum concentrations of cephaloridine, cephradine and cephazolin after administration of 0.5 g intravenously.

Time after injection (hours)	Number of subjects	Mean serum concentrations ± SD (µg/ml)		
		Cephaloridine	Cephradine	Cephazolin
1/4	15	38.04 ± 2.35	40.12 ± 4.71	37.33 ± 2.80
1/2	15	25.54 ± 3.25	27.46 ± 4.04	25.90 ± 3.41
3/4	15	18.05 ± 2.22	19.42 ± 2.62	18.04 ± 1.79
1	15	14.35 ± 1.55	15.32 ± 1.53	14.18 ± 2.06
1 1/2	15	10.64 ± 1.40	12.24 ± 1.71	10.93 ± 1.18
2	15	8.06 ± 0.92	8.90 ± 0.97	8.02 ± 1.13
3	15	5.66 ± 0.61	5.99 ± 0.75	5.89 ± 0.75
4	15	3.48 ± 0.71	4.74 ± 0.85	3.32 ± 0.67
5	15	1.94 ± 0.27	3.06 ± 0.54	1.90 ± 0.28
6	15	0.75 ± 0.32	1.09 ± 0.35	0.80 ± 0.21

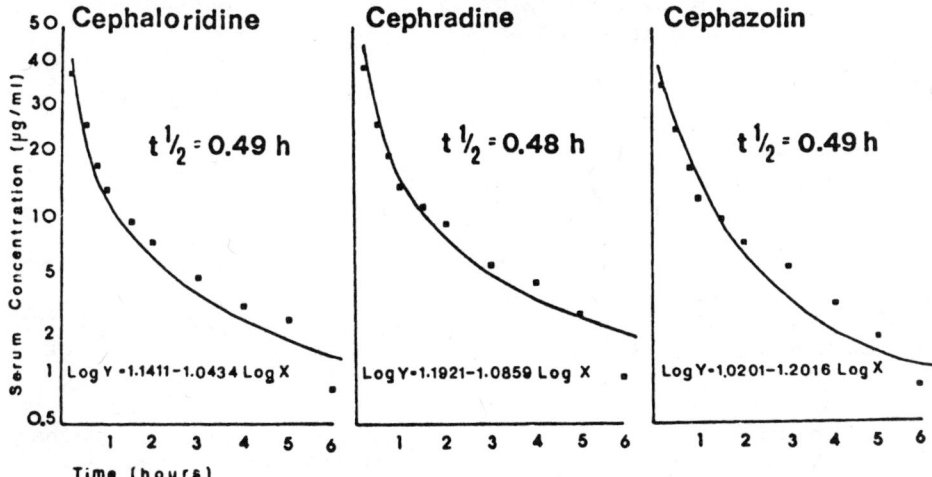

Fig.3. Fitted regression curves on the mean serum concentrations of cephaloridine, cephradine and cephazolin after intravenous administration of 0.5 g. t 1/2 = the mean serum half-life.

The mean serum levels, a quarter of an hour after intravenous injection, are 38.04 ± 2.35 µg/ml for cephaloridine, 40.12 ± 4.71 µ/ml for cephradine and 37.33 ± 2.80 µg/ml for cephazolin. Again the mean serum levels of cephradine are greater than those of cephaloridine and cephazolin.

The mean serum half-lives of cephaloridine, cephradine and cephazolin, after intravenous administration, are 0.49, 0.48 and 0.49 hours respectively.

Figures 2 and 3 show the elimination of cephaloridine, cephradine and cephazolin from the blood serum as a function of time after intra-muscular or intravenous injection.

The extent of binding of cephaloridine, cephradine and cephazolin to human serum proteins as determined in blood serum samples taken one hour after the intramuscular injection by an ultrafiltration procedure, varied from 28.63 ± 3.75% for cephradine to 41.03 ± 2.64% for cephaloridine and 70.36 ± 4.27% for cephazolin (table 3).

Table 3. Extent of binding of cephaloridine, cephradine and cephazolin to human serum proteins

Antibiotic	percentage bound to serum protein
Cephaloridine	41.03 ± 2.64
Cephradine	28.63 ± 3.75
Cephazolin	70.36 ± 4.27

The mean urine concentrations and the amounts of cephaloridine, cephradine and cephazolin recovered after intramuscular or intravenous injection of 0.5 g are illustrated in tables 4 and 5.

The average recovery of cephaloridine, cephradine and cephazolin during the first two hours in the urine samples reached 62.5, 61.4 and 64.6 per cent respectively after intramuscular administration. The average recovery of the above cephalosporins was 88.9, 88.4 and 91.5 per cent respectively after 24 hours.

For the same periods of time the average recovery of cephaloridine, cephradine and cephazolin in the urine of volunteers who received an intravenous injection amounted to 67.4, 62.5 and 69.1 per cent respectively during the first two hours and 90.5, 88.4 and 92.5 per cent respectively after 24 hours.

All cephalosporins reach similar concentrations in the urine after intramuscular or intravenous injection except for the first two hours after intravenous administration, when the mean urine concentrations and the amounts recovered are higher than those after intramuscular injection.

DISCUSSION

Among the available semisynthetic compounds of cephalosporins some are almost completely absorbed from the gastrointestinal tract, such as cephradine (Gadebusch et al. 1972), and some are poorly absorbed, such as cephaloridine and cephazolin (Nishida et al. 1969).

The indications for administering cephalosporins by the intramuscular or intravenous route include the cases where the drug cannot be administered orally or those conditions when a rapid elevation of the antibiotic in the blood is desired. It should be noted that there is great advantage for the therapy with semisynthetic compounds to be continued by oral route after the reasons for parenteral administration have been eliminated.

ABSORPTION AND EXCRETION STUDIES OF CEPHALOSPORINS

This comparative study of cephaloridine, cephradine and cephazolin reveals the following:

1. Satisfactory serum levels of cephaloridine, cephradine and cephazolin are obtained after intramuscular or intravenous administration of a single dose of 0.5 g upto six hours. All three drugs reach peak serum levels half an hour after the intramuscular injection (15.38 $\pm$ 2.63 µg/ml for cephaloridine, 16.74 $\pm$ 2.41 µg/ml for cephradine and 14.47 $\pm$ 2.38 µg/ml for cephazolin). The mean blood serum levels of cephradine are greater than those of cephaloridine and cephazolin (table 1). Our data of cephaloridine and cephazolin are similar to those of other investigators (Gower et al.1973, Nishida et al.1969).

2. The mean blood serum level of cephradine, a quarter of an hour after intravenous injection (40.12 $\pm$ 4.71 µg/ml) is higher than that of cephaloridine (38.04 $\pm$ 2.35 µg/ml) and cephazolin (37.33 $\pm$ 2.80 µg/ml) and during the period studied (table 2).

3. The elimination of cephalosporins from the blood serum as a function of time after intramuscular or intravenous injection, seems to be regulated by the same factors and follows a negative exponential curve (figures 2 and 3).

4. The mean blood serum half-lives of cephaloridine, cephradine and cephazolin after intramuscular or intravenous injection are 1.07, 1.18 and 1.22 hours and 0.49, 0.48 and 0.49 hours respectively.

5. The extent of binding of cephaloridine, cephradine and cephazolin to human serum proteins varied from 28% for cephradine to 41% for cephaloridine and 70% for cephazolin (table 3).

6. Comparison of the urinary concentrations of cephaloridine, cephradine and cephazolin after intramuscular or intravenous injection shows that therapeutically useful levels are obtained upto at least six hours after a single dose of 0.5 g (tables 4 and 5). All cephalosporins reach similar urine concentrations except for the first two hours after intravenous injection, when the mean urine concentrations and the amounts recovered are higher than those after intramuscular injection.

7. The recovery of cephaloridine, cephradine and cephazolin in the 24 hours urine, after intramuscular or intravenous injection is 88.9, 88.4 and 91.5 and 90.5, 88.4 and 92.5 per cent respectively.

Table 4. Mean urine concentrations and amounts of cephaloridine, cephradine and cephazolin recovered after administration of 0.5g intramuscularly.

Cephaloridine

Collection period (hours)	Concentration Mean ± SD (μg/ml)	Amount recovered (mg)	(%)
0 - 2	2,206.5 ± 114.8	312.5	62.5
2 - 4	1,127.3 ± 100.2	105.4	21.1
4 - 6	206.8 ± 22.7	19.3	3.8
6 - 12	12.8 ± 3.1	6.5	1.3
12 - 24	1.6 ± 0.7	1.1	0.2
		444.8	88.9

Cephradine

Collection period (hours)	Concentration Mean ± SD (μg/ml)	Amount recovered (mg)	(%)
0 - 2	2,044.5 ± 108.5	307.1	61.4
2 - 4	1,108.2 ± 95.2	99.5	19.9
4 - 6	215.6 ± 20.3	23.0	4.6
6 - 12	22.1 ± 4.2	10.5	2.1
12 - 24	2.4 ± 0.3	2.1	0.4
		442.2	88.4

Cephazolin

Collection period (hours)	Concentration Mean ± SD (μg/ml)	Amount recovered (mg)	(%)
0 - 2	2,213.2 ± 109.4	323.0	64.6
2 - 4	1,147.4 ± 98.7	111.5	22.3
4 - 6	202.5 ± 27.6	16.0	3.2
6 - 12	15.2 ± 4.9	6.1	1.2
12 - 24	0.8 ± 0.2	1.0	0.2
		457.6	91.5

Table 5. Mean urine concentrations and amounts of cephaloridine, cephradine and cephazolin recovered after administration of 0.5 g intravenously.

Cephaloridine

Collection period (hours)	Concentration Mean ± SD (µg/ml)	Amount recovered (mg)	(%)
0 - 2	2,340.5 ± 121.2	337.4	67.4
2 - 4	1,009.7 ± 93.1	81.3	16.2
4 - 6	214.5 ± 46.3	22.5	4.5
6 - 12	15.4 ± 4.7	11.7	2.3
12 - 24	0.7 ± 0.2	0.9	0.1
		453.8	90.5

Cephradine

Collection period (hours)	Concentration Mean ± SD (µg/ml)	Amount recovered (mg)	(%)
0 - 2	2,127.3 ± 105.6	312.6	62.5
2 - 4	955.7 ± 85.6	92.5	18.5
4 - 6	226.2 ± 32.1	25.1	5.0
6 - 12	12.6 ± 3.4	10.9	2.1
12 - 24	1.1 ± 0.3	1.8	0.3
		442.9	88.4

Cephazolin

Collection period (hours)	Concentration Mean ± SD (µg/ml)	Amount recovered (mg)	(%)
0 - 2	2,491.4 ± 115.3	345.7	69.1
2 - 4	993.2 ± 92.4	88.1	17.6
4 - 6	207.3 ± 41.8	19.8	3.8
6 - 12	16.7 ± 6.3	8.5	1.7
12 - 24	0.8 ± 0.4	1.1	0.2
		463.2	92.5

SUMMARY

Satisfactory concentrations of cephaloridine, cephradine and cephazolin in blood serum of healthy male volunteers were obtained after intramuscular or intravenous administration of single doses of 500 mg. The maximal level in serum was 16.74 ± 2.41 μg/ml for cephradine, 15.38 ± 2.63 μg/ml for cephaloridine and 14.47 ± 2.38 μg/ml for cephazolin and was obtained half an hour after intramuscular injection. The levels of cephradine, cephaloridine and cephazolin a quarter of an hour after intravenous injection were $40.12 \pm 4.71, 38.04 \pm 2.35$ and 37.33 ± 2.80 μg/ml respectively. The recovery of cephradine, cephaloridine and cephazolin in the 24 hours urine after intramuscular or intravenous injection was 88.9, 88.4 and 91.5 and 90.5, 88.4 and 92.5 per cent respectively. The extent of binding of cephradine, cephaloridine and cephazolin to human serum proteins varied from 28% for cephradine to 41% for cephaloridine and 70% for cephazolin.

REFERENCES

Brotzu,G.(1948).Richerche su di un nuove antibiotico.Lav.Ist.Ig. Cagliari.Cited by Abraham,E.P.(1962).The cephalosporins. Pharmac.Rev.14,473-500.

Gadebusch,H.H.,Miraglia,G.J.,Basch,H.I.,Goodwin,C.,Pan,S and Renz, K.(1972).Cephradine.A new orally absorbed cephalosporin antibiotic.Advan.inAntimict.Antineopl.Chemother.1,2,1059.1062.

Gower,P.E.,Dash,C.H.and O'Callaghan,C.H.(1973).Serum and blood concentration of sodium cephalexin in man given single intramuscular and intravenous injections.

Logaras,G.and Paradelis A.G.(1973).Absorption and excretion studies of the antibiotic cephradine in human subjects.In.Progress in Chemotherapy.Proceedings of 8th International Congress of Chemotherapy.(Ed.G.Daikos,Athens,1974).Vol.1,pp

Nishida,M.,Matsubara,T.,Murakawa,T.,Mine.Y.,Yokota,Y.,Kuwahara,S and Goto,S.(1969).In vitro and in vivo evaluation of cephazolin,a new cephalosporin C derivative.Antim.Agents and Cehmother. pp.236-243.

O'Callaghan,C.H.,Tootill,J.P.R.and Robinson,W.D.(1971).A new approach to the study of serum concentrations of orally administered cephalexin.J.Pharm.Pharmac.23,50-57.

OCULAR PENETRATION AND CLINICAL EVALUATION OF

CEFTEZOLE FOR OCULAR INFECTIONS

Masao Oishi

Kenji Nishizuka, Mariko Motoyama and Takeshi Ogawa
Niigata Univeristy of Medicine, 1 Asahi-machi
Niigata-shi, Niigata-ken, Japan

SUMMARY

Intraocular penetration of Ceftezole (CTZ) was investigated in rabbit eye. The peak of aqueous humor level, 1.36 ug/ml, attained at one hour after intramuscular injection of 50mg/kg CTZ, and decreased rapidly to 2 hours. Aqueous/serum ratio in one hour was 7.4%.
After intravenous injection of 50mg/kg, the peak of aqueous level, 2.8ug/ml, revealled at 1/2 hour. The aqueous/serum ratio was 11.79%.
Compared with those of Cefazolin (CEZ), aqueous humor level of CTZ was seemd to be higher than that of CEZ. However, CEZ showed higher value of blood concentration.
Intramuscular or intravenous injections of 1.0g CTZ one or two daily revealled good effects on ocular infections, such as hordeolum, dacryocystitis, keratitis and endophthalmitis. No severe side ffects like allergic reactions were observed, and no abnormal finding in hepatic and renal tests were recognized.

Ceftezole (CTZ) has been synthesized as an analogous compound of Cefazolin (CEZ). It is a new member of the Cephalosporin group and is under development in the research laboratories of the Chugai Pharmaceutical Co. Ltd.
CTZ has a wide antibacterial spectrum for both gram positive and negative bacteria as in the case of CEZ. It possesses bactericidal action and sows antibacterial acitivity toward gram negative bacteria which are especially susceptible to Cephalosporin drugs.
The results of basic research on this drugs were repor-

ted at the 14th Interscience Conference on Antimicrobial Agent and Chemotherapy in San Francisco in 1974.

We have studied on ocular penetration and clinical experiments for ophthalmic use of CTZ, and report these results as follows.

1. Intraocular penetration

Adult white rabbits (body weight : 2.5～3.5kg) were used to investigate the intraocular penetration of CTZ.

1) Aqueous humor concentration

(1) Intramuscular injection

Fig.1 shows the results after a single intramuscular injection of 50mg/kg of CTZ. The CTZ had already penetrated into the aqueous humor one half hour after injection. A peak of 1.36μg/ml was reached after one hour, and after 2 hours, there was a concentration of 0.57μg/ml in the aqueous humor. However, after 4 hours, no CTZ could be found. The blood concentration measured simultaneously reached a peak of 32.24μg/ml after one half hour. Thereafter, it decreased rapidly reaching 0.36μg/ml after 4 hours. None could be found after 6 hours. The aqueous/serum ratio at the peak of the aqueous humor level was 7.14%.

This ratio was higher than that of CEZ (5.8%) and Cephalothin (6.8%) but lower than that of Cephaloridine (30.9%).

When the secondary aqueous humor concentration was measured one hour after the injection, a high penetration of 9.5μg/ml was obtained. This was about 7 times that obtained for the primary aqueous humor. The aqueous/serum ratio was also high : 51.77%.

(2) Intravenous injection

Fig.2 shows the aqueous humor and blood concentration when rabbits were injected once in the ear vein with 50mg/kg of CTZ. After 15 minutes, 2.73μg/ml had already penetrated into the aqueous humor and after one half hour, the maximum concentration of 2.8μg/ml was reached. Thereafter, there was a gradual decreased to 1.93μg/ml after one hour and 0.63μg/ml after 2 hours. After 4 hours, no CTZ could be found.

The blood concentration reached a peak of 39.0μg/ml after 15 minutes and thereafter, rapidly decreased. After 2 hours, it was 2.6μg/ml and after 4 hours, no CTZ could be detected. The aqueous/serum ratio at the aqueous humor level peak was 11.79%.

(3) Comparison with CEZ

The concentrations in the aqueous humor and blood after intramuscular injection of 50mg/kg were compared in a cross over with CTZ.

Aqueous humor penetration of CTZ was better than that of CEZ and a higher concentration was achieved but these high values were maintained for only a short time and tended to decrease much sooner than those of CEZ. However, CEZ showed higher value of blood concentration than that of CTZ.

2) **Ocular tissue concentration**
(1) Intramuscular injection

The ocular tissue concentration of CTZ one hour after a single intramuscular injection of 50mg/kg was measured.

There were relatively high concentration in the outer parts of the eye and lower level in the inner parts.

No drug was found in the vitreous body, the optic nerve and the lens.

(2) Intravenous injection

The ocular tissue concentration one half hour after a single intravenous injection of 50mg/kg of CTZ was very high in the outer parts of the eye and also rather high in the inner parts. There was no penetration in the lens.

In comparison of the intramuscular and intravenous injection, the concentrations were higher in the outer parts of the eye in both cases while those in the inner parts of the eye tended to be lower. There were higher concentrations with intravenous than intramuscular injection.

5. Clinical results

The clinical results are shown in Tab.1. Twenty patients were treated with CTZ injection. They consisted of 5 cases of external hordeolum, 4 of internal hordeolum caused by staph.aureus or staph.epidermidis, 2 of chronic or acute dacryocystitis by staph.aureus, α- streptococcus or GNB, one of corneal infiltration by obligate anaerobes, 3 of corneal ulcers by staph.epidermidis, corynebacterium or GNB, each one of corneal abscess by staph.epidermidis, orbital phlegmone by staph.aureus and endophthalmitis by staph.epidermidis and GNB.

Daily doses of 0.5g for children and 1.0g for adults were given intramuscularly once or twice a day. Serious cases were given 2.0g once a day intravenously or by dripping.

There were 5 cases of excellent, 11 cases of good, 3 of fair and only one case none. The efficacy rate was 80.0%.

The clinical results for different types of bacteria are shown in Tab.2. There was wide ranging efficacy against staph.aureus, staph.epidermidis and GNB. CTZ was also effective against anaerobic bacteria and fairly effective against α- streptococcus.

There were no notable side effects such as allergic reaction and no abnormalities in hepatic or renal function tests

From the results of the basic and clinical research, it can be considered that CTZ is effective against the ocular infections which respond to treatment with the conventional Cephalosporin type drugs.

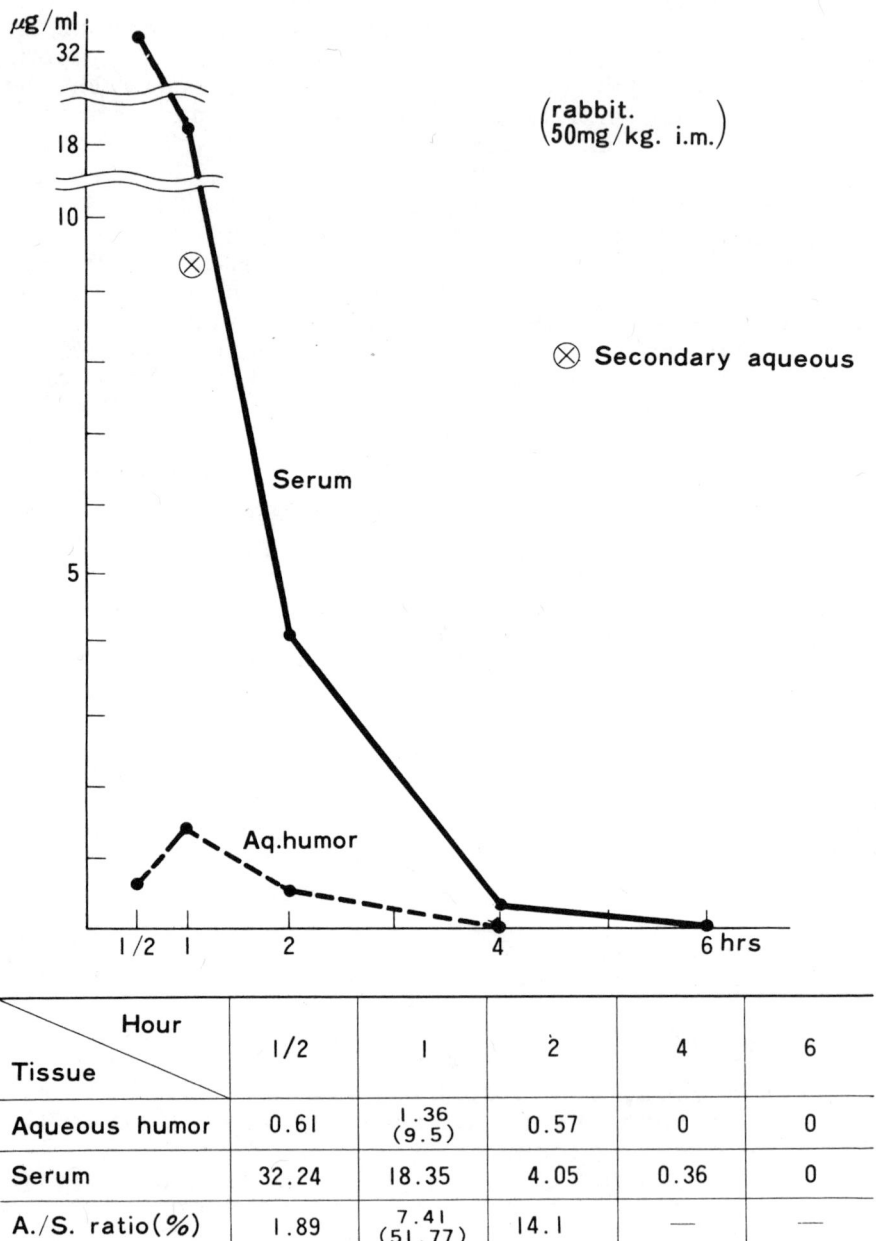

Hour Tissue	1/2	1	2	4	6
Aqueous humor	0.61	1.36 (9.5)	0.57	0	0
Serum	32.24	18.35	4.05	0.36	0
A./S. ratio(%)	1.89	7.41 (51.77)	14.1	—	—

Fig. 1. Aqueous Humor and Serum Level of CTZ.

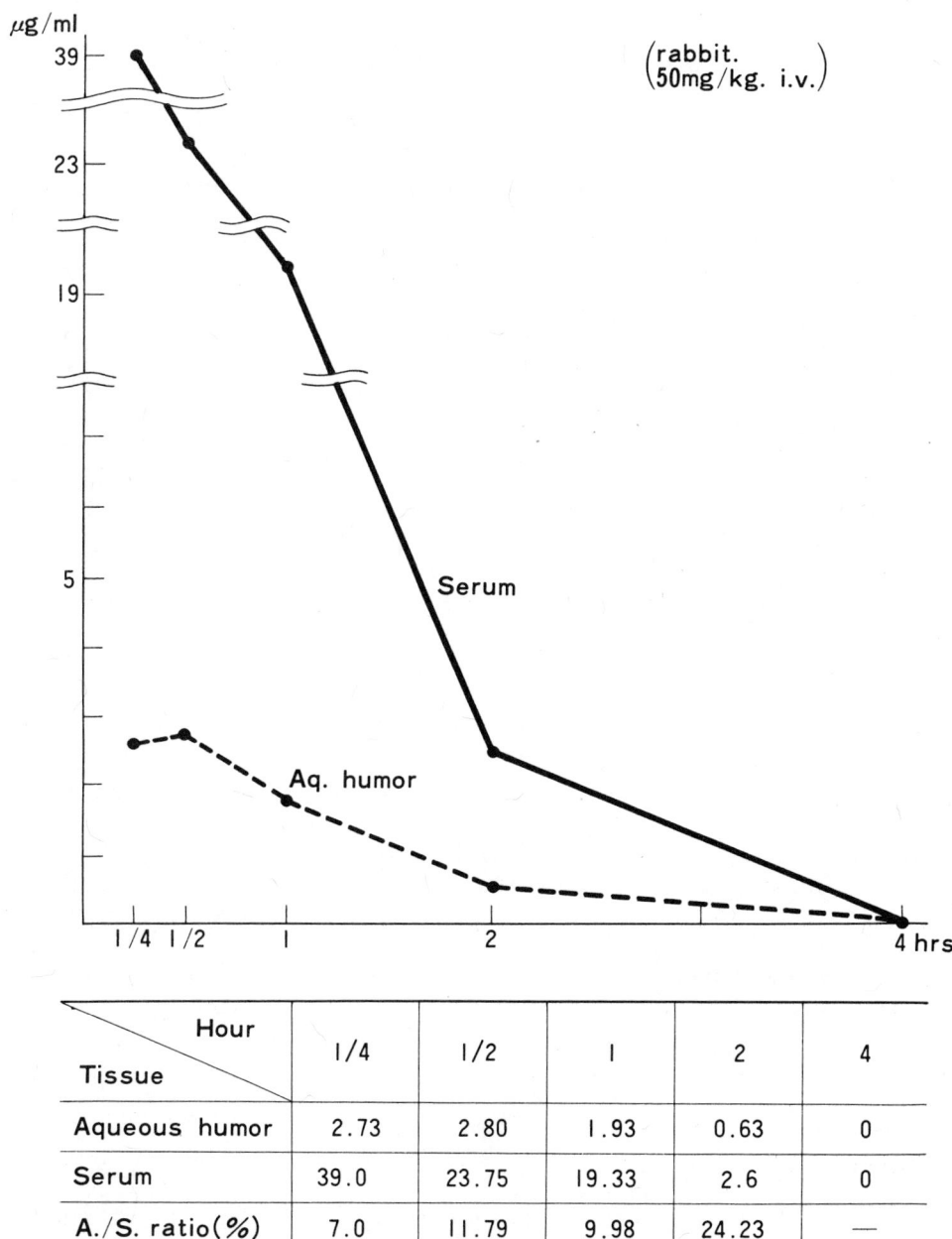

Hour Tissue	1/4	1/2	1	2	4
Aqueous humor	2.73	2.80	1.93	0.63	0
Serum	39.0	23.75	19.33	2.6	0
A./S. ratio(%)	7.0	11.79	9.98	24.23	—

Fig. 2. Aqueous Humor and Serum Level of CTZ.

Table 1. Clinical Results Classified by Diagnosis

Diagnosis	Effect				Total
	Excellent	Good	Fair	Poor	
External Hordeolum	2	3			5
Internal Hordeolum	1	1	1	1	4
Chronic Dacryocystitis		1	1		2
Acute Dacryocystitis	1		1		2
Corneal Infiltration		1			1
Corneal Ulcer		3			3
Corneal Abscess		1			1
Orbitalphlegmone	1				1
Endophthalmitis		1			1
Total	5	11	3	1	20

Table 2. Clinical Results Classified According to Causative Organisms

Organisms	Excellent	Good	Fair	Poor	Total
Staph. aureus	3	2	1	1	7
Staph. epidermidis	2				2
α-Streptococcus			1		1
Corynebacterium		1			1
GNB		2	1		3
Anaerobe		1			1
Staph. epidermidis, GNB		3			3
Total	5	9	2	1	18

PRELIMINARY STUDIES OF THE PENETRATION OF CEPHACETRILE (CELOSPOR®)

INTO HUMAN CEREBROSPINAL FLUID

      H.G. Meyer-Brunot*, C. Schenk* and A.V. Lomar**

    * Research Department, Pharmaceuticals Division,
      CIBA-GEIGY Ltd., Basle, Switzerland
  **Emilio Ribas Hospital, São Paulo, Brazil

Investigations carried out in 1973 by M.B. Corrêa Lima et al. (1) afforded the first conclusive demonstration in a relatively large number of cases that cephacetrile penetrates into the cerebrospinal fluid of patients with purulent meningitis. In purulent meningitis the meninges become more permeable to the substances and also to serum proteins and substances bound to them. In the normal course of healing, their permeability diminishes again. If the meningitis is associated with some disturbance retarding the excretion of an antibiotic, e.g. renal isufficiency, the resultant elevation of the serum concentration can lead to an increase in the concentrations in the CSF, since there is a state of equilibrium between the serum-water and the CSF-water (cf. Fig. 2).

From the pharmacokinetic point of view, the space occupied by the cerebrospinal fluid may be regarded as a "deep compartment", which is to say that the rates of entry and exit of a substance are slower than the rates of elimination of the same substance from the body. Graphically (cf. Fig. 1) this manifests itself in the intersection of the serum and CSF concentration curves. Immediately after the administration of the substance the CSF concentration curve is lower than the serum-water concentration curve. Once it has passed its maximum, the concentration in the CSF declines more slowly than the concentration in the serum-water, so that in the final phase of elimination it can be higher than the plasma-water concentration. It is rather difficult to collect the experimental data required to make a kinetic analysis of the course of the concentrations of a substance in human CSF, on the one hand for technical reasons and on the other because of the ethical considera-

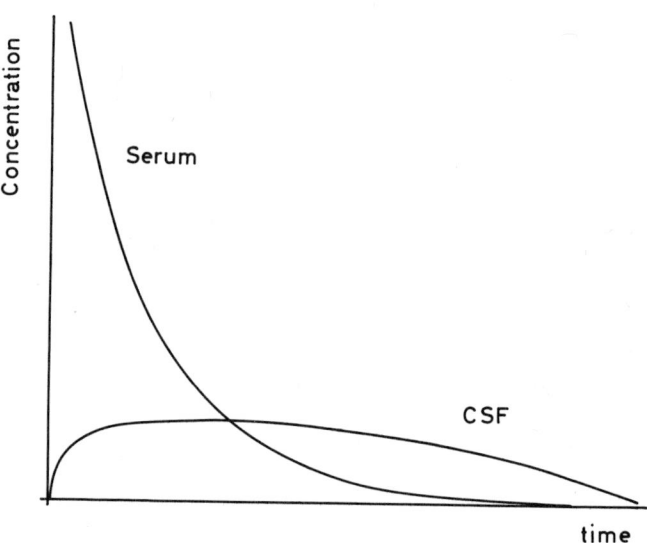

Fig. 1 Theoretical course of concentration curves in serum and CSF after i.v. administration of Celospor.

tions (repeated lumbar punctures). Despite these difficulties it proved possible to accumulate enough data to enable us to ascertain the pattern of the concentrations of Celospor in the CSF of patients with purulent meningitis. To ensure uniformity in the analysis of the samples all the microbiological determinations were performed centrally in Basle.

Fig. 2 shows the drug concentrations determined on the first day of treatment in ten patients (9 adults and 1 child) with bacterial meningitis after a single intravenous dose of 3 g. of Celospor. Samples of blood and CSF were taken 30 min and 1, 4, and 6 hrs after the administration of the drug, in such a way that at the most two lumbar punctures were made in each patient. It should be noted that the CSF concentrations are plotted on a scale five times greater than that of the serum levels. If the intervals are taken into account, it is evident that these measured values follow roughly the same pattern as the theoretical curves depicted in Fig. 1. The intersection of the curves emerges clearly from the diagram. Thirty minutes after the administration of the dose the CSF concentrations have already almost reached their maximum, amounting to between 5 and 10 mcg./ml.; after one hour they range from 6 to 12 mcg./ml. and after six hours concentrations of 2 - 6 mcg./ml. are still present. Since the M.I.C. (minimum inhibitory concentration) of the compound for the causative

PENETRATION OF CEPHACETRILE INTO CEREBROSPINAL FLUID 301

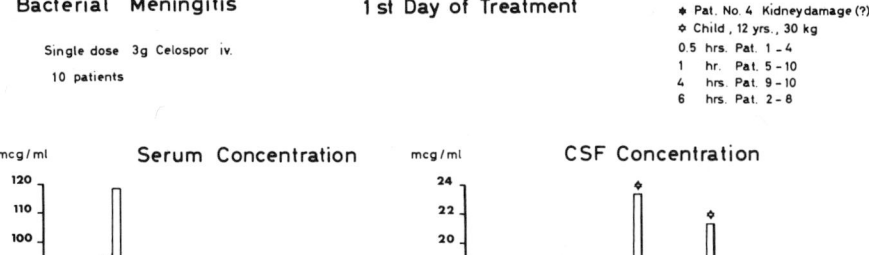

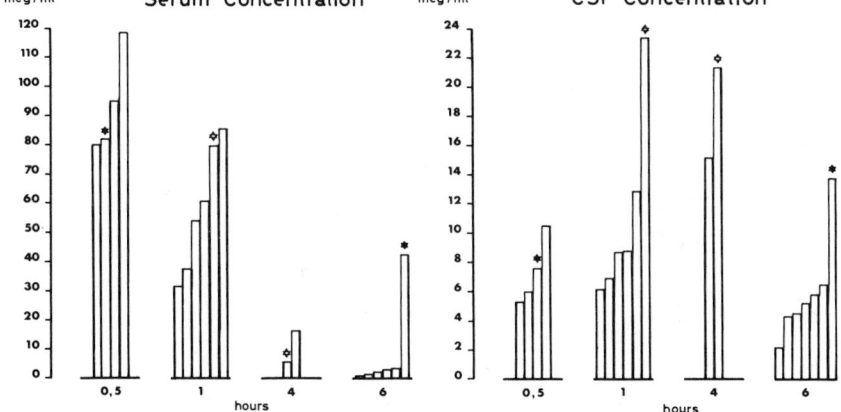

Fig. 2 Concentrations in serum and CSF of 10 patients with bacterial meningitis on 1st day of treatment, 30 minutes and 1, 4 and 6 hours after i.v. injection of 3 g. Celospor. From: Lomar, Fanous, Batt (3).

meningococci, pneumococci and staphylococci is between 0.1 and 1.0 mcg./ml., the CFS still contains therapeutically active concentrations. Gladtke and v.Hattingberg (2) have pointed out that in cases of meningitis the protein content of the CSF is also elevated, and substance bound to the proteins is inactive. Even granting the validity of this observation, the concentrations of Celospor in the CSF are still adequate. The protein content of the serum is normally between 65,000 and 85,000 mg./l. and that of the healthy CSF 180 - 300 mg./l.. In the CSF patients with meningitis it may rise to 8,000 mg./l., but is often much lower, i.e. at the most roughly 10% of the serum protein content. Conceding that 20% of the CSF concentration of Celospor may be inactive - which would correspond to the amount bound in the serum - what remains is still in excess of the M.I.C..

Fig. 3 shows the concentrations measured on the fifth day of treatment in eight of the ten above mentioned patients, who had in the meantime been given Celospor in a dosage of 3 g. four times daily i.v. at intervals of six hours. The serum concentrations display the same pattern as on the first day; the CSF concentrations are slightly lower (3 - 7 mcg./ml. after 30 minutes and 1 hour and

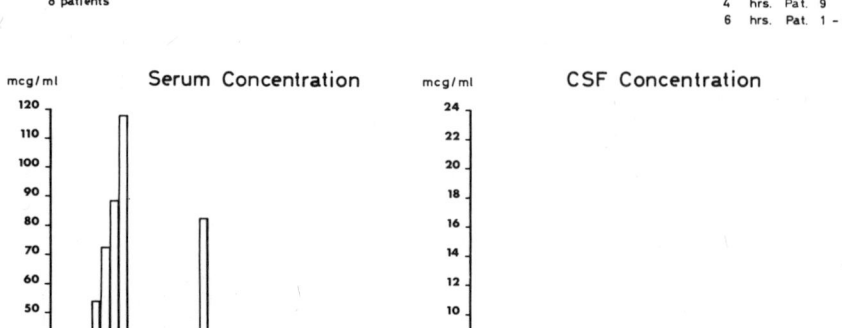

Fig. 3 Concentrations in serum and CSF of 8 of the patients inluded in Fig. 2 on 5th day of treatment, 30 minutes and 1, 4 and 6 hours after i.v. injection of 3 g. Celospor.

1 - 3 mcg./ml. after 6 hours), which is consistent with the decrease in the permeability of the meninges as healing progresses. The CSF concentrations are, however, still above the M.I.C. for the causative cocci.

In the table at the foot of Fig. 4 are listed the steady-state concentrations of Celospor found in the serum and CSF of three patients with purulent meningitis during a continuous intravenous infusion of the drug. As is evident from the curves, after the priming dose the CSF concentration rises during the infusion until it attains a constant equilibrium level. This equilibrium level can be defined for any given substance by the partition quotient q = CSF conc./serum-water conc.. In the three cases in question, the partition quotient of Celospor is consistently in the region of 0.4, which means that the steady-state concentration in the CSF is, on the average, 40% of the concentration in the serum water.

Since the risk of re lapse must be borne in mind, the CSF concentrations of Celospor in subjects with healthy meninges are shown for comparison in Fig. 5. In the lower panel of the figure, the concentrations measured in two cases after an intravenous infusion of Celospor are plotted. As can be seen from the curve, it takes 4 - 6

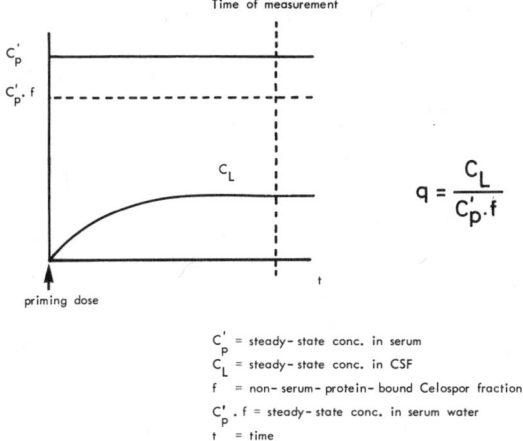

Patient treated by	Age in yrs.	Day of illness	iv.-infusion g/day	steady-state conc.		f = 0.79 q	q mean
				serum mcg/ml	CSF mcg/ml		
H. Arnold	19	1	12	18.2	6.2	0.431	0.395
P. Spring	59	4	10	27	8.6	0.403	~ 0.4
G. Wyss	75	11	6	13.4	3.7	0.350	

Fig. 4 Steady-state concentration of Celospor® in serum and partition quotient q = CSF conc./serum-water conc. in 3 patients with purulent meningitis.

hours until adequate levels are reached, but thereafter the concentrations continue to rise to levels similar to those observed in cases of meningitis. The upper panel depicts the values recorded after the intermittent administration of 2 g. Celospor i.v. every six hours. One hour after the first dose, only traces of Celospor were detected in the CSF; one hour after the fourth dose the concentrations ranged from 3 - 6 mcg./ml.. Under these conditions also, the rise in the CSF concentrations was much slower in persons with healthy meninges than in patients with meningitis. All in all, these findings show that, provided high enough doses are administered, adequate concentrations of Celospor can be reached even in the CSF of healthy persons, so that the risk of relapses occurring owing to the presence of insufficient antibacterial concentrations at the site of infection should be minimal.

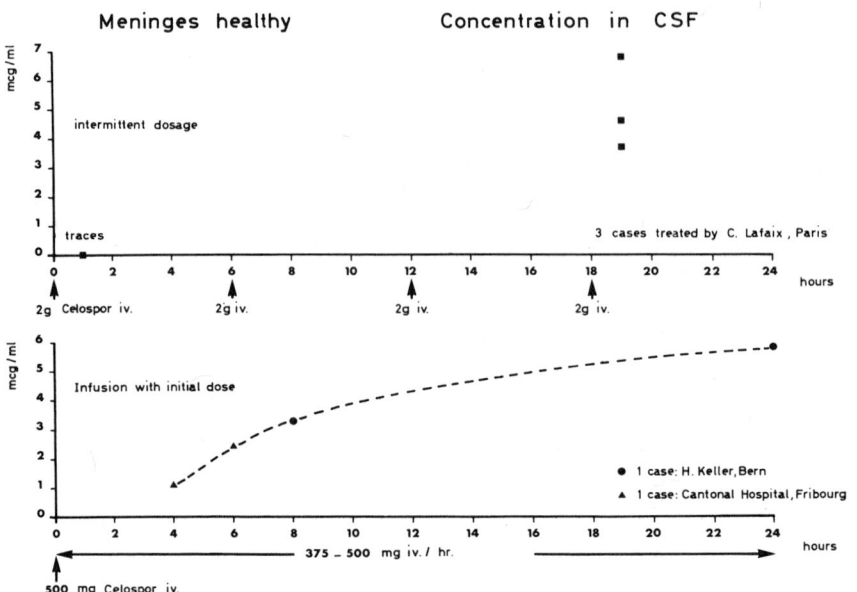

Fig. 5 Concentrations in the CSF of 3 healthy volunteers after intermittent i.v. administration of 2 g. Celospor (upper panel) and of 2 patients during continuous i.v. infusion at a rate of 375-500 mg./hr. after an initial i.v. dose of 500 mg..   From: Keller, Lafaix (3)

References

(1) M.B. Corrêa Lima, E.C. Neto, J. Gorinstein and I. Casz
    A Folha Médica 66, 309 - 316, 1973

(2) E. Gladtke and H.M. von Hattingberg
    Pharmakokinetik, Springer-Verlag, Berlin·Heidelberg·New York
    1973, p. 9

(3) H. Arnold, Freiburg i.Br., Germany
    R. Batt, Bern, Switzerland
    V. Fanous, Kairo, Egypt
    H. Keller, Bern, Switzerland   } personal communications
    C. Lafaix, Paris, France
    P. Spring, Basel, Switzerland
    G. Wyss, Basel, Switzerland

TISSUE CONCENTRATIONS OF CEFAZOLIN IN MAN

E. Sinagowitz, K. Pelz*, A. Burgert, W. Kaczkowski,
H. Sommerkamp, M. Westenfelder

Dept. of Urology * Dept of Microbiology
University of Freiburg, W. Germany

SUMMARY

The antimicrobial efficacy of cefazolin was tested in human patients undergoing urological operations. Concentrations in serum and homogenized skeletal muscle were determined by means of the agar well diffisuion method using a spore suspension of Bacillus subtilus ATCC 6633. Measurements in tissue homogenates were regarded as sufficient for evaluation of antimicrobial activity provided the right standard solution fluid and the amount of retained blood is considered. 2 g of cefazolin given in a short infusion of 25 min reached a peak concentration in muscle tissue of 20 ug/g. This concentration is high enough to inhibit nearly all strains of E.coli, Klebsiella, Salmonella, Shigella and the main part of Proteus mirabilis.

Cefazolin is known as cephalosporin C derivate with a wide range of activity against gram-positive and gram-negative microorganisms. As compared to cephalothin its activity against E.coli, Klebsiella and Salmonella is higher (Nishida et al, 1969; Naumann and Reintjens, 1974; Knothe, 1974; Hoffmann and Vomel, 1974). An elimination half-time of about 2 hours provides high serum levels and therefore allows longer dosage intervals (Naumann and Reintjens, 1974; Regamay et al, 1974). It is assumed that the high protein binding rate of 70-86% (Regamay et al, 1974; Naumann and Reintjens, 1974) leads to lower cefazolin levels in plasma water, the latter being considered the only effective fraction (Bergeron et al,1973; Scholtan, 1968). But in order to evaluate the antimicrobial activity of cefazolin at the site of infection we tested its activity in human tissue.

MATERIAL AND METHODS

Cefazolin was administered to 18 patients undergoing urological operations in different modes of application:

4 patients received a 1 g i.v. injection;

3 patients 2 g in a 2 hours infusion; and

11 patients 2 g in a short infusion of 25 min.

Blood samples and muscle tissue specimens were taken simultaneously at prefixed intervals. Only well perfused muscle tissue was removed in very small pieces from the operation wound and the psoas muscle. Muscle was homogenized with phosphate buffer saline in a 1:1 ratio.

In order to get measureable concentrations the supernatant of the muscle homogenate was diluted with phosphate buffer saline, the test serum was diluted with serum obtained from the same patient before application of cefazolin. The concentrations were determined biologically by means of the agar well diffusion method according to Klein (1957) in the modification as described by Vomel and Hoffmann (1974). The medium was Bacto Antibiotic Medium 1 (Penassay Seed Agar from Difco) inoculated at a temperature of $70^{\circ}C$ with a spore suspension of Bacillus subtilis ATCC 6633 diluted 1:1000. After an incubation time of 21 hours at $37^{\circ}C$ the diameters of the inhibiting zones were measured by means of vernier callipers by two persons in order to avoid reading errors. Finally the concentrations were determined graphically using the standard curves obtained in the same assay.

RESULTS

It is important to select the correct solution fluid for preparing the standard curve. Fig.1 presents the comparison of standard curves obtained with different solution fluids. The curves obtained with the supernatant of muscle homogenate and phosphate buffer saline are corresponding whereas the position of the serum curve indicates that higher tissue concentrations would be determined than actually exist. Thus we used phosphate buffer saline for determination of tissue concentrations, since such amounts of muscle as needed were not available.

Following a suggestion by Rosin et al (1974) the amount of retained blood in the tissue specimens was estimated comparing the tissue:blood ratio of haemaglobin and cefazolin (Fig.2). Whereas the relative haemaglobin content remained nearly stable the tissue:serum ratio of cefazolin showed marked differences with a peak of 45% at 2 hours. These results suggest that the systematic error due to retained blood seem to be very low.

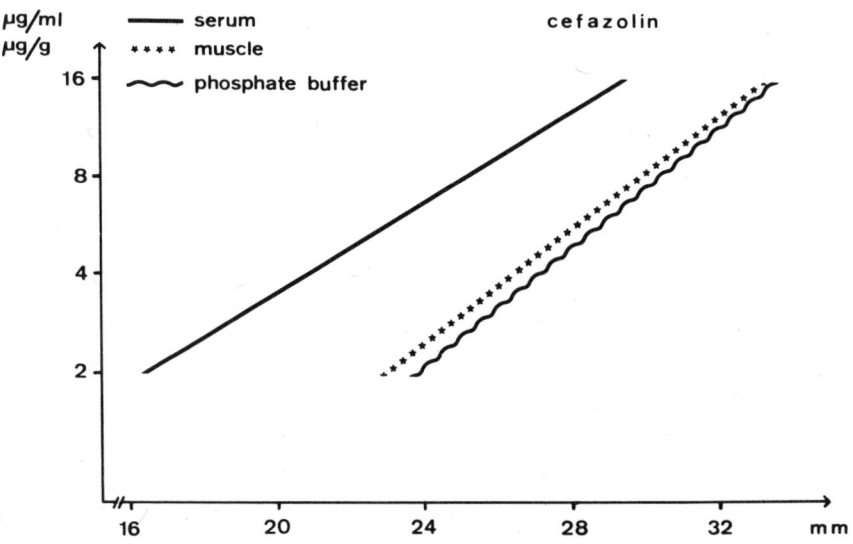

Fig.1 Standard curves determined with human serum, human muscle tissue, and phosphate buffer solution.

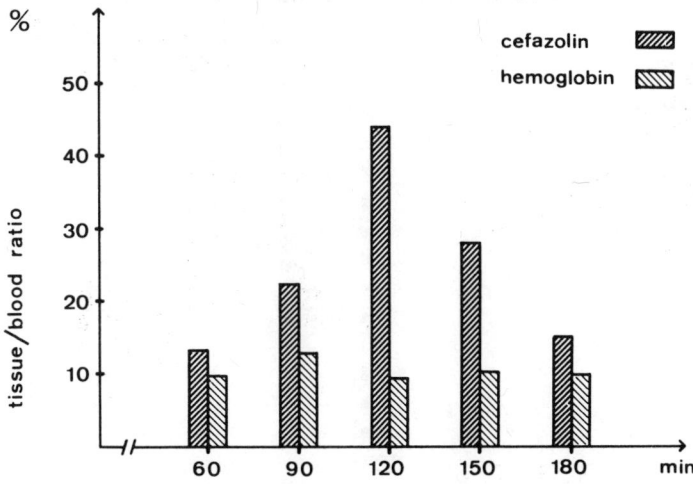

Fig. 2 The ratio tissue:blood of haemaglobin and cefazolin in human muscle tissue.

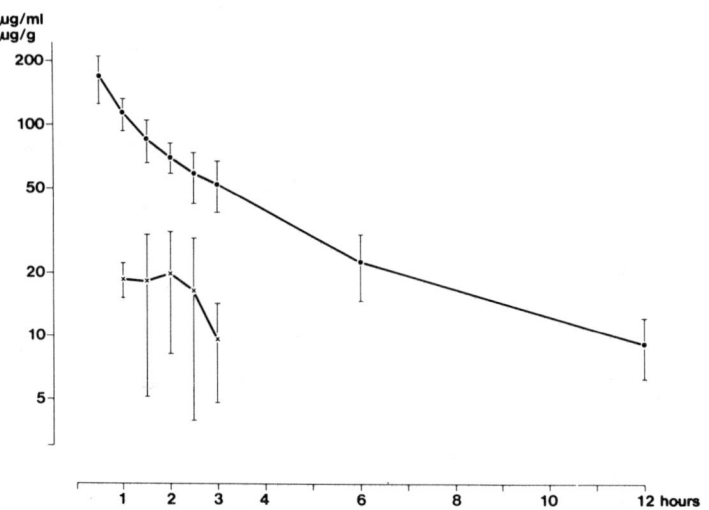

Fig. 3 Serum and muscle tissue concentrations in man after a short infusion of 2 g of cefazolin in 25 min (11 patients, mean value ± standard deviation)

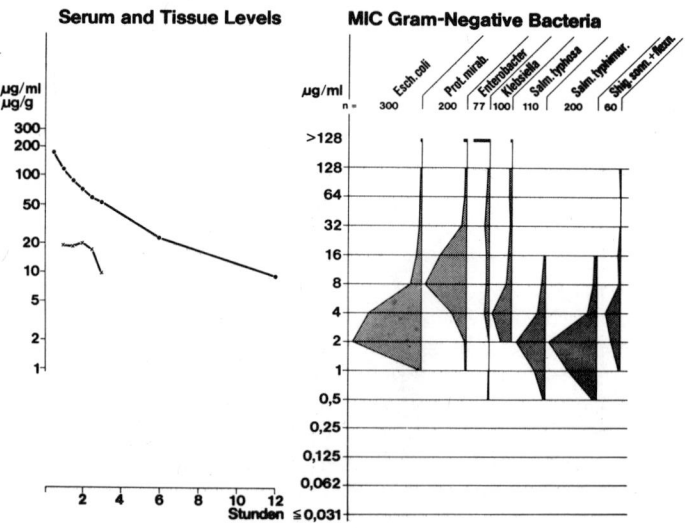

Fig. 4 MIC values of gram-negative bacteria (Knothe, 1974) compared to serum and tissue levels of cefazolin

Due to the mode of application the serum and tissue levels of cefazolin showed a different behaviour. One hour after an iv injection of 1 g of cefazolin the serum concentration was 80 ug/ml, after 6 hours it was still 15 ug/ml. The tissue concentration was increasing to 11.5 ug/g after 2 hours and then declining slightly.

After an infusion of 2 g cefazolin in 2 hours the peak concentration in serum was reached in 2.5 hours with 146 ug/ml, the level after 6 hours was 31 ug/ml. In muscle the highest concentration of 22 ug/g was reached after 3 hours.

30 min after start ofa short infusion (25 min) of 2 g cefazolin the serum level was 171 ug/ml (Fig. 3) which decreased in 6 hours to 22.5 ug/ml. The highest concentration in muscle was reached after 2 hours with 20 ug/g.

DISCUSSION

The optimal method for measuring tissue concentrations of chemotherapeutic drugs is still controversial. Naber et al (1973) suggested levels in the lymph fluid - at least for the kidney - as representative for tissue concentrations. Chisholm et al (1973) regarded the fluid collected in tissue cages according to Guyton (1963) as an equivalent of interstitial fluid. Tan et al (1972) used a skin window for sampling interstitial fluid, and Simon et al (1973) used the fluid in an artificial skin blister for evaluation of tissue concentrations.

We regard measurements of drug concentrations in tissue homogenates as sufficient enough provided the right standard solution fluid and the amount of retained blood is taken into consideration.

Comparing the modes of application of cefazolin we preferred the infusion of 2 g cefazolin in a short time of 25 min despite the recommendation of 2 g cefazolin in a 2 hours infusion (Vomel and Hoffmann, 1974) since no marked differences in serum and tissue concentrations were observed. Another important reason for this preference is the easier supervision of the infusion time by the staff.

Comparing the serum and tissue levels with the MIC values of the main gram-negative bacteria according to Knothe (1974) Fig.4) it becomes evident that cefazolin given in a dosage of 2 g in 25 min two times a day will reach nearly all strains of E.coli, Klebsiella, Salmonella, Shigella and the main part of Proteus mirabilis.

REFERENCES

Bergeron, M.G., Brusch, J.L., Barza, M. and Weinstein, L. (1973) Antimicrobial Agents and Chemotherapy, 4, 396-401.

Chisholm, G.D., Waterworth, P.M., Calnan, J.S. and Garrod, L.P. (1973) British Medical Journal, 1, 569-573.

Guyton, A.C. (1963) Circulation Research, 12, 399-414.

Hoffmann, R. and Vömel, W. (1974) Infection, 2 (Suppl.1),6-17.

Klein, P : Bakteriologische Grundlagen der chemotherapeutischen Laboratoriums-Praxis, Springer, Heidelberg, 1957.

Knothe, H. (1974) Infection, 2 (Suppl.1), 1-5.

Naber, K., Madsen, P.O.,Bichler, K-H., Sauerwein, D. (1973) Infection 1, 208-213.

Naumann, P. and Reintjens, E. (1974) Infection 2, 19-24.

Nishida, M., Matzubara, T., Murakawa, T., Mine, Y., Yokota, Y., Kuwahara, S. and Goto, S. (1969) Antimicrobial Agents and Chemotherapy, 236-243.

Regamay, C., Gordon, R.C. and Kirby, W.M.W. (1974) Archives of Internal Medicine, 133, 407-410.

Rosin, H., Rosin,A-M and Krämer, J. (1974) Infection 2, 3-6.

Scholtan, W. (1968) Antibiotica et Chemotherapia, 14, 53-93. (Karger, Basel/New York).

Simon, C., Malercyzk, V., Brahmstaedt, E. and Toeller, W. (1973) Deutsche Medizinische Wochenschrift, 98, 2448-2450.

Tan, J.S., Trott, A. and Phair, J.P. (1972) The Journal of Infectious Diseases, 126, 492-497.

Vömel, W. and Hoffmann, R. (1974) Infection, 2 (Suppl.1), 40-48.

CEPHAZOLIN SODIUM - AN IN VIVO AND IN VITRO EVALUATION OF 100 PATIENTS WITH URINARY TRACT INFECTIONS IN A DISTRICT GENERAL HOSPITAL

Diana M. D. Rimmer

Department of Microbiology
Hillingdon Hospital
Middlesex, England

Cephazolin sodium is a semi-synthetic cephalosporin antibiotic given by the intramuscular or intravenous route. Peak serum levels of 38 mcg/ml have been obtained following an intramuscular dose of 500 mg. of cephazolin, recordable serum levels persisting for up to eight hours later. Approximately 60 - 80% of an intramuscular dose is excreted in the urine in the biologically active form in the first six hours. Urine levels of 1000 mcg/ml have been recorded following a single 500 mg. intramuscular dose.

One hundred patients were treated with cephazolin sodium for urinary tract infection. The sole criterion for inclusion in the trial was two urine samples yielding more than 100,000 bacteria per ml. of urine, on successive days. Clean catch mid-stream specimens or catheter specimens were refrigerated and processed within 2 - 3 hours of collection. Bacteria were counted using the filter paper strip technique (Leigh & Williams, 1964).

Disc antibiotic sensitivity testing was carried out by the Stokes method, using Oxoid Diagnostic Sensitivity Test Agar and 30 mcg. cephazolin discs (Stokes, 1968). Minimum inhibitory concentrations of cephazolin sodium for the urinary pathogens was determined by a serial dilution method on solid media.

After obtaining consent of the clinician in charge, patients fulfilling the basic criterion were admitted to the trial. The course of cephazolin lasted for five days and consisted of 500 mg. doses given intramuscularly at 12 hourly intervals. Urine samples were collected on the 3rd, 5th, and 8th days after the start of the course, and a follow-up specimen collected between 3rd - 6th week after the start of the course. Note was taken as to whether other antimicrobial agents had been administered during the follow-up period.

The criterion of cure was absence of the infecting organism on the 8th day and in the follow-up specimen.

The age range for trial patients was 22 - 94 years with an average age of 65 years. Sixty-five percent of the patients were females, 35% were males.

In 48 of the patients the urinary tract infection was associated with catheterisation. This group further subdivided into 42 patients where infection followed a single catheterisation and six patients who had long-term, in-dwelling catheters. Of the remaining 52 patients not catheterised, a further 18 had conditions associated with predisposition to urinary tract infection (diabetes mellitus, urinary tract abnormalities, etc.).

The organisms isolated are presented (Table 1). Two patients included in the trial had mixed infections, one with significant numbers of both Escherichia coli and Proteus, and another with Escherichia coli and Streptococcus faecalis, therefore 102 organisms were identified.

All the organisms were reported as sensitive on routine disc sensitivity testing. The range of minimum inhibitory concentrations of cephazolin for the isolates was recorded (Table 2). Eighty-nine percent of the M.i.c.'s for Escherichia coli fell in the range 2.5 - 20 mcg/ml.

Clinically, the patients were divided into two groups - those with symptoms of urinary tract infection and those without.

Eighty-nine patients had symptoms of infection. Eleven of the 89 had loin pain and pyrexia as well as frequency and dysuria, and in one patient the organism was simultaneously isolated from blood and urine. Five of this group showed no clinical response to the course of antibiotic. Two of the five had indwelling catheters whereas the other three had at no time been catheterised.

Eleven patients were symptomless throughout the trial.

Bacteriologically, the patients were assessed on the 8th days and at follow-up between the 3rd and 6th weeks.

On the 8th day (Table 3), the infecting organism had been eliminated from 83% of the patients, 11% still had a significant growth of the initial pathogen, 4% had a mixed growth of organisms, including significant numbers of the original organism and 2% showed reinfection with an entirely different bacterium.

TABLE 1

ORGANISMS ISOLATED

Organisms	Number
Escherichia Coli	55
Proteus Spp.	28
Streptococcus Faecalis	7
Klebsiella Pneumoniae	3
Staphylococcus (Coag.pos.)	5
Micrococcus	4

TABLE 2

RANGE OF M.I.C. OF CEPHAZOLIN FOR INFECTING ORGANISMS

Mcg/ml	1.25	2.5	5	10	20	40	>40
Escherichia Coli		├──────────────────────────┤					
Proteus Spp.				├──────────────────┤			
Streptococcus Faecalis			├────────┤				
Klebsiella Pneumoniae				├────────┤			
Staphylococcus (Coag. Pos.)	├────────┤						
Micrococcus	├────────┤						

Of the original 100 patients, 21 were lost to follow-up, and nine died between completion of the course and the 3rd week (Fig. 1). No death was attributed to cephazolin sodium. Seven deaths were due to bronchopneumonia, one to myocardial infarction and one to "natural causes".

Urines obtained during the 3rd - 6th weeks from 53 of the remaining 70 patients, i.e. 75%, showed complete elimination of the original infecting organism. In 25% of the 70 patients the infecting organism was still present in significant numbers.

During the trial two patients with well-documented penicillin allergy were treated with cephazolin with no untoward effects. Another patient developed an urticarial rash on the buttocks, over the sacral area and around the knees on the 6th day. She was apyrexial. The rash responded to antihistamines within four days. No other local or systemic reactions to the drug were noted.

In conclusion, a random group of 100 patients in a general hospital were treated with cephazolin sodium for proven urinary tract infections. Sixty-six percent had conditions predisposing to urinary tract infection. Under these somewhat difficult conditions the original infecting organism remained absent from the urine of 75% of the 70 patients followed in the 3rd - 6th week period. This compares very favourably with response to other antimicrobial agents currently used in urinary tract infections.

REFERENCES

Leigh, D.A. & Williams, J.D. (1964). Method for the detection of significant bacteriuria in large groups of patients. J. Clin. Path., $\underline{17}$:498

Stokes, E.J. (1968). Clinical Bacteriology, 3rd Edition, p.179. London. Arnold.

TREATMENT OF BACTERIAL PNEUMONIA WITH CEFAZOLIN

Malcolm T. Foster, Jr.

University of Nebraska Medical Center

Omaha, Nebraska, USA

INTRODUCTION

Cefazolin, a relatively new and recently marketed cephalosporin antibiotic, has many pharmacological properties and an antibacterial spectrum which should make it an ideal agent in a patient with suspected bacterial pneumonia.

Previous studies have shown that intramuscular cefazolin produces relatively high blood levels, has a relatively long half life, and modest protein binding. Tissue penetration is good except for the central nervous system and the prostate gland.

Sensity studies have previously shown that all strains of Diplococcus pneumonia and most strains of Staphlococcus aureus, Klebsiella, and Escherichia coli are sensitive in vitro to levels readily obtained by modest intramuscular doses. Most bacterial pneumonias in ambulatory patients are caused by one of these organisms.

The cephalosporin antibiotics are generally considered a safe group of antibiotics. The most troublesome side effects are the development of allergy and the slight possibility of cross allergenicity with the penicillins.

STUDY DESIGN

In the current study 30 consecutive patients with suspected bacterial pneumonia were treated with cefazolin 1000 milligrams administered intramuscularly every 12 hours. The drug was continued for two days after the patient became afebrile, but for a minimum of five days. The drug was to be stopped only if an adverse reaction occurred or if determined that cefazolin was an inappropriate antibacterial agent, either by in vitro antibiotic sensity results or failure to effect a clinical response.

Patients entered into this study presented to the emergency room of a large intercity charity hospital. Criteria for admission included fever, chills, cough, increased sputum production, and a pulmonary infiltrate on chest roentenogram. Children and pregnant women were excluded by design. There were no other exclusions because of condition or underlying disease(s).

Before, during, and after therapy each patient had a sputum culture, chest roentenogram, complete blood count, urinalysis, and an automated twelve channel chemical screen designed to monitor liver, renal, and other vital organs for possible drug toxicity.

RESULTS

A total of thirty consecutive patients who satisfied the above criteria for suspected bacterial pneumonia were entered into this study. Twenty-nine of the thirty responded promptly. A single patient remained febrile and was switched to ampicillin when a cefazolin resistant, ampicillin sensitive organism was demonstrated.

Bacteriology

Ten patients had infection with Diplococcus pneumonia and all responded.

Three patients had Staphlococcus aureus in their sputum and responded.

Ten patients grew normal flora and they responded as well. At least two of these had aspirated and had presumed aspiration pneumonia.

Two patients grew pure cultures of Hemophilus influenzae, one resistant and the other sensitive to cefazolin. As stated above, one responded clinically and one did not respond, requiring a change to ampicillin. The response on ampicillin was likewise very slow, suggesting local factors such as poor drainage or atelectasis may have been operative.

One patient each grew Aeromonas, Pseudomonas, and indole positive Proteus organisms. In each of these cases the organism was clearly resistant to cefazolin, but by the time this information was known the patients had improved clinically and it was elected not to change drugs.

Underlying Diseases

Most of these patients were elderly and either had singularly or in combination alcoholism, diabetes mellitus, ischemic heart disease, or chronic obstructive airway disease. Two patients had significant renal disease. The one patient who grew <u>Pseudomonas</u> had severe pulmonary carcoidosis. In fact only one patient was thought to be free of significant underlying disease. Analyses of these cases does not show any influence by the primary disease process except the one case of chronic airway disease mentioned previously. None of these patients were leukopenic, which may be seen in patients who fail to respond to antibiotic therapy for their infections.

Rate of Response

The defervescence of fever, clearing of the chest roentenogram, and decrease in leukocytosis indicated a rapid rate of response. The total duration of therapy ranged from 3 to 18 days with an average of 7.4 days.

Superinfection

In no case did superinfection occur. Nor did any pathogen persist and emerge resistant to cefazolin.

Clinical or Biochemical Toxicity

None of the patients experienced any clinical abnormality despite careful daily questioning by the investigator. By chance, none of the patients reported prior penicillin alergy, so no observations could be made about cross sensitization.

Only one patient had a biochemical abnormality develop while on therapy, a transient rise in creatine phosphokinase (CPK), which might possibly have been secondary to the intramuscular injections.

None of the patients had any change in their renal function including two patients with significant renal failure.

DISCUSSION

Bacterial pneumonia remains a very common and often lethal disease. In the past most cases were due to infection with <u>Diplococcus</u> pneumoniae and occasionally <u>Klebsiella</u> or <u>Staphlococcus</u> aureus. Currently however, the changing pattern of bacterial infections with the emergence of hospital acquired infections, antibiotic resistant infections, and Gram negative organisms as significant pathogens requires a critical reappraisal of the management of suspected bacterial pneumonias.

The current study suggests that cefazolin is an appropriate agent in suspected bacterial pneumonia. However, the variety of organisms isolated serves as a reminder that definitive bacteriological studies are necessary.

The Gram stain of the sputum or transtracheal aspirate still remains a useful tool for the clinician, not because it identifies the organism, but rather because it alerts him when either a mixed flora is present or that Gram negative organisms predominate. Used in this manner the Gram stain can be most helpful until the results of sputum and blood cultures are known.

Clinicians are often puzzled by the patient with an apparent bacterial pneumonia and an appropriate and prompt response when an antibiotic is administered, but failure to isolate a pathogen. This is evident in the current study. Some possible explanations could be that a patient has aspiration pneumonia, or infection with anaerobic or other fastidious organisms, or non-bacterial pathogens such as viruses or indeed the process might be a non-infection such as a pulmonary embolus. On occasion a patient with no demonstrable pathogen in the sputum will have a positive blood culture and prior antibiotic therapy is yet another possible explanation for failure to isolate a pathogen.

Equally frustrating is the patient that fails to respond when an appropriate antibiotic is administered. Some of the possible explanations include: the organism isolated is not the real pathogen; the antibiotic does not reach the site of infection; metastatic infection, abscess formation, or empyema has occurred; or there is inadequate drainage of pus or persistent atelectasis. Superinfecting organism or mixed infection, underlying disease or obstruction, drug fever, emergence of resistant organisms or formation of L forms are also possible mechanisms for failure.

When the aforementioned are considered it is not surprising that the choice of an appropriate antibiotic is difficult. Penicillin Gr V has stood the test of time and is the drug of choice for pneumococcal pneumonia. Cephalosporins such as cefazolin might be indicated for: _Klebsiella_ infections, _Staphlococcal_ infections, infection with mixed flora, and patients allergic to penicillin.

The current study indicates that cefazolin is both effective and safe in suspected bacterial pneumonia.

IDENTIFICATION OF BETA-LACTAMASES BY ANALYTICAL ISOELECTRIC FOCUSING

M. Matthew and A.M. Harris

Microbiology Department, Glaxo Research Ltd.

Greenford, Middx. U.K.

SUMMARY

Analytical isoelectric focusin gives a direct visual comparison of beta-lactamases, down to extremely low levels of activity, from very crude intracellular preparations. It differentiates between enzymes that are biochemically and immunologically indistinguishable. The genus of the host strain does not affect the isoelectric focusing pattern of an R-factor-mediated beta-lactamase. This can therefore be used in epidemiological studies to monitor the transfer of resistance. Chromosomal beta-lactamases appear to be genus, species and subspecies specific; separation of the enzymes by isoelectric focusion could therefore be used as an aid to taxonomic grouping.

INTRODUCTION

Isoelectric focusing(Vesterberg,1973) is a method of separation in which electrophoresis is used to produce a pH gradient in a mixture of ampholytes. One obtains a very high degree of resolution because focusing is caused by forces that act against diffusion, and enzymes are therefore concentrated during their separation. The technique has been used in the analytical mode for the separation of beta-lactamases on thin layers of polyacrylamide gel (Matthew et al, 1975). Different enzymes produced by various strains can be seen as patterns of bands that can easily be recognised and compared.

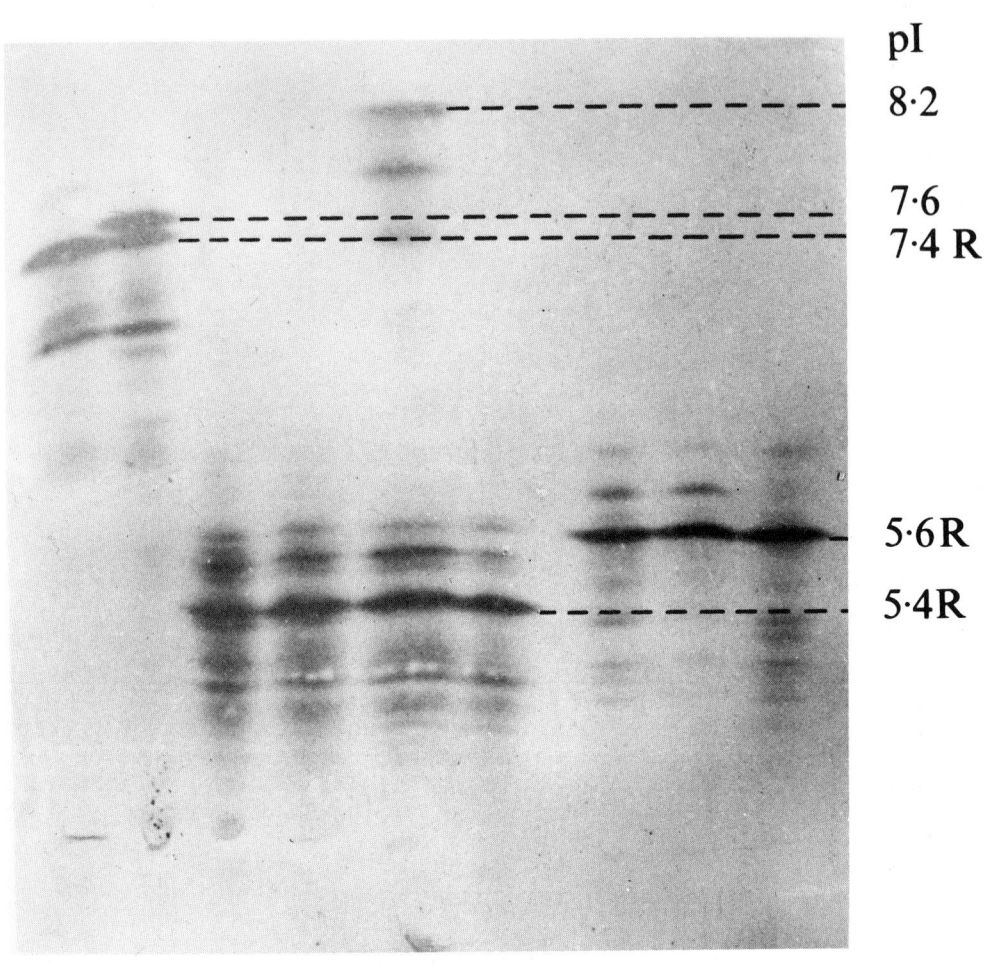

Figure 1

The technique and its application to the separation of beta-lactamases

Samples are loaded as drops of liquid on the surface of the gel; then, during electrophoresis, the enzymes migrate and align themselves as sharp bands at their isoelectric points (pI). Focused enzymes are located by damping the surface of the gel with a solution of a yellow chromogenic cephalosporin that changes colour to pink when the beta-lactam bond is broken (O'Callaghan et al, 1972). This reveals a pattern of beta-lactamase bands (Fig. I - IX), in which an enzyme usually appears as a group of bands consisting of one main band a number of satellite bands (Fig. IX). The pattern is qualitatively identical to that revealed by the conventional starch/iodine/penicillin stain and radically different from the pattern obtained with a protein stain (Matthew et al, 1975). An almost identical picture of a beta-lactamase can be obtained whether the enzyme is highly purified or contained in a completely crude preparation of broken cells. When a focused gel is stained for beta-lactamase, the bands appear gradually. By the time the weakest bands have appeared, the strongest bands have diffused, so that a complete record is obtained by taking serial photographs. In this way, samples with a 16,000-fold range of activity can be compared on a single plate. The method will detect about 0.0002 i.u. enzyme so that bands of beta-lactamase have been seen in preparations of bacteria from genera such as Haemophilus, Neisseria and Streptococcus, that are generally considered not to produce the enzyme. Preparations of 'beta-lactamase negative' mutants of Bacillus licheniformis (Ward and Per-ins, 1973), Enterobacter cloacae (Goldner et al, 1969) and Escherichia coli (Burman et al, 1973; Nguyen-Disteche et al, 1973) have also shown beta-lactamase bands after isoelectric focusing.

The method clearly separates R-factor and chromosomally-mediated beta-lactamases produced by a single strain. This is shown in the figure for strains of Klebsiella aerogenes (Fig. II, enzymes with pI 7.4 and 7.6) and Ent.cloacae (Fig.V, enzymes with pI 5.4 and 8.2). The chromosomal enzymes of the other strains in the figure are so weak that they are not visible in this early photograph. However, two groups of beta-lactamase bands were always seen in preparations from about two hundred strains known to carry transmissible R-factors.

If the beta-lactamase bands of samples run in adjacent tracks are confluent, like those of the enzyme specified by the TEM R-factor, with main band pI 5.4 (Fig. III-VI), this is very strong evidence that the enzymes are identical. The enzymes specified by the R-factors from E.coli, R_{GN14} and Rl, also have bands confluent with those of this pI 5.4 group and their published properties are identical with those of the TEM enzymes (Yamagishi et al, 1969; Richmond and Sykes, 1973; Dale and Smith, 1971). It seems probable that one may be able to predict the properties of a beta-lactamase if it is identical in isoelectric focusing with an enzyme that has already been characterised. In contrast, when enzymes that are focused in adjacent tracks have bands that are non-confluent, this is equally strong evidence that the enzymes are not identical; e.g. (Fig. I and II) the enzyme mediated by R_{GN238}, pI 7.4 is not confluent with the K.aerogenes chromosomal beta-lactamase, pI 7.6.

Isoelectric focusing will distinguish between pairs of beta-lactamases that appear to have identical biochemical properties and substrate profiles and that cross-react with antiserum to one of the enzymes. Separation of one such pair, the beta-lactamases specified by the TEM and RPl R-factors (Sykes and Richmond, 1970) is shown in the figure (VI, VII). The pairs of chromosomal beta-lactamases from Ent.cloacae P99 and 214 (Fleming et al, 1963; Hennessey, 1967) and E.coli D31 and 214T (Burman et al, 1968; Smith, 1963) also have similar biochemical properties and cross-react with antiserum to one of the pair: each pair of enzymes has been separated by isoelectric focusing.

Enzymes with close pI values were always checked for identity or non-identity by running them in adjacent tracks.

Beta-lactamases specified by R-factors

The isoelectric focusing pattern of a beta-lactamase is identical, irrespective of the genus of the host strain carrying the R-factor; e.g. in the figure, the enzymes specified by R_{GN238} (I and II), R TEM (III-VI) and RPl (VII-IX). The beta-lactamase pattern is not altered when the R-factor is integrated into the bacterial chromosome (Fig. VIII and IX). It is therefore impossible to say whether an enzyme is chromosomally or R-factor mediated unless the necessary genetic experiments have been done to prove R-factor or chromosomal transfer.

R-factor-mediated beta-lactamases had been divided by their substrate profiles into two groups (Datta and Kontomichalou, 1965; Hedges et al, 1974). These were the TEM-like enzymes and the oxacillin-hydrolysing enzymes. The latter were further divided into two sub-groups, typified by the beta-lactamases specified by R_{GN238} and R1818 (Dale and Smith, 1974). Isoelectric focusing has demonstrated the existence of two kinds of TEM-like enzyme (Fig. VI and VII). This method has also shown the existence of a third type of oxacillin-hydrolysing enzyme (Matthew, unpublished results). It has a substrate profile similar to that of the R1818 enzyme and is typified by the beta-lactamase specified by R55 (Dale and Smith, 1974).

Drs. N. Datta and R.W. Hedges kindly gave us over a hundred R-factors that specified beta-lactamase. They had been collected from different genera all over the world and had been transferred for the purpose of comparison, into an E.coli K12. Just over 70% specify the TEM-type enzyme and the very similar RP1-type enzyme is specified by another 10% of the R-factors.

As well as showing which particular beta-lactamase is responsible for resistance, isoelectric focusing can be used in epidemiological studies for observing the transfer, between species, of plasmids that specify beta-lactamase. Presumably the method could also be applied to other R-factor specified enzymes, such as those that inactivate aminoglycosides.

Chromosomally-mediated beta-lactamases

These have been seen as a single group of bands in about two hundred and fifty strains from all twenty six gram-negative and gram-positive genera so far examined. The organisms were identified by the methods of Cowan and Steel (1965). It has not been possible to transfer resistance from any of the strains, which are considered to produce only chromosomal beta-lactamases. There is a great variety of these enzymes which have isoelectric points ranging from 3.9 to 8.7 (Matthew and Harris, unpublished results). The distribution of isoelectric points is not related to the substrate profile or other biochemical properties of the beta-lactamases.

The chromosomal beta-lactamases appear to be genus, species and sub-species specific, and strains that produce identical beta-lactmase have always had identical bacterial chracteristics. In the genus Klebsiella, which contains many variable biotypes, the strains can easily be group by the isoelectric focusing patterns of the beta-lactamases they produce. Since it seems probable that beta-lactamases may be universally produced by bacteria, separation of the enzymes by analytical isoelectric focusing could be used in bacterial taxonomy.

REFERENCES

Burman, L.G., Park, J.T., Lindström, E.B. and Boman, H.G. (1973) J.Bacteriol, 116, 123-130.

Cowan, S.T. and Steel, K.J. (1965) Identification of Medical Bacteria, pp.76-82. Cambridge: Cambridge University Press.

Dale, J.W. and Smith, J.T. (1971) Biochem.J., 123, 507-512.

Datta, N. and Kontomichalou, P. (1965) Nature, London, 208, 239-241.

Fleming, P.C., Goldner, M. and Glass, D.G. (1963) Lancet, i, 1399-1401.

Goldner, M., Glass, D.G. and Fleming, P.C. (1969) J.Bacteriol., 97, 961.

Hedges, R.W., Datta,N., Kontamichalou, P. and Smith, J.T. (1974) J.Bacteriol., 117, 56-62.

Hennessey, T.D.G. (1967) J.Gen.Microbiol., 49, 277-285.

Matthew, M., Harris, A.M., Marshall, M.J. and Ross, G.W. (1975) J.Gen.Microbiol., 88, 169-178.

Nguyen-Disteche, M., Pollock, J.J., Ghuysen, J-M., Puig, J., Reynolds, P., Perkins, H.R., Coyette, J. and Salton, M.R.J. (1973) Eur.J.Biochem., 41, 457-463.

O'Callaghan, C.H., Morris, A., Kirby, S.M. and Shingler, A.H. (1972) Antimicrobial Agents and Chemotherapy, 1, 283-288.

Richmond, M.H. and Sykes, R.B. (1973) Adv.Microb.Physiol., 9, 31-88.

Smith, J.T. (1963) J.Gen.Microbiol., 30, 299-306.

Sykes, R.B. and Richmond, M.H. (1970) Nature, London, 226, 952-954.

Vesterberg, O. (1973) Science Tools, 70, 22-28.

Ward, J.B. and Perkins, H.R. (1973) Biochem.J., 135, 721-728.

Yamagishi, S., O'Hara, K., Sawai, T. and Nitsuhashi, S. (1969) J.Biochem. (Tokyo), 66, 11-20.

THE COMBINED EFFECT OF PROTEIN-BINDING AND BETA-LACTAMASES ON THE ACTIVITY OF PENICILLINS AND CEPHALOSPORINS

SYDNEY SELWYN and CHARLES LAM

Department of Bacteriology, Westminster Medical School

London, SW1P 2AR, United Kingdom

Although the practical significance of protein-binding by antibiotics remains controversial, its potential importance is underlined by the therapeutic need for maximal tissue levels, especially with bacteriocidal drugs of the penicillin and cephalosporin groups. Yet, despite startling variations in protein-binding among members of the two groups, the effects of this parameter on antibiotic action have been largely ignored by investigators. Similarly, the therapeutic implications of wide differences in resistance to beta-lactamases among these antibiotics have long awaited a fully comparative and realistic evaluation. Studies have therefore been conducted into these two potential impediments to adequate antibiotic therapy, both individually and when combined. Parallel experiments were performed on benzylpenicillin, ampicillin, amoxycillin, methicillin, cloxacillin, flucloxacillin, carbenicillin, cephaloridine, cephalothin, cephalexin, cephradine and cephazolin.

MATERIALS AND METHODS

Two strains of Staphylococcus aureus were studied in detail: a penicillin-sensitive derivative of '663' originally provided by Glaxo Laboratories Limited (663d) and a penicillin-resistant wound isolate (WS 7). Two clinical isolates of Proteus mirabilis were also used; one was penicillin-sensitive (WP 5) and the other was penicillin-resistant (WP 8).

All liquid cultures, including tube dilution series, were in peptone water; for tests on protein-binding pooled heat-inactivated normal human serum was added in increasing amounts to a maximum of 95%.

Serum samples were screened before being pooled, to eliminate occasional specimens which were antibacterial. Bacterial inocula were approximately 10^5 colony-forming units per ml. of fresh medium. "Antibiotic Agar No. 1" (Oxoid) was the standard solid medium.

The penicillins used were a gift from Beecham Research Laboratories, the cephalosporins from Eli Lilly & Co., except for cephaloridine (from Glaxo Laboratories) and cephradine (from E. R. Squibb & Sons). Five β-lactamase preparations were used: "Neutrapen" containing 800,000 units per vial (Riker Laboratories), "β-lactamases, Batch No. 5" of unspecified potency (Whatman Biochemicals) - both from Bacillus cereus strains, 'TEM' from Escherichia coli, 'K 1' from Klebsiella aerogenes and 'P 99' from Enterobacter cloacae. The last three were gifts from Glaxo Laboratories. All were made up in solution to the same concentrations (equivalent to 80,000 units per ml.), and doubling dilutions were made after 30 minutes at $21^\circ C$. In plate tests a band of medium was spread with 50 units of enzyme per sq. cm. immediately adjacent to a line on which discs were to be placed. The plates were incubated at $30^\circ C$.

In vivo tests were performed on the 'Sutcliffe' strain of mice weighing approximately 25 gm. These were injected intraperitoneally with 10 x LD_{50} of the test bacteria suspended in 5% hog gastric mucin (donated by Glaxo Laboratories). Doubling dilutions of antibiotics were administered subcutaneously 1 hour and 5 hours after infection in batches of 5 mice per dilution. ED_{50} values were calculated by the standard Reed and Muench method.

RESULTS

The ratios of bactericidal concentration (MCC) in 95% serum to minimum inhibitory concentration (MIC) in the absence of serum are presented in Table 1 for all 12 antibiotics against the four test organisms. Cephalexin and cephradine had the lowest mean ratios and were the only antibiotics that possessed exactly the same MIC values in serum-free peptone water as in 95% serum. The actual MIC values for these two drugs were, however, relatively high (2, 8, 8 and 32 µg/ml against 663d, WS7, WP 5 and WP 8, respectively).

The results of tube and plate tests for susceptibility to the β-lactamases agreed very closely. The mean reduction in zone sizes are also included in Table 1. When realistic amounts of the enzymes were used (not exceeding 1 unit per µg of antibiotic) Neutrapen inactivated all the penicillins, the least affected being flucloxacillin (82% loss). Cephaloridine was almost completely destroyed, and a substantial loss occurred in the activity of cephalothin and cephazolin. However, cephalexin lost only 7% of its activity and cephradine was unchanged. The same trend was found using the Whatman preparation from B. cereus and the 'TEM'

TABLE 1.   SERUM PROTEIN-BINDING AND SUSCEPTIBILITY TO β-LACTAMASES AMONG PENICILLINS AND CEPHALOSPORINS

ANTIBIOTIC	Ratio of MCC in 95% serum: MIC in 0% serum					Mean* loss in activity
	Staph.		Proteus		Mean	
	663d	WS 7	WP 5	WP 8		
Penicillin G	4	16	2	$\frac{1}{\infty}$	>25	89
Ampicillin	4	8	2	∞	>25	74
Amoxycillin	4	8	2	∞	>25	72
Carbenicillin	8	16	8	∞	>25	67
Methicillin	4	16	8	∞	>25	44
Cloxacillin	8	32	16	∞	>25	39
Flucloxacillin	8	16	16	∞	>25	36
Cephaloridine	2	32	2	16	13	65
Cephalothin	4	16	4	64	22	39
Cephalexin	1	8	2	16	7	20
Cephradine	1	8	2	16	7	17
Cephazolin	8	32	8	32	21	45

$\frac{1}{\infty}$ = MCC in 95% serum not attainable

* mean % reduction in zone radii produced by the five β-lactamases.

enzyme from Esch.coli. Cephalexin and cephradine were affected by the K 1 enzyme to a lesser extent than any of the other antibiotics (27%).

A summary of the results of in vivo tests on the antibiotics is presented in Table 2. Because each of the penicillins was ineffective in vivo against two of the four test organisms, the cephalosporins performed better overall. Cephalothin, however, was relatively disappointing throughout, requiring more than twice the dose of the other cephalosporins against both Staph. aureus strains and it was ineffective (needing more than 100 mg/kg) against the penicillin-resistant Pr. mirabilis. Cephazolin was also rather disappointing in vivo, being about half as active as cephaloridine

TABLE 2. MEAN IN VIVO ACTIVITY OF ANTIBIOTICS IN INTRAPERITONEAL INFECTIONS DUE TO STAPHYLOCOCCI AND PROTEUS

Antibiotic	Mean ED_{50} (mg/kg/dose)	In vivo efficacy[+]
Penicillin G	>57	*
Ampicillin	>54	*
Amoxycillin	>53	*
Carbenicillin	>53	*
Methicillin	>74	*
Cloxacillin	>62	*
Flucloxacillin	>58	*
Cephaloridine	18.8	187
Cephalothin	51.4	*
Cephalexin	21.7	660
Cephradine	15.5	1025
Cephazolin	32.2	79

[+] Mean ratio (MIC in 0% serum : ED_{50}) x 1000 to give whole numbers

* At least one ED_{50} value not attainable (>100 mg/kg)

except against the penicillin-resistant Pr. mirabilis when it was only slightly less active on a weight-for-weight basis. Both cephalexin and cephradine in terms of ED_{50} were slightly less active in vivo than cephaloridine against penicillin-sensitive organisms but were slightly more active against penicillinase-producers.

DISCUSSION

The substantial degree of susceptibility of 'penicillinase-resistant' penicillins to various β-lactamases is not generally appreciated. However, similar results with enzymes derived from Gram-positive bacteria have been reported using techniques different from those employed by us.[1,2]

Among the β-lactam antibiotics the MIC in serum-free media has little value in prophesying the outcome of treatment. In contrast, the MCC in 95% serum and comparative data on the susceptibility to β-lactamases taken together correlate very well with the ED_{50} values obtained in mice. As shown, the two antibiotics with among the poorest 'routine' MIC values performed remarkably well in these experimental infections, and cephradine was moderately but consistently more active than cephalexin in vivo. The direct relevance of these findings to human infections has yet to be determined, but a further point in favour of cephradine is the recent finding that the 'volume of distribution' of this drug in man is higher than for other cephalosporins.[3]

Acknowledgements

We are grateful to the Westminster Hospital and Medical School Research Committee for financial support, and we wish to thank Dr. R. B. Sykes and Mr. D. M. Ryan of Glaxo Laboratories and Dr. T. K. Clarke of E. R. Squibb & Sons for helpful advice.

REFERENCES

1. Waterworth, P. (1973), J. Clin. Path., 26, 596.

2. Lacey, R. W., & Lewis, E. L. (1975), J. med. Microbiol., 8, 337.

3. Weliky, I., & Zaki, A. (1974), Proc. 8th Internat. Congr. Chemother. (Athens, 1973), Vol. 1, p. 582.

BACTERIAL BIOTRANSFORMATION OF AMPICILLIN, AMOXICILLIN AND OXACILLIN IN VITRO AND IN URINE OF PATIENTS WITH BACTERIURIA

Magda Arr, Hedvig Graber, T.Perenyi, E.Ludwig

Dept. of Medicine and Clinical Pharmacology

Municipal Hospital Peterfy, Budapest, Hungary

It is a well-known fact, that therapy of urinary tract infections (UTI) involves several problem and often needs the close teamwork of clinician and microbiologist. The aim of our study was to improve microbiologic methods and thus give more help to therapy.

Hundred clinical isolates of E.coli were tested for their lactamase activity and susceptibility to various penicillins.

MATERIALS AND METHODS

lactamase activity was tested semi-quantitatively after incubating the strain with benzylpenicillin, ampicillin and amoxicillin for 18 hours and a chromatogram was made on HF 254 silica gel layer. The spots were detected by iodine-starch solution. The enzyme activity was considered "high", when only the hydrolyzed form could be detected, "low" when both the parent compound and its hydrolyzed form were visible and "no activity" when the compound remained intact. The enzyme was inhibited by an equal amount of oxacillin. In vitro sensitivity of the strains was tested by the disc and cup metthods and in some cases by measuring the MIC. Intact ampicillin was measured by the modified method of Smith, the hydrolyzed form by Novick's microiodometric technique (5,10).

RESULTS.AND DISCUSSION

Among the 100 E.coli strains 29 had high enzyme activity ("strong destroyers"); low activity was found in 29 strains against benzylpenicillin, in 11 against ampicillin and in 12 against amoxicillin ("weak destroyers").

Lactamase could be inhibited totally in 25% and partially in 62% of the strains with high activity against benzylpenicillin. Of the strong destroyers of ampicillin 25% could be totally and 68% partially inhibited. From the weak destroyers 30% was completely inhibited, all the others suffered partial inhibition. Oxacillin totally inhibited the degradation of amoxicillin in 27% of the strong, 17% of the weak destroyers, and partially in the rest of them.

The sensitivity of the strains was tested against benzylpenicillin, ampicillin, amoxicillin and to their combinations with oxacillin and dicloxacillin (6,7). Only four strains having no lactamase activity at all were found resistant to all antibiotics. However all the 29 strongly degrading strains were resistant against the combinations, even those whose activity could be inhibited. In strains with low enzyme activity inhibition lead to increasing susceptibility.

Figure 1 shows the increase in sensitivity upon the effect of oxacillin and dicloxacillin, respectively. It can be seen, that nearly all the resistant strains with low enzyme activity became susceptible and the sensitivity of the enzyme negative strains increased. On Figure 2 the same data are to be seen for ampicillin: susceptibility of weak destroyers was considerably increased by the combinations.

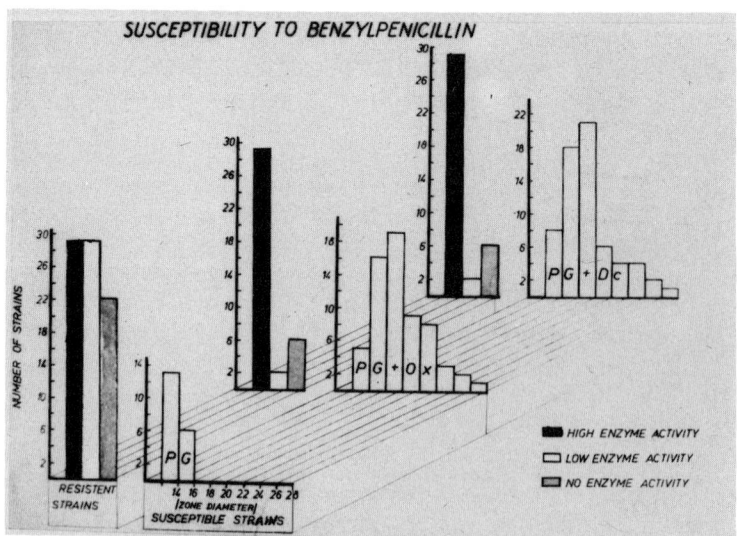

Fig.1.(see text).

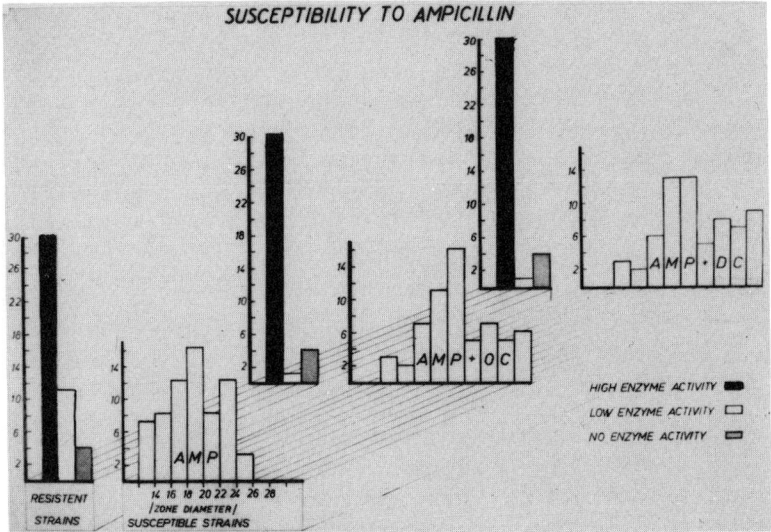

Fig.2.(see text).

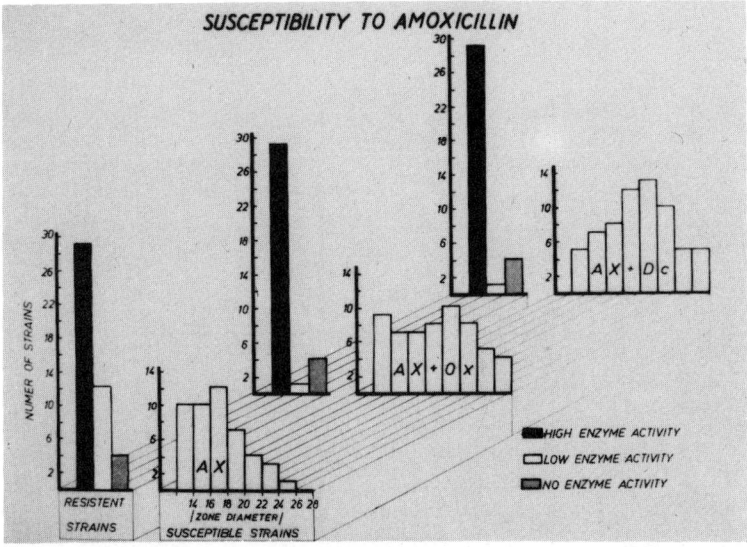

Fig.3.(see text).

As beta-lactamases of Gram negative pathogens are cell-bound (1-4,8,9) the activity of disrupted cells is higher. Twenty % of ampicillin was degraded by the living cells of an E.coli strain with low enzyme activity, however, 70% of the drug was degraded by the same concentration of ultrasonically disintegrated cells.

Some representants of the strains were analyzed in detail. Two E.coli strains were investigated in the presence of 10 ug/ml ampicillin, oxacillin and in the simultaneous presence of both antibiotics, and the possible decrease in concentration of the antibiotics as well. By one of them ampicillin disappeared from the system in 6 hours; in the presence of oxacillin it only decreased slightly. Growth of bacteria was not influenced in either system. By the other strain the concentration of ampicillin decreased by 20% in six hours, in the presence of oxacillin it remained stable. Growth of bacteria was slightly inhibited by ampicillin, but completely blocked by the combination.

We studied the activity of crude enzyme extracts of various strains and its inhibition by oxacillin in the function of time. Fig.5: equal amount of oxacillin entirely inhibited the decomposition of benzylpenicillin, ampicillin and amoxicillin by the enzyme preparation of E.coli 668 -while that of No.1805 was only partially blocked.

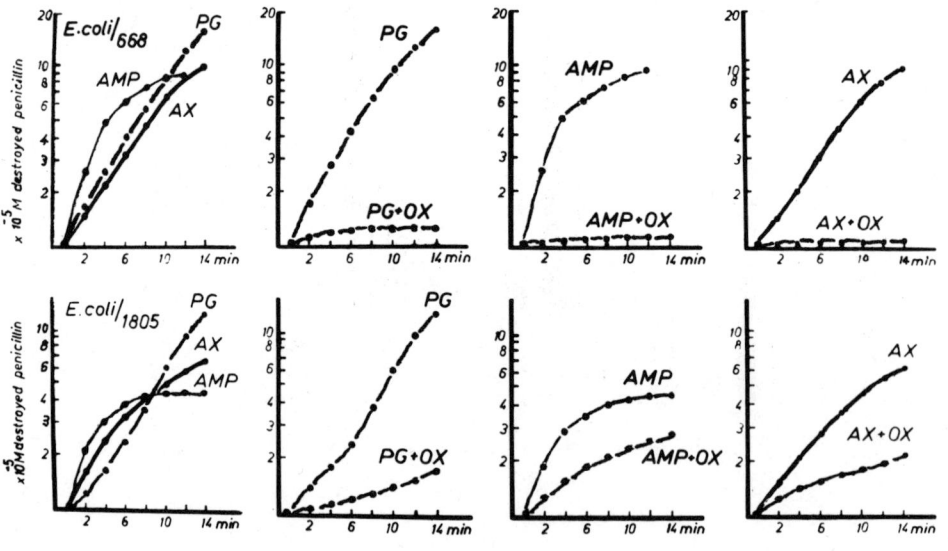

Fig.4. Inhibition effect of oxacillin.(Test 0.2 umol antibiotic; enzyme concentration:E.coli 668:9,6 ug protein, E.coli 1805:48,0 ug protein; pH:5,9; Temp.:20 C.).

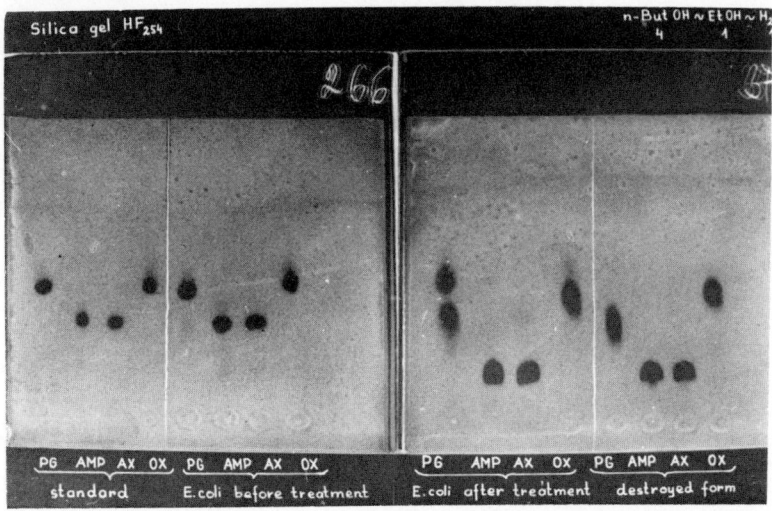

Fig.5. Chromatogram of E.coli isolated from patient's urine before and after treatment (see text).

We tried to evaluate our results from the clinician's aspect. The combination of amino penicillin and oxacillin was administered to some patients with chronic UTI. The therapeutic results were mostly favorable in cases where the original pathogen had low enzyme activity, or no activity at all, -and its in vitro susceptibility could be increased by the combination.

However, the microorganism of some patients altered during treatment and lactamase producing, resistant strain grew instead of the enzyme negative, sensitive isolate. Fig.5. Chromatogram of the lactamase activity of an E.coli strain isolated from patient's urine before and after a 10 day-long treatment with ampicillin and oxacillin. The strain was susceptible to the combination and lactamase negative before therapy, while after it, high enzyme activity and resistance developed. In such cases, of course, treatment was changed. In cases, where in spite of in vitro inhibition of enzyme activity, the strain remained resistant, the combination failed to improve the result of the therapy:the microorganism remained resistant in vivo as well. Our in vitro studies may forecast the chances of successful combined therapy:good results are to be expected, where the pathogen has only a low enzyme activity which can be inhibited.

At the same time our data prove that precise bacteriological analysis of the cases may contribute to better therapeutic results.

REFERENCES

1. Hamilton-Miller,J.M.T.:J.gen.Microbiol.41.175.1965. 2. Hamilton-Miller,J.M.T.et al:Nature.2o8.235.1965. 3. Hennessey,T.D.:J.gen.Microbiol.49.277.1967. 4. Neu,H.C.:Appl.Microbiology.17.383. 1969. 5. Novick,R.P.:Biochem.J.83.236.1962. 6. O'Callagham,C.H. and A.Morris:A.A.C. 6.442.1972. 7. Sabath,L.D.:A.A.C.2lo.1967. 8. Sabath,L.D. et al: Biochem.J.96.739.1965. 9. Smith,J.T.:J.gen.Microbiol.30.299.1963. lo. Smith,J.W.G. et al:Analyst.92.247.1967.

SUBSTRATE PROFILES OF β-LACTAMASES AGAINST NEWER β-LACTAM-ANTIBIOTICS

B. Wiedemann, V. Krcmery and H. Knothe

Institut für Medizinische Mikrobiologie der Universität
Frankfurt,
West Germany

In recent years it has become common to classify enzymes of gram-negative bacteria, which inactivate β-lactam-antibiotics, by means of their substrate profiles, i.e. their relative activity towards a set of substrates (β-lactam-antibiotics). One such classification which acquired a general recognition is that of Jack and Richmond. However several new derivatives of both semisynthetic Penicillins and cephalosporins have been introduced since. Therefore it seems important to investigate the possible application of substrate profiles to evaluate the relative stability of some newly introduced substances towards β-lactamase, which are mostly coded by R-factors from hospital strains in the Frankfurt area.

The bacterial strains were clinical isolates of different hospitals in Frankfurt. The sensitivity against some of the drugs used is listed in Table 1.

Table 1. MIC of strains tested

	E.coli Ampicillin resistant	E. coli Cephalotin resistant	E. coli Mecillinam resistant	Serratia marcescens
Ampicillin	128	128	16-128	128
Amoxycillin	128	128	16-128	128
Mecillinam	1	2	4- 64	0,2 128
Cephalotin	32	256	32	128

We included eleven ampicillin resistant strains of E.coli with an MIC of 128 μm/ml or more. All the strains of E.coli included in a second group were resistant to Ampicillin and Cephalotin. Five strains were moderately resistant to Mecillinam. These strains differed in their sensitivity to the other tested antibiotics. Finally we tested five strains of Serratia marcescens resistant to ampicillin and cephalosporin but different in their sensitivity against Mecillinam. We used the iodometric method for the determination of the substrate profiles as described by Jack and Richmond. In this brief report we are not going into details of different substrate profiles and we are not trying to describe new classes of enzymes, although it seems to us that there exists a great variety of enzymes in nature which can be subdivided in more and more subgroups, the more substrates are tested. We want to concentrate on the activity of enzymes on Ampicillin and ampicillin-like substances like Amoxycillin and Mecillinam.

The first group of ampicillin-resistant strains produced enzymes which inactivated a larger amount of Ampicillin than of Penicillin. As some decomposed only minor amounts of Cephaloridine they can be grouped into class III of the classification of Jack and Richmond. In these groups of strains Amoxycillin was shown to be a good substrate for their ampicillinases, since the rate of its decomposition was nearly as high as that of Ampicillin. Although the rate of inactivation of the amidinopenicillin, Mecillinam, seems to be less than that of Ampicillin, the difference is not clear enough to explain the difference in the sensitivity. Similarly, two ureido penicillins tested, still were good stubstrates to all enzymes, although these substrates were more stable than Ampicillin and Amocycillin. The different cephalosporins included in this study reacted differently. While Cephaloridin was inactivated to a similar extent as Mecillinam, Cephoxitin proved to be very stable. Other cephalosporins were in an intermediate state, like Cephalotin and Cephaloxin.

Table 2. β-lactamase activity of Ampicillin-resistant E.coli

Group	IIb	IIIa	IIIa?
Number of strains	2	7	2
Penicillin	100	100	100
Ampicillin	122	226	200
Amoxycillin	61	183	103
Mecillinam	67	105	70

Table 3. β-lactamase activity of Cephalotin-resistant E.coli

Penicillin	1000	100	100	100
Ampicillin	218	370	75	163
Amoxycillin	250	400	147	204
Mecillinam	187	290	141	78

Four strains of E. coli, which were resistant to Cephalotin (table 3) show their good hydrolysing ability against Cephaloridin and other cephalosporins but again, cephoxitin was the most stable substrate. Although all these strains were sensitive to mecillinam, the β-lactamase destroyed this antibiotic to a similar extent as Ampicillin or Amoxicillin.

Since we have been especially interested in the activity of mecillinam, we included some mecillinam-resistant strains in this study (Table 4), but it turned out to be difficult to find E. coli strains resistant to this drug. So we used moderately resistant strains of E.coli. Again, there was no correlation between resistance to mecillinam and the activity of enzymes against this drug. 1, there is no marked difference between low and high resistant strains, and 2, there is no difference between the enzymes of this group with the enzymes of other groups of bacteria. The final group of enzymes tested were those from Serratia marcescens (table 5). The behaviour of the enzymes of these strains were strikingly different from those of E.coli strains. Three strains produced an enzyme extremely active against Carbenicillin, while all the other enzymes had a very low activity against Carbenicillin. More over these enzymes are very active against all the substrates tested. Some even destroyed Oscacillin. The other two strains which were able to transfer resistance to ampicillin and cephalosporins to E.coli and other recipient bacteria, were less active against

Table 4. β-lactamase activity of Mecillinam resistant E.coli

	low resistance[1]	high resistance[2]
Penicillin	100	100
Ampicillin	148	167
Amoxicillin	179	176
Mecillinam	129	137

[1] mean of three strains [2] mean of two strains

Table 5. β-lactamase activity of Serratia marcescens

	non-transferable resistance[1]	transferable resistance[2]
Penicillin	100	100
Ampicillin	124	101
Amoxycillin	45	108
Mecillinam	13	62

[1] mean of three strains [2] mean of two strains both resistant to Mecillinam

Carbenicillin but very active against Penicillins and cephalosporins. Here for the first time there seems to be difference in the activity of the β-lactamases of resistant and sensitive strains against mecillinam. But again a difference from 13 to 62 will not be any evidence of the correlation between resistance and enzyme activity against mecillinam.

By using substrate profiles as a measure for the usefulness of an antibacterial drug one has to be very careful. Not only that the iodometric assay of the cephalosporins is useful only for comparative studies involving a single substrate and is unsatisfactory for absolute measurements (Richmond and Sykes) but also an instability of a drug atainst β-lactamases does not conclusively mean that the drug must be inactive against the bacteria producing the enzyme. In contrast mecillinam is very active against many strains of E.coli, while the enzymes of sensitive strains destroy the drug. According to the hypothesis of Richmond and Sykes the activity of Mecillinam, despite the sensitivity of the drug against β-lactamases, may be due to the fact that mecillinam can leak through the cell wall avoiding strategically located β-lactamases on special routes of entry to the target of the drug. But this remains to be proved.

BETA-LACTAMASE RESISTANCE OF CEPHAZOLIN

AND OTHER CEPHALOSPORINS

C.S. Goodwin and Joyce P. Hill

Division of Hospital Infection

Clinical Research Centre, Harrow, Middlesex HA1 3UJ

During the first few hours of interaction between an antibiotic and a bacterial culture different changes may occur with strains that have similar minimal inhibitory concentrations of that antibiotic. Continuous turbidimetric monitoring of cultures of bacteria in the biophotometer is particularly suitable for recording the interaction between β-lactam antibiotics and bacteria that produce β-lactamases. We have studied the activity of some cephalosporins in the biophotometer relating the results to the MICs for dense populations of bacteria, and to the exact concentration of organisms at the time of addition of the antibiotic.

MATERIALS AND METHODS

Four strains of <u>Escherichia coli</u> and one of <u>Klebsiella pneumoniae</u> were isolated from clinical lesions at Northwick Park Hospital. β-lactamase activity was detected by using a chromogenic cephalosporin. The time required for a colour change from yellow to red - as the β-lactam ring is cleaved - was noted.

Minimum inhibitory concentrations of cephazolin, cephaloridine and cephalothin were estimated by serial dilution of each antibiotic in Sensitest Agar (Oxoid), and a multiple inoculator that delivered approximately 0.01 ml of a suspension of 1×10^5 or 2×10^7 bacterial/ml.

Bacterial cultures that were monitored in the biophotometer were grown in a medium with an osmolality of 325 mOsmol/kg. Six independent bacterial cultures, at 37°C and continuously stirred, were each grown from 0.04 ml of an overnight broth culture inoculated into 8 ml of medium to produce a concentration of approximately 3×10^6 bacteria/ml. Antibiotic was added during the early or mid-phase of logarithmic growth; before the addition of antibiotic a viable count was performed on the culture. Antibiotic assays were performed at intervals after addition of the antibiotic.

RESULTS

β-lactamase Activities and MICs

The times required for a colour-change of the chromogenic cephalosporin by the bacterial strains are shown in table I. Escherichia coli strain nos. 17 and 150 were rapid producers of β-lactamase, strain no. 55 was a moderately-fast producer and strain no. 72 was slow. The MICs with two different inocula are in table II; the larger inoculum was the concentration of organisms that was found at the time of antibiotic addition in the biophotometer experiments. Among the strains of E. coli the larger inoculum with cephazolin resulted in a 2-fold increase, with cephaloridine a 4-fold increase, and with cephalothin a 2 to 3-fold increase of the MIC. This smaller inoculum effect for cephazolin may indicate that it is more stable than other cephalosporins to bacterial β-lactamase.

In uninoculated culture medium at $37^{\circ}C$ the antibiotic concentration decreased slowly during 24 hours; with cephaloridine 32 μg/ml after 4 hours it had decreased to 30 μg/ml. However, in

Table I. Times for colour-change of chromogenic cephalosporin

Bacterial strains		Minutes					
		2	5	10	30	60	120
E. coli	17	−	+				
	55	−	−	−	+		
	72	−	−	−	−	−	+
	150	−	−	+			
Klebsiella	21	−	−	−	−	+	

the presence of E. coli strain no. 150 after 2 hours cephaloridine could not be detected (table IV); but after 4 hours with cephazolin 32 µg/ml the concentration was still 4·5 µg/ml. With E. coli strain no. 150 the times to lysis and recovery after antibiotic addition are shown in table III; at the time of antibiotic additon the concentration of organisms was found to be 2×10^7 orgs/ml. With cephaloridine 32 µg/ml although lysis of the E. coli occurred after 10 minutes the organism recommenced growth after only $2\frac{1}{2}$ hours; but with cephazolin 32 µg/ml the organism did not regrow for 8 hours after antibiotic addition. With other antibiotic assays a similar correlation was found between the time to recovery and the disappearance of the antibiotic from the culture medium. With cephaloridine 128 µg/ml - 8-fold

Table II. Minimum inhibitory concentrations (µg/ml) with different inocula

Bacterial strains		Inoculum 1×10^5 orgs/ml			Inoculum 2×10^7 orgs/ml		
		C'zolin	C'loridine	C'lothin	C'zolin	C'loridine	C'lothin
E. coli	17	2	2	4	4	12	12
	55	1	2	8	2	8	16
	72	1	2	4	2	8	12
	150	2	4	4	4	16	8
Klebsiella	21	1	2	2	1	4	2

Table III. Times to lysis and recovery of E. coli strain no. 150 after antibiotic addition.

Antibiotic	MIC*	Result	Concentration of antibiotic (ug/ml) at indicated time (hours) after its addition				
			8	16	32	64	128
Cephaloridine	16	Lysis	+NL	0·25	0·25	0·25	0·25
		Recovery		1	2·5	3	3·5
Cephazolin	4	Lysis	0·75	0·5	0·25		
		Recovery	3·5	6	8		

* Inoculum 2×10^7 orgs/ml   + NL = No lysis

Table IV. Antibiotic concentrations after addition of 32 µg/ml to E. coli 150

	Antibiotic concentration (µg/ml) at:			
	Hours after antibiotic addition			
Antibiotic	0	1	2	4
Cephaloridine	26	1·5	–	–
Cephazolin	32	25	12	4·5

Table V. Times to lysis and recovery of E. coli strains no. 17 and 55 after antibiotic addition

Strain	Antibiotic	MIC*	Result	Concentration of antibiotic (µg/ml) at indicated time (hours) after its addition			
				2	4	8	16
E. coli 17	Cephaloridine	12	Lysis		NL	0·5	0·25
			Recovery		...	4	5
	Cephazolin	4	Lysis		NL	NL	(0·75)
			Recovery		...	...	3
E. coli 55	Cephaloridine	8	Lysis		0·5	0·25	0·25
			Recovery		6	16·5	20
	Cephazolin	2	Lysis	1·5	0·75	0·5	
			Recovery	8	15	20	

( ) = partial lysis

Table VI. Times to lysis and recovery of E. coli strain no. 72 and Kleb. pneumoniae strain no. 21 after antibiotic addition

Strain	Antibiotic	MIC*	Result	Concentration of antibiotic ($\mu g/ml$) at indicated time (hours) after its addition			
				2	4	8	16
E. coli 72	Cephaloridine	8	Lysis		0·5	0·25	0·25
			Recovery		5·5	14	20
	Cephazolin	2	Lysis	(1·5)	(0·75)	0·5	
			Recovery	11·5	20	20	
Klebsiella 21	Cephaloridine	4	Lysis		0·75	0·5	0·5
			Recovery	4	8		11
	Cephazolin	2	Lysis	1·5	1	0·75	
			Recovery	3	16	20	

( ) = partial lysis

more than the MIC - E. coli strain no. 150 regrew after only $3\frac{1}{2}$ hours, but with cephazolin 16 $\mu g/ml$ - 4-fold more than the MIC - the organism did not regrow for 6 hours. In other experiments, not reported here, E. coli strain no. 150 was found to produce 2 β-lactamases, the chromosomal type Ib, and the R-factor-mediated type IIIa, according to the classification of Richmond & Sykes. Type IIIa β-lactamase is widespread among enterobacteria and it is significant that cephazolin was apparently more resistant than cephaloridine to this enzyme and to the chromosomal β-lactamase. The resistance of cephalothin to the β-lactamase of this strain appeared to be intermediate between cephaloridine and cephazolin; with a concentration of cephalothin 32 $\mu g/ml$ the organism regrew after $4\frac{1}{2}$ hours. However, when antibiotic was added to a slightly greater concentration of organisms - 5×10^7 orgs/ml - with cephazolin 16 $\mu g/ml$ the organism regrew after only $3\frac{1}{2}$ hours; with cephalothin 32 $\mu g/ml$ the organism regrew after 2 hours.

With most strains of E. coli, with an antibiotic concentration equivalent to the MIC with the larger inoculum similar delays were found, although with the same concentration of antibiotic cephazolin delayed recovery for longer than cephaloridine, such as with E. coli strain no. 55 (table V). However with E. coli strain no. 17 cephazolin appeared to be less active than cephaloridine (table V).

With E. coli strain no. 72 (table VI) with concentrations equivalent to the MICs similar delays were found. With Klebsiella pneumoniae strain no. 21 at twice the MIC cephazolin restrained regrowth for 16 hours and cephaloridine for 8 hours (table VI), probably indicating that cephazolin was more resistant than cephaloridine to the β-lactamase of this group of organisms.

CONCLUSION

Our results are consistent with those of a recent report by Greenwood & O'Grady, who did not relate their results to MICs with an inoculum equivalent to the concentration in the biophotometer, but who reported that cephazolin induced rapid lysis of dense populations of enterobacteria at a lower concentration than other cephalosporins, and its stability to β-lactamases was generally considerably greater than that of other cephalosporins.

INTERACTIONS OF NEW CEPHALOSPORINS WITH SOME CEPHALOSPORINASES

Roger Labia

Ecole Normale Superieure (ER 156 CNRS)

24, rue Lhomond, 75231 Paris Cedex 05, France

INTRODUCTION

Bacterial strains resistant to one, or few, β lactam antibiotics generally produce β lactamases which are the enzymes able to cleave an amide bond in penicillins and cephalosporins and make the penicilloic thus obtained completely inactive. Recently Richmond and Sykes (1973) reported a classification of β lactamases essentialy based on the profile of activity of these enzymes on various substrates and reaction with various inhibitors.

The catalytic activity of an enzyme appears to be one of its most important characteristic. In kinetic studies of β-lactamases, computerized microacidimetry (Labia et al. 1973), allows accurate and reproducible determinations of Michaelis Menten constants Km and Vmax and also the ratio τ = Km/Vm directly proportional to the antibiotic half-life at " low" concentrations (Labia 1974).

This technique avoids many of the disadvantages of other methods and reveals the real catalytic aptitude not only against penicillins but also against cephalosporins (Kazmierczak et al. 1973).

Bacterial resistance to cephalosporins involves cephalosporinases, so we compared the interactions of some new cephalosporins with three cephalosporinases producing bacterial strains.

MATERIALS AND METHODS

Bacterial Strains

All strains are sensitive to carbenicillin and resistant to cephalotin. E. coli was given by Dr. Philippon (Hôpital Cochin, Paris), Proteus morganii was given by Dr. Chabbert (Institut Pasteur, Paris) and Enterobacter cloacae by Dr. Pitton (Genève).

Enzymatic extracts

The bacterial strains are grown and treated as described previously (Labia et al. 1975). Enzyme induction is performed with 500 µg/ml of penicillin G.

Affinity chromatography

This purification is performed as the technique described previously (Labia et al. 1975)

Antibiotics

We used the following antibiotics : Penicillin G (Laboratoires Rhône Poulenc Specia), Ampicillin, Carbenicillin (Laboratoires Beecham Sevigné), Cephalotin, Cephaloridin, Cefazolin, Cefamandole (Laboratoires Eli Lilly France).

Determination of kinetic constants

The reaction kinetics are monitored by the computerized microacidimetric method (Labia et al. 1973) using a Mettler pH stat and Wang 600 " mini computer ".
τ = Km/Vm, called " enzymatic stability of the substrate (Labia 1974), is also determined for each antibiotic.

Minimal inhibitory concentration (MIC)

MIC are measured by Steers (1959) technique, with Mueller Hinton medium.

Table I : E. coli

	Km (µM)	Vm (rel.)	τ (rel.)	MIC (µg/ml)
Penicillin G	5	19	87	-
Cephalotin	29	100	100	254
Cephaloridin	490	250	670	16
Cefazolin	330	121	960	16
Cefamandole	21	3,1	2300	2

RESULTS

In the four cephalosporins studied cephalotin has the shorter half life, we can see than MIC are also higher for this antibiotic with the three strains, Muggleton et al. (1967) comparison of cephalotin and cephaloridin shows that cephalotin MIC is generally higher that cephaloridin MIC.

- Cephaloridin and cefazolin have always a similar behaviour, as τ and MIC are generally very similar. These results are in good agreement with microbiological evaluation from Nishida et al. (1970) which shows than cefazolin is slightly more active than cephaloridin. An another hand cefazolin presents a pharmacocinetic advantage (higher plasmatic level and longer half life) and a very lower nephrotoxicity. On the microbiological point of view the difference between these two antibiotics is small, that is shown in tables I, II, III.

Cefamandole appears to be relatively resistant to β lactamases, that is in good agreement with bacteriological evaluation of Neu (1974) which shows than this antibiotic appears to be active on cephalosporinase producing strains as for example Serratia or Proteus.

The enzymes caracterised here present some analogy with enzymes described previously such as E. coli 214 T and 419 studied by Dale and Smith (1971) or Proteus morgani described in 1965 by Ayliffe.

The very low hydrolysis of penicillin G by β lactamases from E. cloacae is in good agreement with observations of Hennessey (1967), Hennessey and Richmond (1968) and Ross and Boulton (1973).

The observations reported here shows than computerized microacidimetry provides a good solution in the determination of β lactamases Michaelis Menten constants either of the penicillinase or cephalosporinase group.

The ratio τ = Km/Vm appears to be a very pertinent parameter as a good correlation can be found between τ and MIC as shown on figure I. Other problems are also involved in bacterial resistance to β lactam antibiotics such as "crypicity factors" (Richmond and Curtis 1974) and also specific activity of the β lactamase. This last problem is not very easy to study particularly in the case of inducible β lactamases, as all antibiotics have not the same induction properties. We are now studing these aspects.

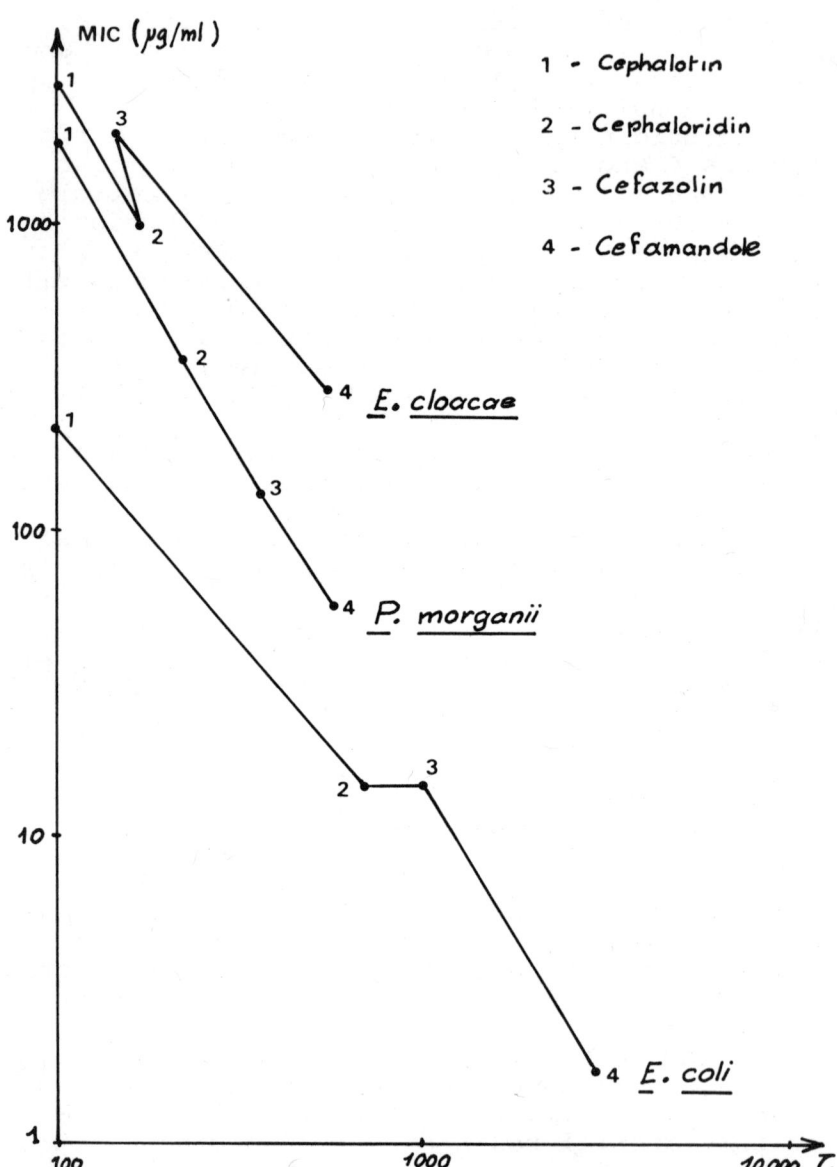

Figure 1. Relationship between τ and MIC

Table II : **Proteus morganii**

	Km(μM)	Vm(rel.)	τ(rel.)	MIC(μg/ml)
Penicillin G	2,5	18	55	-
Cephalotin	25	100	100	2000
Cephaloridin	86	188	182	200
Cefazolin	130	190	290	100
Cefamandole	70	56	500	56

Table III : **Enterobacter cloacae**

	Km(μM)	Vm(rel.)	τ(rel.)	MIC(μg/ml)
Penicillin G	-	1	-	-
Cephalotin	60	100	100	3000
Cephaloridin	236	240	165	1000
Cefazolin	200	250	134	2000
Cefamandole	6	2	500	300

Table III shows in the case of Enterobacter cloacae than penicillin G hydrolysis is very low, that don't allows a precise determination of Vmax for this antibiotic. Cephalotin hydrolysis is about a hundred time higher and may be measured with a good accuracy and reproducibility.

In order to get a regular reproducibility in the kinetic constants of cephalosporins for all strains we gives the maximum velocities of enzymatic hycrolysis as a relative unit with cephalotin as a reference (Vm = 100). Km is an absolute constant expressed in μM. τ = Km/Vm is also a relative unit given also with cephalotin as a reference τ = 100.

DISCUSSION

Each of the three bacterial strains studied here produces only one β lactamase. All these enzymes present a lot of common characteristics :
- no detectable hydrolysis of carbenicillin, this is in good agreement with the fact than the producing strains are sensitive to carbenicillin ;
- very low, if any, hydrolysis of ampicillin ;
- high hydrolytic activity of cephalotin.

REFERENCES

- Ayliffe G.A.J. Cephalosporinase and penicillinase activities of gram negative bacteria. J. gen. Microbiol., 40, 119-126 (1965).

- Dale J.W. and Smith J.T. Some relationships between R-Factor and chromosomal β lactamases in gram-negative bacteria. Biochem. J., 123, 507-512 (1971).

- Hennessey T.D. Inducible β lactamase in Enterobacter. J. gen. Microbiol., 49, 277-285 (1967).

- Hennessey T.D. and Richmond M.H. The purification and some properties of a β lactamase (cephalosporinase) synthetized by Enterobacter cloacae. Biochem. J., 109, 469-473 (1968).

- Kazmierczak A., Philippon A., Chardon H., Labia R. and Le Goffic F. Constantes cinétiques (Km et Vmax) des β lactamases mesurées par une méthode microacidimétrique couplée à l'ordinateur. Ann. Microbiol. (Inst. Pasteur), 124 B, 259-268 (1973).

- Labia R., Andrillon J. and Le Goffic F. Computerized microacidimetric determination of β lactamase Michaelis Menten constants. FEBS letters, 33, 42-44 (1973).

- Labia R. comportement enzyme substrat. Introduction de la notion de stabilité enzymatique dans le cas des β lactamases. C.R. Acad. Sci., 279(D), 109-112 (1974).

- Labia R., Kazmierczak A., Philippon A., Le Goffic F., Faye J.C., Goldstein F.W. and Acar J.F. β Lactamases de Pseudomonas aeruginosa et résistance à la carbenicilline. Ann. Microbiol. (Inst. Pasteur), 126 A, 449-459 (1975).

- Labia R., Philippon A., Le Goffic F. and Faye J.C. Identification de la β lactamase R-TEM chez Pseudomonas aeruginosa. Biochimie, 57, 139-143 (1975)

- Muggleton P.W. and O'Callaghan C.H. The antibacterial activities of cephaloridine : laboratory investigation. Postgrad. Med. J., 43 supp., 17-22 (1967).

- Neu H.C. Cefamandole, a cephalosporin antibiotic with an unsually wide spectrum of activity. Antimicrob. ag. chemother., 6, 177-182 (1974).

- Nishida W., Matsubara T., Murakawa T., Mine Y. and Yokota Y. Cefazolin. A new semisynthetic cephalosporin antibiotic. II In vitro and in vivo antimicrobial activity. J. antibiot., 23, 137-148 (1970).

- Richmond M.H. and Curtis N.A.C. The β lactamases of gram negative bacteria and their possible physiological role. Adv. Microbiol. Physiol., 9, 31-88 (1973).

- Richmond M.H. and Curtis N.A.C. The interplay of β lactamases and intrisic factors in the resistance of gram-negative bacteria to penicillin and cephalosporins. Ann. N.Y. Acad. Sci., 235, 553-568 (1974).

- Ross G.W. and Boulton M.G. Purification of β lactamases on QAE Sephadex. Biochim. Biophys. Acta, 309, 430-439, (1973).

- Steers E., Flotz E.L. and Graves B.S. An innocula replicating apparatus for routine testing of bacteria susceptibility to antibiotics. Antibiot. Chemother. (Basel), 9, 307-310 (1959).

THE ACTIVITY OF HAEMOPHILUS INFLUENZAE β-LACTAMASE

S. Kattan, P. Cavanagh,* J.D. Williams
Department of Medical Microbiology
The London Hospital Medical College
Turner St., London E1 2AD
*Public Health Laboratory Service
Stoke-on-Trent

SUMMARY

H. influenzae β-lactamase was found to closely resemble the E. coli TEM β-lactamase in its substrate profile and rate of hydrolysis of benzyl penicillin, ampicillin and cephaloridine. The permeability barrier to ampicillin and benzyl penicillin observed in the E. coli strain was not detected in the Haemophilus influenzae strain as judged by the activity of whole cell suspensions. It is concluded therefore that this difference is responsible for the smaller amounts of ampicillin required to inhibit β-lactamase producing strains of H. influenzae compared to strains of E. coli producing β-lactamase.

INTRODUCTION

Recently attention has been drawn to severe infections caused by ampicillin resistant strains of Haemophilus influenzae. Moreover, some resistant strains have been shown to produce β-lactamase (Williams et al, 1974).

We have previously demonstrated the substrate profile of this enzyme to be not unlike that of the TEM β-lactamase produced by strains of E. coli and other gram-negative organisms. In this paper we have investigated further the activity of the H. influenzae enzyme and compared it to that of the E. coli TEM β-lactamase.

MATERIALS AND METHODS

Strains

A strain of H.influenzae (4348) producing β-lactamase and requiring 4.0 μgm/ml ampicillin for its inhibition was maintained on chocolate agar and grown overnight in Levinthal broth when required. A strain of E. coli J53 (R6K) producing the TEM β-lactamase and requiring more than 1,000 μgm/ml ampicillin for its inhibition was maintained on nutrient agar and grown overnight in nutrient broth when required.

Enzyme preparations

Supernatants from washed and ultra-sonicated cells, subjected to high speed centrifugation, were used for determinations of β-lactamase activity. Portions of cell suspensions were retained prior to sonication in order to determing the activity of whole cells.

β-lactamase activity

Inactivation of benzyl penicillin, ampicillin and cephaloridine by the enzyme preparations was determined by the iodometric technique of Perret (1954). The amount of antibiotic hydrolysed was calculated by the method of Alicino (1961). Non-specific uptake of iodine was determined in control assays using iodine-inactivated enzyme.

Dry weights

Washed cells of known optical density (OD) were taken to dry weight in an Edwards freeze dryer. The OD/dry weight equivalent was calculated for each strain.

RESULTS

Relative β-lactamase activities

Table 1 shows the relative rates of hydrolysis of ampicillin and cephaloridine compared to that of benzyl penicillin, using sonic extracts of H.influenzae strain 4348 and E. coli strain J53 (R6K). It is clear that the substrate profiles of the H.influenzae and E. coli enzymes are, from our own determinations, identical. Moreover, closer agreement to Jack and Richmond's data (1970) is observed when sonicated cells are clarified by centrifugation, than our previous data has shown using sonic extracts which had not been centrifuged (Kattan et al, 1975).

TABLE I

RELATIVE RATES OF HYDROLYSIS OF THREE ANTIBIOTICS BY H.INFLUENZAE AND E.COLI ꞵ-LACTAMASES

Relative Rate of Hydrolysis*

Antibiotic	H.influenzae ꞵ-lactamase strain 4348	E.coli ꞵ-lactamase strain J53 (R6K) TEM	E.coli TEM[+]
Benzyl penicillin	100	100	100
Ampicillin	174	177	165
Cephaloridine	160	165	145

* compared to that of Benzyl penicillin (= 100%)

+ Jack and Richmond (1970)

Rates of hydrolysis

The rates of hydrolysis of benzyl penicillin, ampicillin and cephaloridine were determined using whole cell suspensions and their sonic extracts.

ꞵ-lactamase activity of the sonic extracts expressed as μmoles of antibiotic hydrolysed/mg dry weight/hour are shown in Table II. It is clear from this data that the activities of the two enzymes are almost identical. Despite the similar rates of hydrolysis by the two enzymes, the minimum inhibitory concentration (M.I.C.) of ampicillin required by the E.coli strain is very much greater than that required by the strain of H.influenzae. In order to clarify this point the ꞵ-lactamase activity of whole cell suspensions must be considered. The data from such determinations is shown in Table III. Rates of hydrolysis are expressed as a % ratio of the activity of sonicated to whole cells. It is apparent that the H.influenzae cell suspension is more active than their sonic extracts. This is probably due to incomplete disruption of the cells and hence loss of enzyme upon sedimentation of the cells, rather than enzyme denaturation during ultra-sonication. The activity of E.coli cells, however, is between 1,000 and 2,000% less than the sonicated preparation, indicating restricted access between substrate and enzyme for benzyl penicillin and ampicillin. Such a permeability barrier was not observed with E.coli cells and cephaloridine. With H.influenzae cells hydrolysis took place to a similar extent using sonic extract and cell suspension alike with

TABLE II

RATE OF HYDROLYSIS BY H.INFLUENZAE AND E.COLI (TEM) β-LACTAMASES

Extract from	μ moles hydrolysed/hour/mg dry cells		
	B.penicillin	Ampicillin	Cephaloridine
E.coli J53 (R6K) TEM	63.8 51.4	91.1	85.2
H.influenzae 4348	68.0 50.3	87.5	80.1

TABLE III

β-LACTAMASE ACTIVITY OF SONICATED CELLS COMPARED TO WHOLE CELL PREPARATIONS

	% Rate of Hydrolysis $\frac{\text{Sonicated preparation}}{\text{Whole cell preparation}}$		
	Antibiotic		
Strain	B.penicillin	Ampicillin	Cephaloridine
E.coli J53(R6K) TEM	1,000 1,861 2,000	1,200	61.6
H.influenzae 4348	186 59 60	71	78.5

all three substrates, indicating that restricted access is not at all the case with the H.influenzae strain.

DISCUSSION

It is apparent from the data presented here that the H.influenzae enzyme resembles the TEM β-lactamase in its substrate profile and in its rates of hydrolysis of benzyl penicillin, ampicillin and cephaloridine. The E.coli enzyme, however, appears much less accessible to benzyl penicillin and ampicillin in intact cells than does the H.influenzae enzyme. It is probable, therefore, that this lack of any permeability barrier to ampicillin in intact H.influenzae cells is responsible for the much lower M.I.Cs of ampicillin required by resistant strains compared to ampicillin resistant E.coli. The β-lactamase producing E.coli cells were as active on cephaloridine as their sonic extracts, as were H.influenzae cells, indicating, as expected, no permeability barrier to cephaloridine in either strain. These findings are consistent with those of Medeiros and O'Brien (1975).

We have shown in a previous report that cephaloridine and cephamandole were equally active on β-lactamase producing and non-producing strains of H.influenzae, although cephamandole was the more active compound. Both compounds were, however, susceptible to β-lactamase attack. It was expected, therefore, that H.influenzae cells would be more freely permeable to cephaloridine and cephamandole than to the two penicillins investigated. The results do not indicate this to be the case with cephaloridine, the percentage ratio of the activity of sonicated to whole cells being slightly greater than that for benzyl penicillin and ampicillin. However, as cephaloridine is significantly less active than ampicillin against H.influenzae its susceptibility to enzyme attack may be of little relevance. Preliminary experiments with cephamandole indicate that the above ratio may be less than those for ampicillin, benzyl penicillin and cephaloridine. It is regrettable that these results are as yet unsubstantiated.

REFERENCES

Alicino, J.F. Iodometric methods for the assay of penicillin preparations. Analytical Chemistry, 18, 619-620 (1946).

Alicino, J.F. Iodometric assay of natural and synthetic penicillins, 6-amino-penicillanic acid and Cephalosporin C. ibid, 33, 648-649 (1961)

Kattan, S., Cavanagh, P., Williams, J.D. Relationship between β-lactamase production by Haemophilus influenzae and sensitivities to penicillins and cephalosporins. The Journal of Antimicrobial Chemotherapy, 1, 79-84 (1975)

Medeiros, A.A., O'Brien, T.F. Ampicillin resistant H.influenzae Type B possessing a TEM-type β-lactamase but little permeability barrier to ampicillin. Lancet, i, 716-718 (1975).

Perret, C.J. Iodometric assay of penicillinase. Nature 174 1012-1013 (1954).

Williams, J.D., Kattan, S., Cavanagh, P. Penicillinase production in Haemophilus influenzae. Lancet, ii, 103 (1974).

AMPICILLIN RESISTANCE AND BETA-LACTAMASE ACTIVITY IN CLINICAL ISOLATES OF SHIGELLA SONNEI

Harold C. Neu and Alice Prince
Division of Infectious Diseases
College of Physicians and Surgeons
Columbia University
New York

There has been a marked increase in the resistance of Shigella sonnei to ampicillin in the past decade. This has been seen in England (Davies et al 1970) New Zealand (Smith et al 1974) and New York (Neu et al 1975). The precise mechanism of resistance has not been defined in each instance, but the studies in London (Davies et al 1970) and those of the strains from New Zealand (Smith et al 1974) suggested that these were two kinds of resistance: low level, nontransmissible; and high level, transmissible. The nontransmissible was due to a β-lactamase that hydrolyzed cephalospoxins rapidly. The transmissible resistance is due to an R-factor mediating a β-lactamase that does not confir cephalosporin resistance. We (Neu 1969) had described similar type of resistance in Escherichia coli and we wished to see if the increased resistance of Shigella to ampicillin that we (Neu et al 1975) had noted in 1972-73 was similar to that seen in England and New Zealand.

Materials and Methods

Shigella sonnei isolates were those we collected from patients hospitalized at both voluntary and municipal hospitals in New York City in the period 1972 to 1974. E. coli K 12 (W 1485), nalidixic acid resistant, was used as a recipient in mating experiments.

Minimal inhibitory concentrations (MIC) were determined by use of a multiple inoculator device which delivered 10^4 colony forming units to Muller Hinton agar plates which contained the antibiotics in two-fold increasing concentrations. Mating experiments were performed by previously described methods (Neu et al 1973). Colicin typing was performed by Dr. John D. Nelson,

Dallas, Texas. Colicin production was tested by the method of Fredericq (1952).

Enzyme extracts were prepared from bacteria grown to late logarithmic phase in Muller Hinton broth. The bacterial cells were separated by centrifugation, washed with phosphate buffer and sonically disrupted. Cellular debris and ribosomal material were removed by centrifugation and the supernatant material dialyzed at $3°C$ for 36h in 25mM potassium phosphate buffer. This material was used for enzyme assays.

B-lactamase was determined by a modification of The Novick microiodometric method with the assay run at pH7.0 at $30°C$ (Neu and Winshell 1970). Inhibition of cephalosporin hydrolysis was determined with cephloridine as substrate following the decrease in absorption at 255nm in the presence of 50mM cloxacillin or 25 mM sodium chloride.

Results

The resistance patterns of the S. sonnei tested were of eight types. Only three of the strains which were resistant to ampicillin alone transferred their resistance to E. coli K 12, W 1485. There were eight strains which were also resistant to cephalothin. Of these strains only one transferred resistance to cephalothin as well as to ampicillin.

The MICs of ampicillin were determined for the resistant strains. There were 29 of the 37 strains tested that had MIC values for ampicillin in excess of 400 ug/ml and the remaining strains had MIC values of 100 to 400 ug/ml for ampicillin. It should be noted that seven of the later strains had carbenicillin MIC values of 12.5 to 50 ug/ml. There were six strains which had cephalothin MIC values greater than 400 ug/ml and twelve strains with MIC values of 25 to 400 ug/ml. It is of interest that none of the strains had a cefazolin MIC in excess of 200 ug/ml and that 26 of the 37 strains were inhibited by 12.5 ug/ml or less.

Three strains were selected for further characterization. One of them failed to transfer resistance to ampicillin, one transferred ampicillin resistance and the third transferred resistance to both ampicillin and cephalothin. A comparison of the B-lactamase activity is given in table 1.

All three were not typeable with standard colicin typing materials. They had come from different hospitals. Strain 2701 was isolated from a patient after therapy with ampicillin. It is seen that strain 2701 has poor activity against ampicillin but hydrolyzes cephalothin as effectively as it does penicillin G. It has no activity against oxacillin and methicillin. In contrast strains 4-18 and 10-101 are more active against ampicillin than

Table 1
Comparison of β-lactamase activity of some extracts of S. sonnei

Substrate	2701	Strain 4-18	10-101
		Percent hydrolyzed	
Penicillin G	100	100	100
Ampicillin	8	152	158
Oxacillin	0	10	24
Methicillin	0	2	0
Cephloridine	57	65	110
Cephalothin	102	13	10

against penicillin G. Both show some activity against oxacillin and only poor activity against cephalothin. Strain 10-101 does hydrolyze cephloridine as well as penicillin G in contrast to strain 4-18.

There was no correlation of the MIC values for various β-lactam antibiotics and the amount of substrate hydrolyzed by a sonic extract of the intact microorganisms. The MIC values of the E.coli strains which had mated with strain 4-18 and 10-101 were similar to the parents. It is of note that the E.coli K 12 (R-10-101) hydrolyzed penicillin G more effectively than did the parent strain, but ampicillin and cephloridine less well.

The inhibition of hydrolysis of cephloridine by cloxacillin and sodium chloride was tested. Strain 2701 showed no inhibition of hydrolysis by cloxacillin whereas both strains 4-18 and 10-101 were inhibited. However, the degree of inhibition was much greater with strain 10-101. Sodium chloride had no effect on strain 4-18, stimulated the activity of 10-101 and had a 50% inhibition of strain 2701. None of the strains were inhibited by parachlormercuribenzoate.

It is apparent that strains 4-18 and 10-101 contain two types of β-lactamase one of which they can transfer to recipient E. coli and one which is no-transmissible.

Discussion

These strains of S. sonnei do not resemble the type of beta-lactam resistance commonly encountered in E. coli. Strain 2701 is similar to some of the strains of Smith et al (1974), but differs in the higher level of resistance. In spite of differences in the method of assay of MIC data our nontransmissible strains were resistant to more than 400 ug/ml of ampicillin. Furthermore strain 2701 had a cephloridine MIC of 25 ug/ml. At the present we do not know the frequency with which strains such as 2701 occur in clinical isolates, but we have found a number of non colicin typeable strains which show similar characteristics. In addition we have found three other types of nontransmissible β-lactamase resistance in S. sonnei. The two transmissible types of β-lactamase illustrated by strains 4-18 and 10-101 are distinct from each other in their specific activities and in their response to cloxacillin or sodium chloride. It is of note that the strains do not transfer all of their β-lactamase activity even though the MIC values of the penicillins and cephalosporins are similar in donor and recipient. Of major difference was the transfer of resistance to cephalothin by strain 10-101. We had not encountered this in a study of shigella (Neu et al 1975) nor in E. coli (Neu et al 1973) nor in a large study of salmonella resistant to ampicillin and cephalothin. In most instances cephalothin resistance appears to be chromosomal in nature. Indeed the poorer hydrolytic activity of the recipient E. coli strain suggests that factors other than hydrolysis of the cephalothin may be important.

Although the majority of our strains of shigella which were ampicillin resistant alone were not mediated by R factor the level of resistance is such that infections could not be cured by ampicillin. It seems that when strains of shigella are multiply resistant to antibiotics; that is, agents of different classes, the resistance to ampicillin is primarily R factor whereas in those strains resistant to ampicillin alone chromosomal resistance is more common. There is no explanation for the development in nature of the later strains.

References

Davies, J. R., Farrant, W. N., and Uttley, A. (1970), Lancet, 2, 1157-1159.

Fredericq, P. (1952), Annual Review Microbiology. 11, 7-22.

Neu, H. C. and Winshell, E. B., (1970), Archives Biochemistry Biophysics, 139, 278-288.

Neu, H. C., Cherubin, C. E., Vogt, M., Huber, P., Glazer, S., and Winter H., (1973), American Journal Diseases of Children, 126, 174-177.

Neu, H. C., Cherubin, C. E., Longo, E. D., and Winter J., (1975), Antimicrobial Agents and Chemotherapy, 7, 833-835.

Smith, J. T., Brenner, D. A., and Datta N., (1974), Antimicrobial Agents and Chemotherapy, 6, 418-421.

INHIBITION OF BACTERIAL CELL WALL SYNTHESIS BY AMPHOMYCIN

S. Ōmura, H. Tanaka, M. Shinohara, R. Ōiwa, and T. Hata

The Kitasato Institute and Kitasato University

5-9-1, Shirokane, Minato-ku, Tokyo, Japan

Summary: Amphomycin and tsushimycin, antibiotics consisting of a fatty acid and a straight peptide-chain, were found to be specific inhibitors of synthesis of bacterial cell wall peptidoglycan. The antibiotics inhibit peptidoglycan synthesis on a step from UDP-MurNAc-peptide to peptidoglycan.

In our research program for new antibiotics we found an antibiotic No. PO-386, which was active against gram-positive bacteria. It was identified with amphomycin, an acid peptide antibiotic isolated by Heineman et al.(1953). The structure of it was determined as shown in Fig. 1. (Bodanszky et al. 1973) Polymyxin and colistin were given as example of the representative antibiotic consisting of a fatty acid and a peptide ring. These antibiotics are more active against gram-negative bacteria than gram-positive bacteria, and exhibit strong toxicity. They were reported to interfere in the function of bacterial cell membrane. (Benedict et al. 1947)(Newton 1953) (Newton 1956) (Chapman 1962)

$$\begin{matrix} CH_3 & CH_3 \\ & \diagdown \\ & CH-(CH_2)_5-CH=CH-CH_2-CO-Asp-MeAsp-Asp-Gly- \\ & \diagup \\ CH_3 & \quad\quad Asp-Gly-Dab-Val-Pro-Dab-\ D-Pip \end{matrix}$$

Dab : Diaminobutyric acid
D-Pip : D-Pipecolic acid

Fig. 1 Structure of Amphomycin

On the other hand, amphomycin containing a fatty acid and a straight peptide-chain is mainly active against gram-positive bacteria and its toxicity is relatively low. Therefore, the mechanism of action of amphomycin or tsushimycin was supposed to be different from those of polymyxin and colistin.

EXPERIMENT AND RESULTS

Whole cells of <u>Bacillus cereus</u> T were used in studying the mechanism of action of amphomycin. The effect of the antibiotic on growth of the organism was examined, before studying the influence of amphomycin on incorporation of synthetic precursors of cell wall, protein and nucleic acids into acid-insoluble fraction. When the antibiotic was added to a culture medium containing 0.5% peptone and 0.5% meat extract before the incubation, growth of the bacteria was completely inhibited by amphomycin in the concentration of over 10 mcg/ml . When it was added at the logarythmic phase of growth, 2.5 hours after the incubation, lysis of the bacteria was observed in the presence of over 10 mcg/ml of the antibiotic, and then even after 24 hours restoration of the growth was not recognized. This shows that amphomycin acts as a bactericide against <u>B. cereus</u> T in the concentration over 10 mcg/ml.

The influence of amphomycin on the biosynthesis of nucleic acid, protein and cell wall of the bacteria was studied according to the Roodyn's method. (Roodyn <u>et al</u>. 1960)

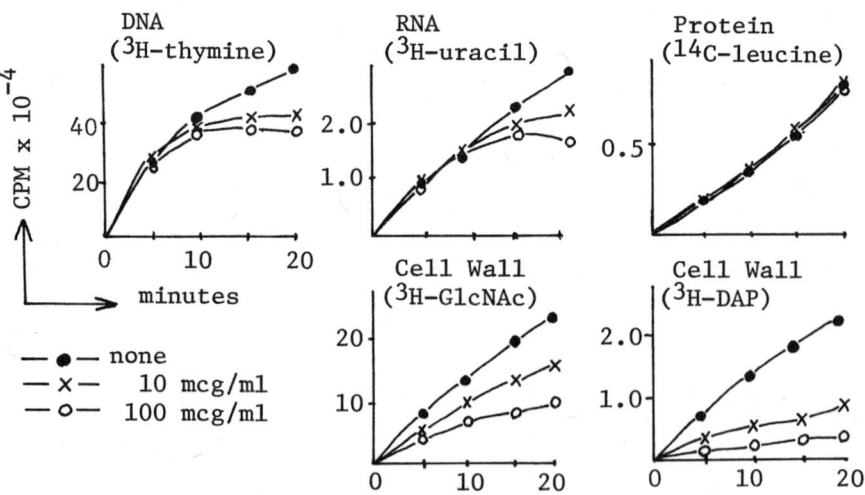

Fig. 2 The Effect of Amphomycin on Nucleic Acid, Protein and Cell Wall Synthesis in <u>B. cereus</u> T.

^{3}H-thymine, ^{3}H-uracil, ^{14}C-D,L-leucine, ^{3}H-N-acetylglucosamine (^{3}H-GlcNAc), and ^{3}H-α,ε-meso-diaminopimelic acid (^{3}H-DAP) were used as the biosynthetic precursors of the macromolecules. The incorporation of them into the acid-insoluble macromolecule fraction was determined quantitatively by the liquid scintilation counting method. As shown in Fig. 2, the incorporation of both ^{3}H-thymine and ^{3}H-uracil into DNA and RNA was not inhibited at all until 10 minutes, but a little extent of inhibition was observed after 10 minutes in the presence of 10 mcg or 100 mcg of amphomycin per ml. On the protein synthesis, any influence was not observed even in the concentration of 100 mcg/ml of amphomycin.

The other hand, the influence on the cell wall synthesis was observed evidently within 5 minutes of incubation time as shown in Fig. 2. At 10 minutes after the begining of incubation, 55% inhibition of incorporation of ^{3}H-GluNAc or 95% inhibition of that of ^{3}H-DAP was observed in the presence of 100 mcg/ml of amphomycin. From these results the primary site of action of amphomycin was suggested to be the inhibition of bacterial cell wall synthesis. As shown in Fig. 2, the incorporation of ^{3}H-DAP was almost inhibited by amphomycin, while that of ^{3}H-GlcNAc was inhibited by half. This gives us suggestion that amphomycin is a specific inhibitor which interfered not with the synthesis of teichoic acid but with that of peptidoglycan alone.

In order to know the site of action of amphomycin on the peptidoglycan synthesis, the accumulation of intermediates of cell wall peptidoglycan was observed using ^{3}H-DAP according to the Lugtenberg's methods. (Lugtenberg et al. 1971) This is, growing cells of B. cereus T was collected after exposuring to the antibiotic. The extract of the cells with boiling water was fractionated by paper chromatographic technique in the solvent system, isobutyric acid and 1M ammonia (5:3). Peptidoglycan, uridine diphosphate-N-acetyl muramyl-peptide (UDP-MurNAc-peptide) and lipid intermediate were analyzed as radio activities on paper chromatograms.

Enduracidin and bacitracin belonging to peptide group antibiotics were used as references of this experiment. They were reported to inhibit the bacterial cell wall synthesis and to cause the accumulation of UDP-MurNAc-peptide, an intermediate of cell wall synthesis. (Matsuhashi et al. 1969), (Stone et al. 1970) As shown in Table 1, a large amount of UDP-MurNAc-peptide was accumulated by the addition of all these antibiotics. The amount of the accumulation with amphomycin was far larger than those both with enduracidin and with bacitracin . The evident inhibition of synthesis of peptidoglycan and the accumulation of a large amount of UDP-MurNAc-peptide suggested that amphomycin inhibits a synthetic step from UDP-MurNAc-peptide to peptidoglycan.

Table 1. Effect of Amphomycin, Enduracidin, Bacitracin and Tsushimycin on the Synthesis of Cell Wall Peptidoglycan in B. cereus T.

	C. P. M.		
	Peptidoglycan	UDP-MurNAc-peptide	Lipid intermediate
	Rf 0.0-0.05	Rf 0.05-0.08	Rf 0.9-1.0
None	6084	133	82
Amphomycin			
10 mcg/ml	381	2242	87
100 mcg/ml	200	2241	113
Enduracidin			
10 mcg/ml	123	313	82
100 mcg/ml	90	800	87
Bacitracin			
10 mcg/ml	4308	432	106
100 mcg/ml	1020	723	111
Tsushimycin			
1 mcg/ml	389	2047	66
10 mcg/ml	213	1895	69
100 mcg/ml	127	1089	80

30 min. 37°C

We also studied the mode of action on tsushimycin and laspartomycin which belong to amphomycin group antibiotic. These antibiotics were active bactericidally aginst B. cereus T and lysis of bacterial cells were observed in the concentration of both 10 mcg/ml and of 100 mcg/ml at one hour after the addition of the antibiotic. The restoration of the growth of cells was observed in the presence of 10 mcg/ml of laspartomycin but was not observed with 10 mcg/ml of tsushimycin. Effect of tsushimycin and laspartomycin on the incorporation of the biosynthetic precursors into acid-insoluble macromolecule fraction was examined by the same method in the experiment with amphomycin. Syntheses of nucleic acid and protein were not inhibited, but that of cell wall was evidently inhibited by tsushimycin. While the incorporation of precursors was inhibited by laspartomycin. Therefore, tsushimycin is a specific inhibitor of cell wall synthesis but laspartomycin is not. As shown in Table 1, tsushimycin derived the accumulation of a large amount of UDP-MurNAc-peptide in B. cereus T, but did not do the increase of lipid intermediate. By the way, tsushimycin has the same peptide chain as amphomycin, and the difference in the structure between them is the fatty aicd moiety alone. From these results, it is concluded that amphomycin and tsushimycin inhibit the bacterial cell wall synthesis on a step from UDP-MurNAc-peptide to peptidoglycan.

It was found that amphomycin and tsushimycin, which consist of a fatty acid and a straight peptide-chain, inhibit the synthesis of cell wall peptidoglycan. It is interesting that the primary site of action of the antibiotics is different from those of polymyxin and colistin which consist of a fatty acid and a peptide ring. We will study further in details about the mechanism of action of these antibiotics.

REFERENCES

1) Heineman, B., Kaplan, M. A., Muir, R. D. and Hooper, I. R. (1953), Antib. & Chemo., 3, 1239.
2) Bodanszky, M., Sigler, G. F. and Bodanszky, A. (1973), Amer. Chem. Soc., 95, 2352.
3) Newton, B. A. (1953), J. Gen, Microbiol, 9, 54.
4) Newton, B. A. (1956), Bacterial. Rev., 20, 14.
5) Benedict, R. G. and Langlyke, A. F. (1947), J. Bacteriol., 54, 24.
6) Chapman, G. B. (1962), J. Bacteriol.,84, 180.
7) Roodyn, D. B. and Mandel, G. (1960), Biochem. Biophys. Acta., 41, 80.
8) Lugtenberg, E. J. J. and Dehaan, P. G. (1971), J. Microbiol. Serol., 37, 537.
9) Matsuhashi, M., Ohara, I. and Yoshiyama, Y. (1969), Agr. Biol. Chem., 33, 134.
10) Stone, K. J. and Strominger, J. L. (1971), Proc. Nat. Acad. Sci., 68, 3223.

EFFECT OF PRIMYCIN ON DNA

A. Caróczy, T.M. Jovin, and F. Hernádi
Departments of Biophysics and Pharmacology
University School of Medicine, Debrecen, Hungary
and
Max Planck Institute of Biophysical Chemistry
Göttingen, West Germany

SUMMARY

The antibiotic primycin in 100 μM concentration almost completely inhibits the temolate function of 100 μM poly/dA-dT/, poly/dG-dC/, poly/dA/, natural phage DNA or calf thymus DNA in enzyme mixture containing E. coli RNA polymerase in excess. The inhibition occures mainly during elongation. The primycin has a similar inhibitory effect in the case of E.coli DNA polymerase I. investigated with different templates.

INTRODUCTION

The antibiotic primycin was isolated from cultures of an actinomyces strain /Vályi-Nagy et al. 1954/. The molecule /Fig.1./ contains guanidine and arabinose groups /Aberhart et al. 1970/. It is active against many gram-positive bacteria and M.tuberculosis. The primycin inhibits the inductive synthesis of tryptophan pyrrolase in rat liver /Vályi-Nagy and Daróczy 1967/, but has no effect on basal enzyme synthesis. It interacts with polynucleotides in vitro by forming easily sedimentable aggregates under certain conditions /Blum 1965/. In present experiments we studied under in vitro conditions the effect of primycin on the template function of DNA and polynucleotides for E.coli RNA polymerase and DNA polymerase I.

METHODS

DNA polymerase I. and RNA polymerase was prepared from E.coli cells as described /Jovin et al. 1969, Zillig et al. 1970, Arndt-Jovin et al. 1975/. Enzyme activities were assayed according to published procedures /Jovin et al. 1969, Burgess 1969/. The solubility of primycin in water is about 50 µg/ml. We used 10 % of 1-2-propylene glycol in every enzyme mixture to prevent precipitation. We did not observe any significant decrease in enzyme activity caused by this concentration of propylen glycol. The primycin was produced at the Dept.of Pharmacology, Debrecen /Hungary/ and in the Chinoin Pharmaceutical Works, Budapest /Hungary/.

RESULTS AND DISCUSSION

Investigating the action of primycin on E.coli RNA polymerase under the same conditions as stated by Burgess /Burgess 1969/ there is no observable effect on enzyme activity. In such circumstances the template DNA is present in excess in the enzyme mixture. Decreasing the DNA concentration, the primycin inhibits the ^{14}C-ATP incorporation. When the calf thymus DNA is present in 15 µM concentration the 75 µM primycin almost completely inhibits the ^{14}C-ATP incorporation /Fig.2./. The inhibition

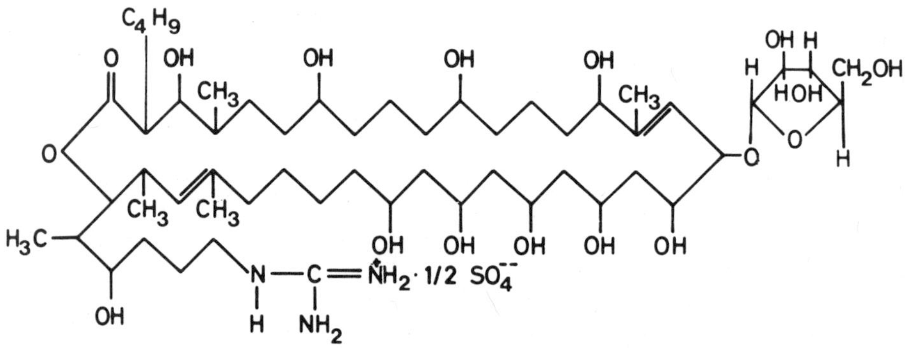

Fig.1. Structure of primycin /Aberhart et al. 1970/.

varies as a function of the concentration of template DNA besides that of primycin. The extent of inhibition does not vary with time from 10 to 60 minutes. The inhibition can not be suppressed by elevation of RNA polymerase concentration. Decreasing the enzyme concentration the inhi-

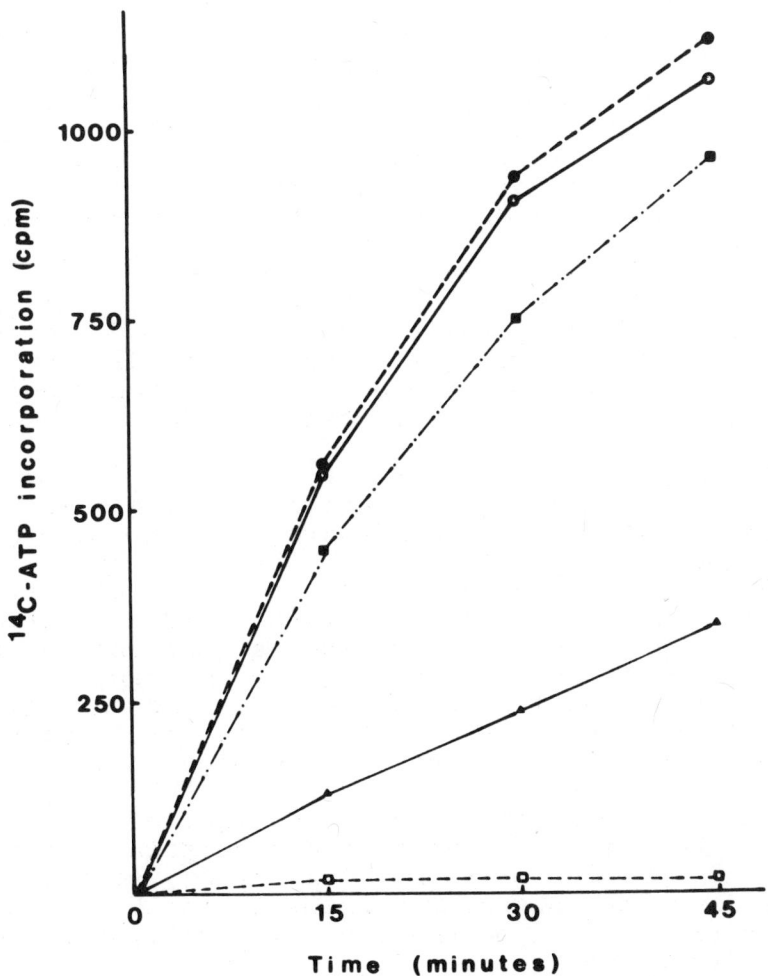

Fig.2. The effect of primycin on ^{14}C-ATP incorporation by E.coli RNA polymerase. The reaction was carried out of 37°C in a mixture /Burgess 1969/ contained 500 mµM RNA polymerase holo enzyme, 15 µM calf thymus DNA, 10 % propylene glycol and different concentrations of primycin. The concentration of primycin was /µM/: ●──●, without primycin; ○──○ , 25; ■──■ , 37.5; ▲──▲ , 50 and □──□, 75.

bition leaves unchanged. On the basis of these results we can say that the primycin does not inhibit the RNA synthesis at the enzyme site, but inhibits the synthesis at the template DNA site.

We investigated the effect of primycin on the RNA synthesis, i.e. ^{14}C-ATP incorporation using different template DNA. The inhibition was essentially the same with core enzyme, holo enzyme and enzyme containing x factor. The inhibition was not stronger when the template was intact phage DNA. So the specific initiation does not seem to be the inhibited step.

To decide whether the initiation or elongation is inhibited we investigated the γ-^{32}P-ATP incorporation. The primycin even in 125 μM concentration was not able to inhibit the γ-^{32}P-ATP incorporation in higher degree than 50 %, while in such circumstances the ^{14}C-ATP incorporation was completely inhibited.

To investigate the elongation separately we used $\lambda\phi$80 phage DNA in 10 μM concentration with holo enzyme in 40 mμM concentration. The ^{3}H-CTP was added to the enzyme mixture only after increasing the concentration of KCl from 0.1 M to 0.4 M. The rate of the ^{3}H-CTP incorporation was unchanged in the next 30 minutes, but the incorporation was completely inhibited by 100 μM primycin. On the basis of these results we can say that the primycin slightly inhibits the RNA synthesis at the initiation step, but completely inhibits the elongation.

Under in vivo conditions the effect of primycin seemed to be similar to that of actinomycin D. Actinomycin D requires G-C base pairs for its action, so does not act on poly/dA-dT/ template. The primycin inhibits the ^{3}H-UTP incorporation by RNA polymerase using poly/dA-dT/ or poly/dA/ template as well /Fig.3./.

The primycin proved to be an inhibitor using poly /dG-dC/ template, too. So we can say that the primycin does not require special base pairs or bases for its action and does not require the double stranded form of the template.

We studied the in vitro effect of primycin not only on the RNA synthesis, but on the DNA synthesis by E.coli DNA polymerase I., too. The primycin proved to be an inhibitor also in this case /Fig.4./. The incorporation of ^{3}H-dTTP was inhibited as a function of the concentration of the template besides that of primycin. The enzyme concentration did not alter the inhibition by primycin. The

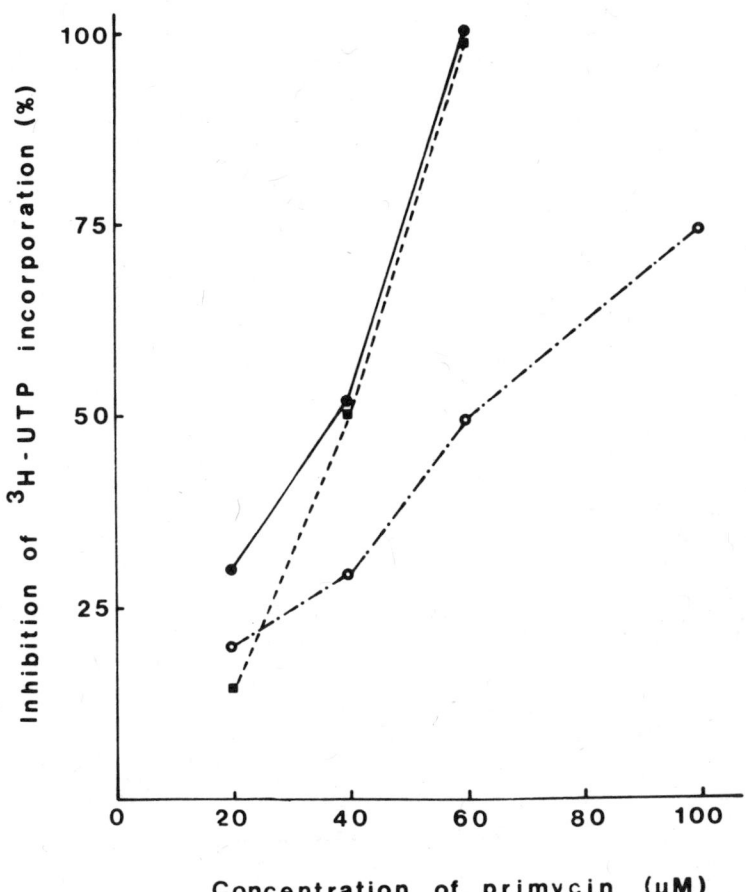

Fig.3. Inhibition of RNA polymerase activity by different concentrations of primycin. The activity was measured as ^{3}H-UTP incorporation within 30 minutes. The reaction was carried out at 37°C in a mixture /Burgess 1969/ contained 200 mµM RNA polymerase holo enzyme, 10 % propylene glycol and templates in different concentrations: ■--■ , poly /dA-dT/ 20 µM; ●——● poly/dA/ 20 µM; ○—·—○ , poly/dA/ 100 µM.

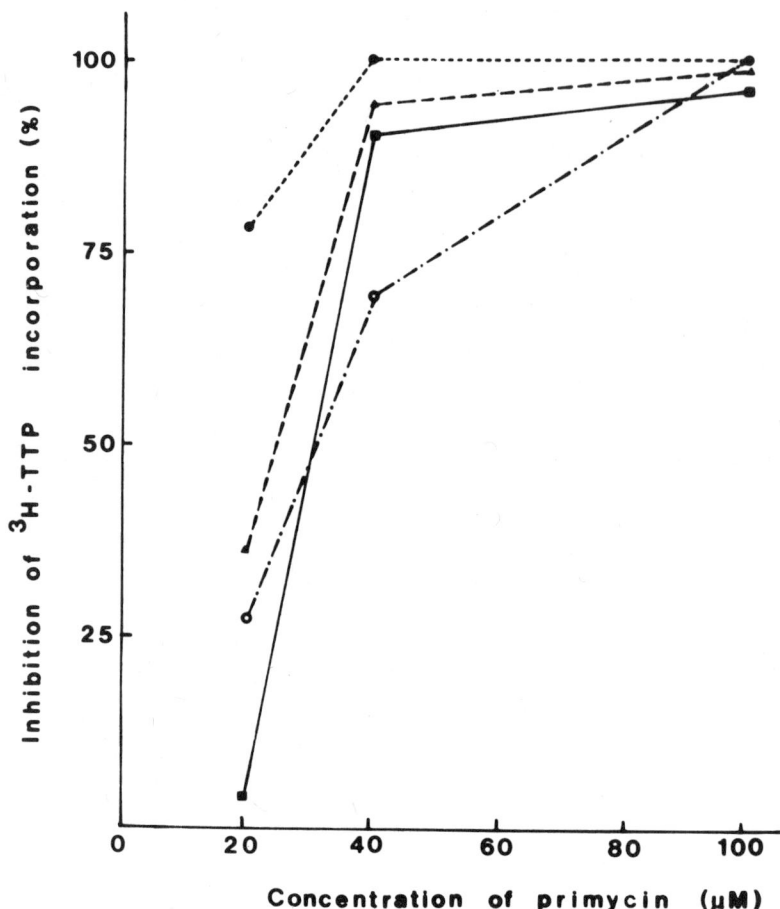

Fig.4. Inhibition of DNA polymerase activity by different concentrations of primycin. The activity was measured as ^{3}H-dTTP incorporation /Jovin 1969/, in the presence of 10 % propylene glycol, with different template concentrations: ●——●, calf thymus DNA 15 μM; ○——○, calf thymus DNA 75 μM; ▲——▲, poly/dA-dT/ 180 μM; ■——■, poly/dA/· oligo/dT/ 90 μM.

primycin was active using calf thymus DNA, poly/dA-dT/ and poly/dA/.oligo/dT/ template as well. The primycin proved to be as active in the inhibition of DNA synthesis as in the inhibition of RNA synthesis.

REFERENCES

Aberhart,J., Fehr,T., Jain,R.C., deMayo,P., Motl,O., Baczynskyj,L., Gracey,D.E.F., MacLean,D.B. and Szlágyi,I. /1970/, J.Amer.Chem.Soc., 92, 5816

Arndt-Jovin,D.J., Jovin,T.M., Bahr,W., Frischauf,A-M. and Marquardt,M. /1975/, in press

Blum,J.J. /1965/, Arch.Biochem.Biophys., 111, 635.

Burgess,R.R. /1969/, J.Biol.Chem., 244, 6160.

Jovin,T.M., Englund,P.T. and Bertsch,L.L. /1969/, J.Biol. Chem., 244, 2996.

Vályi-Nagy,T., Uri,J. and Szilágyi,I. /1954/, Nature, 174, 1105.

Vályi-Nagy,T. and Daróczy,A. /1967/, Biochem.Pharm., 16, 1051.

PIPEMIDIC ACID, A NEW SYNTHETIC ANTIBACTERIAL AGENT

P.ADAMOWICZ, J.F.DELAGNEAU, P.de LAJUDIE[*],
M.PESSON and M. REYNIER
Direction des Recherches
LABORATOIRE ROGER BELLON
159, av. du Roule - 92200 NEUILLY - FRANCE

SUMMARY

Pipemidic acid is a broad-spectrum antibacterial agent, effective principally against Gram-negative organisms, Proteus included. It is bactericidal by inhibition of DNA synthesis. It has a protective effect in experimental infections with *E.coli* and *Ps.aeruginosa* and is effective for the treatment of urinary tract infections in man. Its toxicity is low (LD 50 for mice = 5-6 g/Kg) and it is practically free of any side-effect in man. After oral administration, it is excreted mostly through the kidneys, and it reaches high levels in urine. The average recommended dosage is 400 mg twice a day.

Pipemidic acid

The search for new agents effective against gram-negative bacteria has led to the synthesis of about 60 news substances, among which has been selected pipemidic acid (compound 1489 RB) : 8-ethyl 5-oxo 2-piperazinyl 5,8-dihydro pyrido (2,3-d) pyrimidine-6 carboxylic acid.

Pipemidic acid, by its structure, is related to nalidixic acid, oxolinic acid and piromidic acid.

Methods of preparation have been described by PESSON *et al.* 1974a, 1974b, 1974c, and french patent LABORATOIRE ROGER BELLON 1972. Results of the first in vitro and in vivo studies of the new agent have been published lately (de LAJUDIE *et al.* 1974a, 1974b).

We report here more extensive findings on the antibacterial activity of pipemidic acid and the first results of its clinical applications.

METHODS

In Vitro Tests

Pipemidic acid (PPA) and nalidixic acid (NA) have been dissolved in 0,1 N NaOH, and further diluted in water. Bacterial susceptibility tests were done by dilutions in nutrient agar or TSA, inocula of about 10^6 cells being dispensed by means of a multipoint inoculator. In some tests, the activity of PPA was compared with that of the following compounds : ampicillin, carbenicillin, cephaloridin, colistine, gentamycin, sulfamethoxazole-trimethoprim, nitrofurantoïn, nalidixic acid and piromidic acid. The bactericidal effect of PPA was studied by the dilution method (CHABBERT, 1963), with inocula of about 10^6 cells/ml - After 5 and 24 hrs at 37°C, aliquots of 0,1 ml were plated for evaluation of the percentage of survivors from the number of colony-forming units. The resistance rate was determined by the cellophan transfer method of BOUANCHAUD and ACAR, 1969. The mode of action of PPA on DNA synthesis was investigated in *Pr. morganii* cultured in the presence of 14C-thymidine, radioactivity being measured in TCA-precipitated DNA. Correlation between loss of viability and breakage of DNA was studied, after incorporation of 14C-thymidine, addition of PPA and enzymatic treatment, by the radioactivity of fractions obtained by ultracentrifugation in a sucrose gradient. Effect on human and animal cells was studied in TCA - insoluble DNA from cultures of human (Chang) liver cells, and pig and hamster liver cells.

In Vivo Tests

For <u>experimental infections</u>, lethal doses of $E.coli$ or $Ps.aeruginosa$ (5×10^7 to 8×10^7 cells per mouse) were injected intra-peritoneally to female mice weighing 18-20g. Solutions or suspensions of PPA were administered orally or subcutaneously. The animals were observed during 6 days, and the protective dose 50 (PD 50) was then determined by the methods of Reed and Muench 1938 and Liechfield and Wilcoxon 1949.

<u>Pharmacology</u> - <u>Toxicology</u> - Tests for general pharmacology have been conducted by the usual methods, after oral administration of 25 to 200 mg of pipemidic acid. The acute toxicity has been studied in mice, rats and dogs treated by oral and parenteral routes. Toxicity after repeated administration has been determined in Rat (doses of 25, 50 and 100 mg/Kg for 6 weeks, and 15, 75 and 300 mg/Kg for 6 months) and Dog (50, 100 and 200 mg/Kg for 3 months). Behaviour and body weight increase, hematological and biological data, renal and hepatic functions have been analyzed. At the end of the experiments, the animals were killed and their organs subjected to histo-pathological examination. For teratogenetic studies, PPA was administered to rats and mice from the 6th to the 14th day of pregnancy, at doses of 20 and 200 mg/Kg, and to rats from the 5th to the 7th day of pregnancy at a dose of 400 mg/Kg.

<u>Clinical trials</u> - PPA was given orally in 200 mg capsules, the most frequent dosage for adults being 2 capsules twice a day. Side-effects and biological data were carefully recorded. PPA was assayed in biological specimens by the diffusion method with $Pr.morganii$.

RESULTS and DISCUSSION

In Vitro Antibacterial Activity

For 430 laboratory strains and 1569 recent clinical isolates, 73 p.100 and 90 p. 100, respectively, are sensitive to 25 µg/ml or less of PPA. In 5 comparative tests, PPA was more active than either NA or piromidic acid, especially on $Pseudomonas$. Lately, some 40 strains resistant to NA have been found by Y. CHABBERT sensitive to PPA. It compares favorably with most antibiotics or synthetic chemicals commonly used in urinary tract infections.

In peptone water, PPA, NA and piromidic acid have the same bactericidal effect ; in the presence of serum, however, PPA retains it activity, but the two other compounds show a high rate of inactivation.

The mutation rate of *Esch.coli K12* is about 3×10^{-9} with 10 µg of PPA per ml ; for NA, the same rate may be attained, but with a much higher concentration of the selective agent (100-200 µg/ml).

In Vivo Experiments

No effects on nervous central system, vegetative nervous system, or circulatory system have been recorded. Pipemidic acid doesn't interfere with choleresis, diuresis or coagulation.

Acute toxicity is very low, by oral and parenteral routes (DL 50 for mice : 5 and >1 g/Kg respectively).

After repeated administration, pipemidic acid show a good tolerance ; no serious anomalies have been detected.

Pipemidic acid is effective for the treatment of experimental infections with *E.coli* and *Ps.aeruginosa*, and it has a protective effect on *E.coli* infection in mice.

Clinical Trials - Pharmacokinetics

Blood and Urinary levels of pipemidic acid in patients - Urinary levels were determined in three normal subjects who received 1200, 800 or 600 mg of PPA per day during three days. For the group treated with 800 mg/day, the levels never fall below 150-200 µg/ml, and may reach peaks as high as 800-900 µg/ml. No accumulation was detected. No side-effects were recorded.

- Blood and Urinary levels have been determined in renal insufficiency. As could be expected, urinary concentrations of PPA are proportional, and blood concentrations inversely proportional, to creatinine clearance.

Results of treatment of urinary tract infections with PPA. PPA was given orally, at a dosage of 800 mg per day, to 277 patients. Clinical and bacteriological recoveries were obtained in 77 per cent of these, with disappearance of the causative microorganism in 80 per cent. Tolerance was good in 325 patients treated with 800 mg of PPA per day during at least 10 days ; very few side-effects and practically no biological anomaly were detected.

CONCLUSIONS

Pipemidic acid, for its broad spectrum, strong antibacterial activity and high urinary levels, together with its in vivo efficacy and lack of toxicity, ought to take place among the first-ranking agents intended for use in urinary tract infections. Bacteriological and clinical cure may be expected in a few days, without any serious side-effect, with two daily oral doses of 400 mg of pipemidic acid.

LITERATURE CITED

BOUANCHAUD D.H. et ACAR J.F. (1969)
    Path. Biol. 17, 763-767

CHABBERT Y. (1963)
    L'antibiogramme, Ed. de la Tourelle, St-Mandé

LABORATOIRE ROGER BELLON - Brevet français n°2.194.420, priorité du 2 août 1972

LAJUDIE (de) P., ROQUET F., REYNIER M., ADAMOWICZ P. (1974)
    C.R. Acad. Sci. 279B, 1931-1934

LAJUDIE (de) P., HORVATH E., LERICHE B., PATTE S. (1974b)
    J. Pharmacol. Clin. 1, 155-171

LIECHFIELD and WILCOXON (1949)
    J. Pharmacol. 96, 99

PESSON M., LAJUDIE (de) P., ANTOINE M., CHABASSIER S., RICHER D., GIRARD P. (1974a)
    C.R. Acad. Sci. 278, C1169-1171

PESSON M., ANTOINE M., CHABASSIER S., GIRARD P., RICHER D. (1974b)
    C.R. Acad. Sci. 278, C 717-719

PESSON M., ANTOINE M., CHABASSIER S., GEIGER S., GIRARD P. RICHER D., LAJUDIE (de) P., HORVATH E., LERICHE B., PATTE S. (1974c)
    Eur. J. Med. Chem. - Chimica Therap. 9, 585-590 et 591-596

REED L.J. and MUENCH H. (1938)
    Am. J. Hyg. 27, 493-497

CLINICAL STUDIES OF PIPEMIDIC ACID IN THE FIELD OF PEDIATRICS

Susumu Nakasawa, Ei Tanaka and Hajime Sato

Clinic of Pediatrics, Tokyo Metropolitan Ebara Hospital
and Department of Pediatrics, Showa University School
of Medicine, Tokyo, Japan.

Pipemidic acid (1) is a new synthetic antibacterial agent having a pyridopyrimidine ring which follows piromidic acid (2). Their chemical structures are shown in Fig. 1. Compared to analogous agents like piromidic acid and nalidixic acid (3), it has some interesting chemotherapeutic properties such as excellent antibacterial potency against gram-negative organisms including Pseudomonas aeruginosa and bacteria resistant to

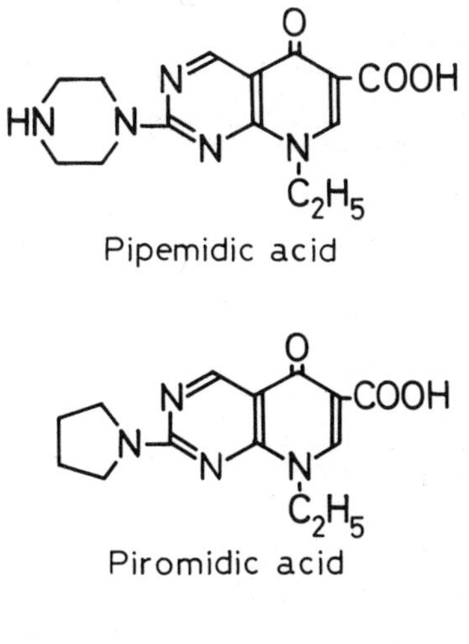

Pipemidic acid

Piromidic acid

Fig. 1. Chemical structures of pipemidic acid and priomidic acid.

nalidixic acid, oral efficacy on experimental animal infections due to gram-negative bacteria including Pseudomonas aeruginosa, which is generally higher than the effect of piromidic acid, nalidixic acid, cephalexin, ampicillin and carbenicillin, and good distribution to tissues, whose levels are generally higher than the plasma level.

The antibacterial spectrum of pipemidic acid and piromidic acid were investigated by the agar dilution method (Table 1). Though some gram-positive bacteria were susceptible to the both agents at relatively high concentrations, the most susceptible to them were gram-negative bacteria. The MIC values of pipemidic acid for most gram-negative bacteria such as Escherichia coli, Shigella, Salmonella, Klebsiella, Proteus, Vibrio, Serratia, Neisseria, Haemophilus, Yersinia and Pasteurella ranged between 1.56 and 6.25 µg/ml, which were generally one fourth or one eighth of the MIC values of piromidic acid. It was noted that 2 strains of Pseudomonas aeruginosa were inhibited by 12.5 or 25 µg of pipemidic acid per ml. The sensitivity of clinical isolates to pipemidic acid and piromidic acid was also examined by the agar dilution method. All of the 48 Shigella strains tested were inhibited by less than 1.56 µg of pipemidic acid per ml

Table 1. Antibacterial spectrum

Organism	MIC (µg/ml)	
	Pipemidic acid	Piromidic acid
Staphylococcus aureus Terajima	25	12.5
S. aureus 209P, JC-1	12.5	12.5
S. aureus No. 50774	25	12.5
Bacillus subtilis PCI 219	6.25	3.13
Corynebacterium pyogenes C-21	25	50
Erysipelothrix rhusiopathiae Agata	100	200
Streptococcus hemolyticus A65	200	400
Diplococcus pneumoniae I Neufeld	200	>400
Listeria monocytogenes LI-2402	200	>400
Escherichia coli K-12	1.56	3.13
E. coli NIHJ, JC-2	1.56	25
E. coli var. communis	3.13	12.5
Shigella flexneri 2a EW10	3.13	25
S. sonnei EW33	1.56	6.25
Salmonella enteritidis No. 1891	1.56	6.25
S. typhimurium S-9	3.13	12.5
Klebsiella pneumoniae No. 13	6.25	50
Proteus vulgaris OX$_9$	6.25	6.25
P. morganii Kono	3.13	25
Vibrio parahaemolyticus S-1	3.13	3.13
Serratia marcescens X100	6.25	50
Pseudomonas aeruginosa Tsuchijima	12.5	100
P. aeruginosa No. 12	25	200
Neisseria meningitidis Osa	1.56	1.56
Haemophilus influenzae Shiga	1.56	1.56
Yersinia enterocolitica MY-79	1.56	6.25
Pasteurella multocida M-17	1.56	0.78
Brucella abortus Kusayanagi	200	>400

Table 2. MICs for Shigella sp.

(48 recent clinical isolates)

Drug	MIC (µg/ml)					
	≥1.56	3.13	6.25	12.5	25	50
Pipemidic acid	48 (100%)					
Piromidic acid			11	20	16 (98%)	1

Table 3. MICs for Salmonella sp.

(47 stock strains)

Drug	MIC (µg/ml)						
	≥1.56	3.13	6.25	12.5	25	50	≥100
Pipemidic acid	24	22 (98%)	1				
Piromidic acid					9	36 (96%)	2

Table 4. MICs for P. aeruginosa

(45 stock strains)

Drug	MIC (µg/ml)					
	6.25	12.5	25	50	100	>100
Pipemidic acid	2	19	17 (84%)	3	4	
Piromidic acid						45 (100%)

Table 5. Urinary excretion of pipemidic acid in children

Patient	Age Sex	Body weight (kg)	Dose (mg/kg)	Urine pooled for 0 to 7 h	
				Concn(µg/ml)	Recovery(%)
U.T.	11 male	37	10	342	91.2
M.M.	8 male	22	17	540	10.1

irrespective of antibiotic-resistance, while 25 µg of piromidic acid per ml was required to inhibit 98% of them (Table 2). In 47 strains of Salmonella species, 98% was inhibited by 3.13 µg of pipemidic acid per ml or lower, while 96% by 25 or 50 µg of piromidic acid per ml (Table 3). The MIC values of pipemidic acid for 45 strains of Pseudomonas aeruginosa ranged from 6.25 to 100 µg/ml and 25 µg of the drug per ml inhibited 84% of them (Table 4). None of the strains were inhibited by piromidic acid even at 100 µg/ml. Plasma, urine and fecal levels of pipemidic acid in children were determined by the thin-layer cup-plate method using Escherichia coli Kp as an indicator organism. Fig. 2 shows plasma levels of pipemidic acid in children given a single oral dose of 10 or 17 mg/kg. The peak plasma levels of 7.4 and 6.8 µg/ml were seen 1 and 3 hours after dosing, and rather high plasma levels were detected even 7 hours later. Urinary excretion of pipemidic acid in the same children is shown in Table 5. Concentrations of pipemidic acid in urine pooled for 7 hours were 342 and 540 µg/ml, and its recoveries were 91.2 and 10.1%. Fecal levels of pipemidic acid in children were around 500 µg/g after oral dosing of 125 mg, 3 times a day for 2 days, and above 600 µg/g after oral dosing of 250 mg, 3 times a day for 2 days (Fig. 3). It is evident from these results that a lot of pipemidic acid is excreted into urine and feces as an antimicrobially active form. Tissue levels of pipemidic acid were determined by radioassay in rats receiving carbon 14-labeled pipemidic acid at a single oral dose of 50 mg/kg. As seen in Fig. 4, most of tissues showed higher pipemidic acid levels than blood. The highest pipemidic acid concentrations were found in kidney and liver followed by lung, muscle, heart and blood. A similar distribution pattern was obtained by whole-body autoradiography of the rat receiving carbon 14-labeled pipemidic acid. Therapeutic results of bacterial dysentery in children treated with pipemidic acid are summarized in Table 6. Causative organisms were all Shigella sonnei in 40 cases treated, most of which were resistant to ampicillin and chloramphenicol. Daily doses of pipemidic acid ranged between 30 and 100 mg/kg, mostly

Table 6. Therapeutic results of bacterial dysentery in children with pipemidic acid

Age-distribution	Cases	PPA-administration		Clinical effects	Rate hardly excluding the germs	Side effects		
		mg/kg/day	Treated days			Liver	Kidney	Others
9 months ~ 13 years and 1 month	40	30-100mg (40-50mg)	5 — 7	100%	7.5%	$\frac{0}{33}$ (0)	$\frac{0}{33}$ (0)	$\frac{0}{40}$ (0)

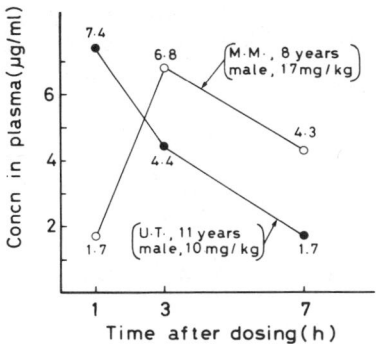

Fig. 2. Plasma levels of pipemidic acid in children.

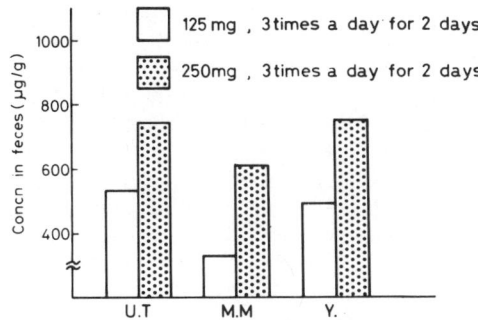

Fig. 3. Fecal levels of pipemidic acid in children.

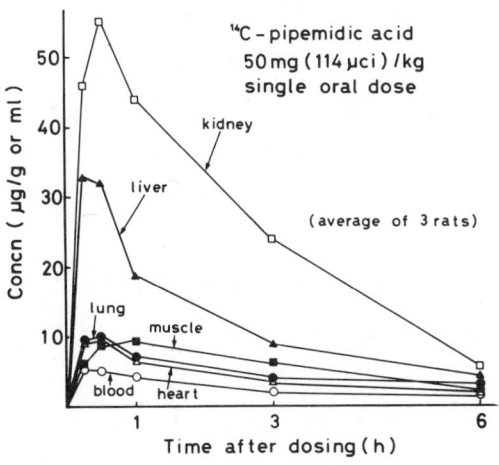

Fig. 4. Tissue levels of pipemidic acid in rats.

between 40 and 50 mg/kg. The administration terms were from 5 to 7 days. All the cases showed the marked improvement in fecal appearances within 4 to 7 days after the initiation of medication, being accompanied by relief of clinical symptoms. By this dosing regimen, the drug failed to eliminate the causative organisms only in 7.5% of the cases. No adverse effect was observed in respect of liver and kidney functions.

The efficacy of pipemidic acid on dysentery especially due to ampicillin-resistant strains was impressive.

LITERATURE

1. Matsumoto, J. and S. Minami: Pyrido[2,3-d]pyrimidine antibacterial agents. 3. 8-Alkyl- and 8-vinyl-5,8-dihydro-5-oxo-2-(1-piperazinyl)pyrido[2,3-d]pyrimidine-6-carboxylic acids and their derivatives. J. Med. Chem. 18:74-79, 1975.
2. Shimizu, M, S. Nakamura and Y. Takase: Piromidic acid, a new antibacterial agent: Antibacterial properties. Antimicrob. Agents Chemother. 1970, 117-122, 1971.
3. Lesher, G. Y., E. J. Froelich, M. D. Gruett, J. H. Bailey and R. P. Brundage: 1,8-Naphthyridine derivatives. A new class of chemotherapeutic agents: J. Med. Pharm. Chem. 5:1063-1065, 1962.

IN VITRO AND IN VIVO STUDIES ON ANTIBIOTICS FROM SKIN MICROCOCCACEAE

S. SELWYN, P. D. MARSH and TUSHNA N. SETHNA

Department of Bacteriology, Westminster Medical School

London, SW1P 2AR, United Kingdom

Primary skin cultures from 1,320 individuals - including 790 healthy people - yielded 173 strains of Micrococcaceae species which possessed considerable antibacterial activity. Inoculation of these antagonistic organisms on to background lawns of representative Gram-positive and Gram-negative bacteria revealed widely varying ranges and degrees of inhibitory effects. Antagonistic strains of Staphylococcus aureus were chiefly confined to bacteriophage Group II and had a narrow spectrum of action limited mainly to Corynebacterium and Streptococcus species. Coagulase-negative staphylococci and micrococci, however, included strains with broad antibacterial spectra. A particularly active and stable inhibitory strain of Staph. epidermidis (biotype 4) was isolated from the forehead of one of us (S.S.). This organism (referred to as 'S6$^+$') was selected for detailed investigation.

ANTAGONISTIC ACTION OF STAPHYLOCOCCUS 'S6$^+$'

The antimicrobial spectrum of activity was tested by direct (simultaneous) and indirect (deferred) competitive growth as in our earlier work.[1] S6$^+$ antagonised all the representative strains of Gram-positive bacteria tested, including species of Bacillus, Clostridium, Corynebacterium, Micrococcus, Staphylococcus and Streptococcus, as well as the principal species of Bacteroides, Bordetella, Brucella, Haemophilus, Mycoplasma, Neisseria and Pasteurella. There was no cross-resistance with standard antibiotics, and the most multiple-resistant Staph. aureus strain we have yet encountered was fully sensitive to the action of S6$^+$. However, members of the Enterobacteriaceae and Pseudomonas genus were generally resistant, as were fungi.

Inhibition zones in deferred tests were between four and give times wider than in the direct tests.

Replicate plating revealed a bactericidal action for the inhibitor, and it could pass through cellophane and dialysis membranes. Time-lapse photographic studies under a plate microscope showed that the inhibitor was produced in substantial amounts by at least the second hour of culture. Further details of the kinetics of the inhibitory effect have been obtained from mixed growth experiments both in standard batch cultures and in a chemostat system for continuous culture. But because liquid cultures do not provide a realistic model of the skin ecosystem, we have recently developed quantitative procedures on solid surfaces for batch culture and continuous culture (Milyani and Selwyn, to be published).

CONCENTRATION AND PURIFICATION OF ANTIBACTERIAL AGENT

Crude extracts of $S6^+$ culture on semi-solid agar had relatively more antibacterial activity than $S6^+$ broth cultures (even when the broth was vigorously aerated). Large-scale batch cultures in sloppy agar (0.2%) were therefore used as the source of further supplies of antibacterial agent. After freezing and thawing, the liquid phase was clarified by centrifugation and membrane filtration. Precipitation of large molecular moieties first with hydrochloric acid and then with zinc chloride did not reduce the titre of inhibitory activity, which was, however, still only about 1 in 8.

Gel filtration of the supernatant was carried out through Sephadex G 15 and G 10 columns. Fractions were collected and tested for antibacterial action and spectrophotometric absorbence at 280 nm. The elution profiles of G 15 and G 10 extracts showed that antibacterial activity was associated with a single homogeneous area in the zone of overlap between the exclusion limits of the two types of Sephadex column. The active area did not exactly coincide with absorption bands - which are mainly a feature of aromatic amino acid-containing compounds.

At this stage the activity of the material had increased by about 1,000 times as compared with the crude extract. It now produced inhibition zones on cultures of Escherichia coli, Klebsiella spp., Pseudomonas aeruginosa and even Candida albicans. Occasional strains of actively swarming Proteus spp. were, however, relatively resistant. The semi-purified extract could pass through cellophane PT 300, was dialysable, stable for 20 minutes at up to 100°C and stable also over a pH range of 1-10. Antimicrobial activity was destroyed by trypsin, papain and pronase but not by pepsin. The agent dissolved in organic solvents as well as in water.

CHEMICAL COMPOSITION AND NATURE OF THE AGENT

Chemical and physical analysis including chromatography and gel filtration show that the inhibitory agent is a polypeptide of about 800 molecular weight. Ninhydrin treatment and quantitative analysis reveal eight main amino acids: aspartate, glutamate, glycine, alanine, cysteine, leucine, valine and proline in the proportions 1.4, 1, 4, 2.6, 0.6, 1.2 and 1. The data are compatible with a relatively small cyclical polypeptide.

The accumulated results show that the agent is not a bacteriophage, bacteriocine, lysozyme or lysostaphin - all of which are well known to occur among organisms in this group. The antimicrobial substance is a true antibiotic which is totally different from any at present in use.

IN VIVO ACTIVITY AND SIGNIFICANCE OF $S6^+$ AND ITS ANTIBIOTIC

Until the yields and purification can be further improved, in vivo work is being confined to ecological studies at the skin surface. $S6^+$ itself can be readily established on normal human or rabbit skin. Initial preparation with chlorhexidine is useful on human skin when high counts of 'resident' bacteria are present. Detailed investigations using the rabbit model show that without the prior use of skin disinfectants $S6^+$ rapidly overgrows and suppresses the relatively small numbers of resident commensals already present. If the skin is occluded with plastic which is impervious to air and moisture, all bacterial growth increases at first as also does any antagonistic effect. This is clearly seen when the skin is inoculated with $S6^+$ together with either Staph. aureus or a skin micrococcus (Table 1). Even when $S6^+$ is inoculated 2 days after the other bacteria it becomes predominant within a day (Table 2).

Direct comparisons between the results of bacterial antagonism by $S6^+$ in vivo and in vitro show that the effects are more pronounced on the skin than on artificial solid media; and, in turn, antagonism occurs more actively on solid media than in comparable liquid media. Presumably these findings are due to the differing extent of dilution and diffusion of the $S6^+$ antibiotic under the various conditions of growth. It was also noted that when $S6^+$ was cultured in vitro, after prolonged growth on the skin it produced antibiotic as actively as it had before its inoculation on to the skin.

TABLE 1
SIMULTANEOUS INOCULATION OF MIXED CULTURES ON OCCLUDED RABBIT SKIN

Inoculum	Log Viable Count* on Day				
	0	1	2	3	5
(Micrococcus Type 7	6.20	1.20(4.38)^x	<1(4.20)	<1(3.94)	<1(3.90)
(S6$^+$	6.48	4.50(5.25)	4.68(5.71)	4.38(5.44)	4.85(5.70)
(Staph.aureus	6.23	4.08(5.51)	3.90(5.30)	3.20(5.23)	2.20(5.00)
(S6$^+$	6.48	4.68(5.25)	4.20(5.71)	4.23(5.44)	4.71(5.76)
Control area (normal flora)	(1.90)	(3.23)	(3.04)	(3.38)	(3.45)

* Colony-forming units per sq. cm. of skin sampled by standard swabbing technique (Selwyn and Ellis [1]).

^{x} Values in parentheses are counts of bacteria when grown separately on skin.

When the semi-purified S6$^+$ antibiotic is applied in a single dose to the skin it exerts a marked antibacterial effect for more than 24 hours. In vitro the antibiotic is produced on media which mimic the harsh conditions of the epidermis - for instance containing 5% sodium chloride and 1% oleic acid, incubated both aerobically and anaerobically. Certainly the presence of organisms like S6$^+$ on patients' skin has been shown in our recent epidemiological work to confer substantial protection against bacterial colonisation and infection of dermatological lesions.[2] Unlike Staph. aureus 'strain 502A' which has been used prophylactically on human skin[3], S6$^+$ has minimal pathogenic potential and produces a powerful antibiotic. Its clinical use on

TABLE 2
CONSECUTIVE INOCULATION OF STAPHYLOCOCCI AND MICROCOCCI ON TO OCCLUDED RABBIT SKIN

Inoculum	Log Viable Count* on Day						
	0	1	2	3	4	5	7
(Staph. aureus	7.54	5.51	5.70	5.23	4.08	3.38	2.94
(S6+	-	-	5.30[1]	5.44	4.94	4.85	4.72
(Micrococcus Type 7	6.87	4.38	4.30	2.90	1.69	<1	<1
(S6+	-	-	4.60[1]	4.50	4.32	4.76	4.85
(S6+	7.17	5.44	5.25	4.30	4.20	4.32	4.76
(Micrococcus Type 7 OR	-	-	4.17[1]	<1	<1	<1	<1
(Micrococcus Type 7 (high dosage)	-	-	6.48[1]	3.90	2.38	<1	<1

* Colony-forming units per sq. cm. of skin
[1] Second organism inoculated 48 hrs. after first one

the skin surface - and perhaps elsewhere - could be an economical means of preventing bacterial infections of burns, wounds, and other lesions, while at the same time satisfying ecological requirements.

Acknowledgements

We wish to thank the Westminster Hospital and Medical School Research Committee and Beecham Products Ltd. for financial support.

REFERENCES

1. Selwyn, S., & Ellis, H., (1972), Skin bacteria and skin disinfection reconsidered, Br. med. J., 1, 136.

2. Selwyn, S. (1975), Natural antibiosis among skin bacteria as a primary defence against infection, Br. J. Derm., 92, in press.

3. Anthony, B. F., & Wannamaker, L. W., (1967), Bacterial interference in experimental burns, J. exp. Med., 125, 319.

ANTIMICROBIAL SUBSTANCES FROM THE LARVAL ISOLATES OF GREATER WAX MOTH, GALLERIA MELLONELLA L.

ADAM PASZEWSKI, JAN JAROSZ

Department of Plant Physiology, Maria Curie-Skłodowska University, Poland

LYSOZYME-LIKE LYTIC ENZYME OF STREPTOCOCCUS FAECALIS

According to the generally accepted hypothesis bacteria and fungi of insects are needed for some physiological processes of the host to extend its own metabolic faculties. The significance of intestinal flora in the digesting process was found in many organisms; also the role of symbionts in the synthesis of biological activity of substances necessary for normal development of insects was pointed out. Bucher and Williams (1967) have reported that the specifically uniform composition of the autochthonous gut flora of G.mellonella is represented by fecal streptococci belonging to Streptococcus faecalis. The bacterium S. faecalis was found in all stages of the insect development and frequently it was the only organism present. Waterhouse (1959) and Dudziak (1975) have observed normal development of Galleria in bacteria-free cultures. The time of complete metamorphosis of the axenic insects was the same as that of those which contained organisms in their intestinal tracts. The digestion of such unusual food as beeswax takes thus place owing to the gut enzymes of Galleria larvae.

The authors suggest a hypothesis that, owing to its bacteriolytic properties, S. faecalis can be considered as a nonspecific component of the humoral defence mechanism of Galleria against microbial infections. The bacterial lysozyme released in the exponential growth phase of S. faecalis (Conover et al., 1966) protects the insect from the multiplicity of organisms absorbed with the food and regulates the formation of a typical gut flora. It would seem that S. faecalis lysozyme-like lytic enzyme, beside the insect lysozyme (Mohrig and Messner, 1968), determines the final composition of the normal gut flora in Galleria larvae. This seems to be the role of S. faecalis in the development of the wax moth, G. mellonella (Jarosz, 1975).

The process of selection progressed with aging of the larvae. Among young larvae one could usually observe mixed small populations (from sterile to 10^3, often to 0.5×10^5 bacteria/larva) with a marked dominance of S. faecalis. The microflora of mature larvae was most frequently represented by large uniform populations of active lytic enterococci (from 10^5 to 10^7, sometimes to 0.3×10^8 cells/insect). Pupal stages and imagines were found to contain the highest percentage of individuals with pure cultures of S. faecalis. The small number or the absence of other organisms in the large Str. faecalis populations suggest that enterococcal muramidase inhibited the growth of the ingested bacteria. The solutions which contained the lytic enzyme inhibited the growth of larval isolates sensitive to egg-white lysozyme, notably Micrococcus, Sarcina and Bacillus spp.

These bacteria constituted the main admixture in S.fae-
calis populations of Galleria larvae. It seems likely
that a similarly sterilizing effect may be excerted by
the enzyme in the gut of the insects, the more so, that
the infectious doses which occur in nature are much lower than those used in the experiment.

In addition to the factors which limit the number
of species and cells of bacteria in the insect gut: the
extremal pH values, digestive enzymes, antimicrobial
substances in the food, anaerobic conditions in the intestinal tract, inappropriate oxydo-redox (Eh)potential,
there should also be included antimicrobial substances
of the intestinal flora.

Paszewski (1959) showed, as mentioned above, that
the preincubation of Mycobacterium sp. ATCC No. 607 in
the presence of extracts from the larvae of the wax moth
leads to a fall in its resistance to penicillin and sulphatiazole. The sensitivity of acid-fast bacilli to
chemotherapeutics is perhaps linked with the effect of
lysozymes in the haemolymph and in the intestinal tract
of Galleria larvae present.

GALLERIN, A NEW POLYPEPTIDE ANTIBIOTIC

Accidental microflora of G. mellonella was not numerous; it was represented mainly by spore-forming bacterium classified as Bacillus spp. Some strains of
Bacillus were able to produce antibiotics. The antibiotic agent active against Gram-positive bacteria and
acid-fast bacilli was separated from B. subtilis strain
53, and it proved to be identical with subtilin(Jarosz,
1973).

The strain 26a of B. subtilis R produced in the synthetic NK/2-Sym's medium two antibacterial factors; bacteriolytic enzyme eluated from Sephadex G-25 column at the ratio $Ve/Vo = 1$, and gallerin, a new polypeptide antibiotic which was eluated at 1.625 void volume. Gallerin-producing strain 26a of B. subtilis was grown in surface cultures at $35°C$ and gave maximum yields after 4 - 5 days. The presence of manganese in the medium at 0.5×10^{-4} M $MnSO_4 \cdot 4H_2O$ concentration stimulated the formation of the antibiotic, but it did not effect antibiotic activity. During fermentation at first the number of cells increased, and during the last stage the activity of the fermentation broth increased rapidly, achieving 400 - 700 units of Sarcina lutea/ml.

Gallerin has been isolated from the fermentation broth by adsorption on Amberlite CG-50 (H^+, 100-200 mesh). The crude substance was eluated by the stepwise pH gradient in the range 0.02-0.05 M hydrochloric acid, and neutralized on weakly basic anion exchange of the Amberlite IR-4B (OH^-, 20-50 mesh) type. Impurities were removed from the eluate by precipitating them with lead acetate (0.05%). The formed adduct of the peptide with picric acid was divided on CM-cellulose buffered with 0.02 M citrate buffer, pH 5.7, and the adsorbed antibiotic was eluated by continuous ionic stength gradient in the range 0.02 - 0.25 M sodium chloride. Further purification was carried out by gel filtration on Sephadex G-50 column.

Gallerin was a thermostabile substance, and it dialyzed through cellophane membranes. It was stable under acid conditions, its activity decreased in alkaline solutions. The antibiotic gave negative reactions with ninhydrin, biuret, Millon, Sakaguchi, Molisch, ferric chloride tests and positive reaction with Folin-Ciocalteu test. The substance is not hemolytic for red blood cells; it is not inactivated by proteolytic enzymes: trypsin, pepsin and pronase P. It acted much more strongly under acid conditions (pH 6.4) than alkalic ones (pH 7.6). The picrate form was soluble in water and lower alcohols. The free base was soluble in water and lower alcohols, and insoluble in acetone (the picrate form was very good soluble in acetone).

The ultraviolet absorption spectrum of free base in water gave end absorption, solutions in 99% methanol showed a characteristic absorption maximum at 207, and very small one at 255 and 280 nm. The IR spectrum suggested a polypeptide type of the antibiotic. This was confirmed by the determination of the amino acid content of this substance. In the hydrolysates lysine 12.8; aspartic acid (asparagine) 9.41; isoleucine 8.81; histidine 6.67; glutamic acid (glutamine) 6.52; phenylalanine 5.53; leucine 4.48; valine 1.51 and cystine 0.96g/16g N, and five amino acids were found in trace.

A small antibacterial activity spectrum was shown by gallerin. It very active against Gram-positive bacteria, notably micrococci and staphylococci (MIC determined by twofold agar dilution method was 0.09-0.39 mcg/ml, pH 6.4), and in this way it was similar to that of the lysozyme activity. Bacteriolytic action was not observed. The minimum inhibitory concentration for acid-fast bacteria: Mycobacterium sp. ATCC 607, Myc. smegmatis I, Myc. phlei was slightly higer (12.0 - - 50.0 mcg/ml). Gallerin was not active against Gram-negative bacteria or fungi even at 300.0 mcg/ml concentration.

The antibiotic at 23 ppm concentration stimulated (by 5%) the increase in body weight of Japanese quails, particularly in comparison with oxytetracycline used at twofold concentration.

REFERENCES

Bucher G. E., and Williams R. 1967. The Microbial Flora of Laboratory Cultures of the Greater Wax Moth and its Effect on Rearing Parasites. J.Invertebr. Pathol., 9, 467-473.
Conover M.J., Thompson J. S., and Shockman G.D. 1966. Autolytic Enzyme of Streptococcus faecalis. Biochem. Biophys. Res. Commun., 23, 713-719.
Dudziak B. 1975. Studies on the Role of Microorganisms in Alimentation of Galleria mellonella L. Ann. Univ. Mariae Curie-Skłodowska, XXX, C, in print.
Jarosz J. 1973. Antibiotic Properties of Bacillus subtilis strain No. 53 Isolated from the Intestinal Flora of Galleria mellonella L. Larvae. Acta Microbiol. Polon., B, 35-42.
Jarosz J. 1975. Lysozymelike Lytic Enzyme of Streptococcus faecalis and its Role in the Larval Development of Wax Moth, Galleria mellonella. J. Invertebr. Pathol., 26, in print.
Mohrig W., and Messner B. 1968. Immunreaktionen bei Insekten. Biol. Zbl., 87, 705-718.
Paszewski A. 1959. Influence of an Enzyme Extract from the Larvae of G. mellonella together with Penicillin or Sulphatiazole on the Growth of M. tuberculosis 607. Ann. Univ. Mariae Curie-Skłodow., 20, 435-438.
Waterhouse D. F. 1959. Axenic Culture of Wax Moths for Digestion Studies. Ann. N. Y. Acad. Sci., 77, 283-289.

ADVANTAGES OF NEW TETRACYCLINE-COMPLEXES IN HUMAN THERAPY

Kahán, I.L., Kulka, F., Vigh, E.

Department of Ophthalmology and I. Department of
Surgery, University Medical School,
Szeged, Hungary

Lipid-soluble tetracyclines such as methacycline /MOTC/, doxycycline /DOOTC/ and minocycline /MINO/ have come to be increasingly used in the past 1o years as a result of their high antibiotic activities, and their high tissue affinities. However, there is a lack of preparations suitable for parenteral administration.
Aqueous solutions with the pH of blood /ph=7,4/, containing high concentrations of the antibiotic /2o-5o mg/ml/, can be prepared from all tetracyclines simply by dissolution in an aqueous solution of tris-/hydroxymethyl/aminomethan: "Tri-tetracyclines" /1,2,3/. The distribution coefficients of the parent compounds between chloroform and water are not significantly altered by the complexing agent /Fig.1/.
In vitro experiments demonstrated the low minimal inhibitory concentrations /MIC/ of the Tri-tetracyclines, which are equal to or lower than those of the parent compounds /Table I/. A total absence of local tissue toxicity was found towards chicken fibroblast cultures / 4 /. The lethal dose /LD_{5o}/ was above 5oo mg/kg for

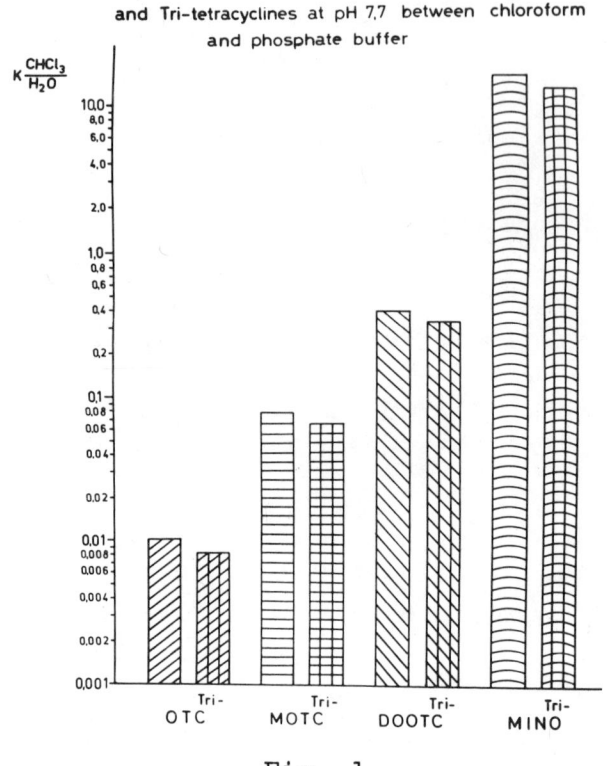

Fig. 1

all i.v. administered Tri-tetracyclines.
On i.v. administration to rabbits, roughly equal serum levels were found for the MOTC and DOOTC complexes, but a much lower level for Tri-MINO /Fig.2/. According to recent findings, however, therapeutic efficacy is correlated more to tissue antibiotic levels. Fig. 3. demonstrates the lung and serum levels 8 hours after administration of different tetracyclines. As a consequence of its higher lung-affinity and nevertheless its rapid excretion, Tri-MOTC was expected to be the antibiotic of choice for the local treatment of thoracic empyema. All but 2 of 14 empyema-patients were treated daily with 5o mg Tri-MOTC /1/12 of the oral dose/

Table I

In vitro activity of tetracyclines and tri-tetracyclines versus Staphylococcus aureus 8357 NCTO 42					
Tetracycline parent compound	Tetracycline	Tri-tetracycline	ΔMIC (tetracycline tri-tetracycline)	Standard error	Probability
Oxytetracycline	0,61	0,47	0,14	0,03	<0,01
Doxycycline	0,53	0,32	0,21	0,05	<0,01
Methacycline	0,44	0,23	0,21	0,04	<0,01
Minocycline	0,30	0,30	-	-	-
Average of MIC values in µg/ml from 8 separate tests					

Table II

Microbiological data of pleural fluids									
Microorganisms	No of cases	Sensitive to				Resistant to			
		OTC	MOTC	DOOTC	MINO	OTC	MOTC	DOOTC	MINO
Proteus	2	1	1	1	ND	1	1	1	ND
Staphylococcus albus haem.	4	1	1	2	ND	3	3	2	ND
Escherichia coli	3	2	2	2	ND	1	1	1	ND
Streptococcus α haem.	1	1	1	1	ND	-	-	-	ND
Mixed microorganisms	2	1	1	1	ND	1	1	1	ND
No growth	1	-	-	-	-	-	-	-	-
Klebsiella	1	-	-	-	1	1	1	1	-
	14	6	6	7	ND	6	6	5	ND
ND = not determined									

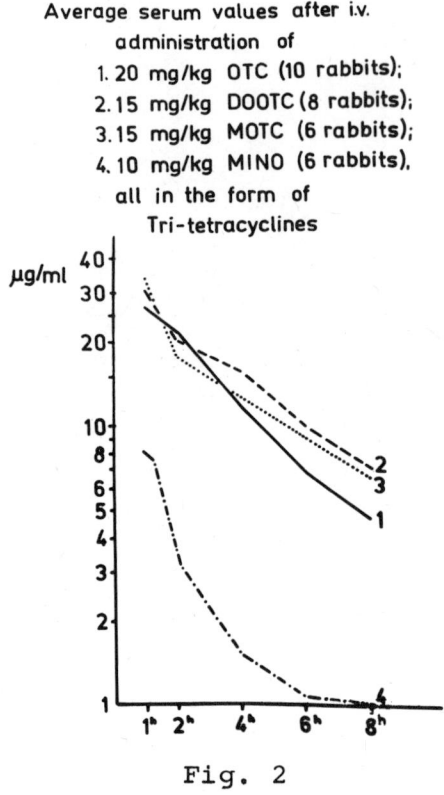

Fig. 2

intrapleurally. The exceptions involved patients whose infective agents cultured from the empyema were sensitive only to Tri-DOOTC or Tri-MINO /Table II/, and these patients were treated with Tri-DOOTC and Tri-MINO, respectively. All patients were in a septic-toxic state, the empyema being on average of 100 days' duration 2-3 days after commencement of local Tri-tetracycline therapy, in 11 patients the temperature fell to a normal level, while the previously purulent exudate became serous, and then disappeared. In spite of local administration, Tri-MOTC gained access into the lungs and the general circulation, as evidenced by chromatography and subsequent bioautography of the urine /4/.

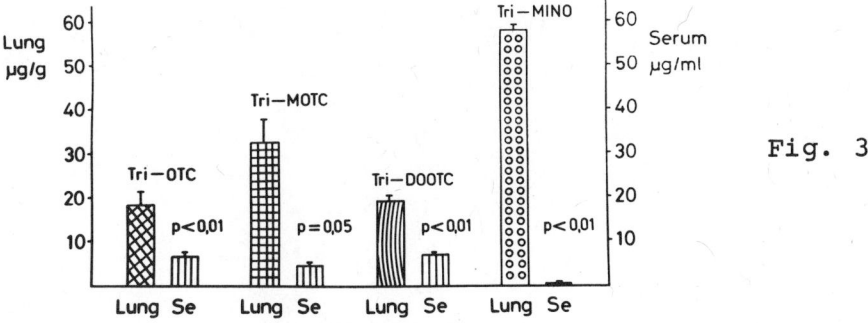

Antibiotic levels in the lung (µg/g) and serum (µg/ml) 8 hr after the i.v. administration of 20 mg/kg OTC, 10 mg/kg MOTC, 15 mg/kg DOOTC and 10 mg/kg MINO in the form of Tri-tetracyclines (6 rabbits in each case).

Fig. 3

In thoracic surgery antibiotic protection is generally performed by i.v. administration. Since DOOTC is known to be the only tetracycline which is not toxic to the kidneys and may be administered even when the patient's condition is poor, Tri-DOOTC was administered i.v. at different intervals before surgery. Altogether 27 patients received Tri-DOOTC, 23 of them prior to thoracic surgery. When a sinlge dose of 200 mg or 100 mg DOOTC was administered i.v. in the form of Tri-DOOTC the mean serum concentrations after 3o minutes were 4.9 ug/ml and 4.0 µg/ml, respectively, and then gradually decreased. Simultaneously the urinary antibiotic output was followed /Fig. 4.a.b./. The antibiotic content of the surgically-removed lung tissue was investigated histochemically and determined quantitatively from the extracts. The antibiotic contents of almost all lung-samples excised 12 hours later exceeded even the highest serum levels measured, and amounted to ten times the serum values in some inflammatory or less-malignant growth-containing lung-specimens /Fig. 5/. In these less-infiltrated carcinomatous pulmonary specimens, the

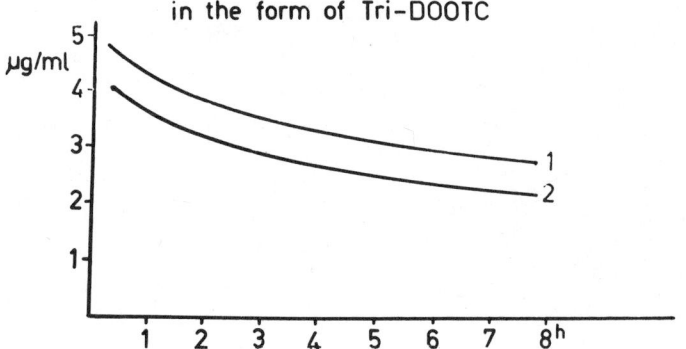

Fig. 4a

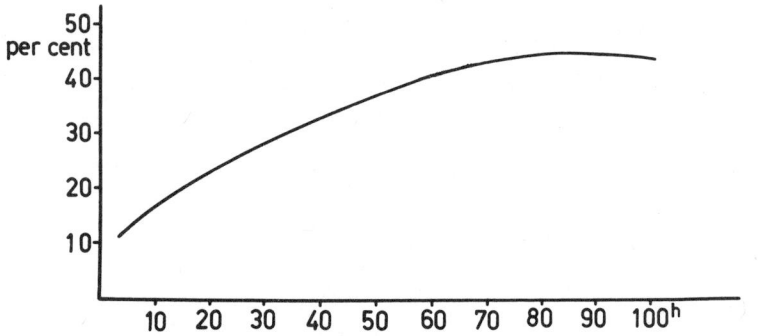

Fig. 4b

fluorescence of DOOTC is located at two different sites: in the alveolar endothelium, and in necrobiotic tumour cells. As even the lowest lung-levels were much higher than the MIC-values, prophylactic administration of Tri-DOOTC before thoracic surgery appears to be justified. The postoperative course was uneventful in every case.

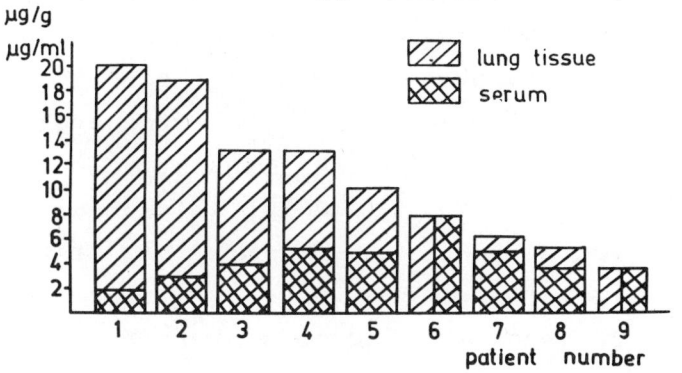

Fig. 5

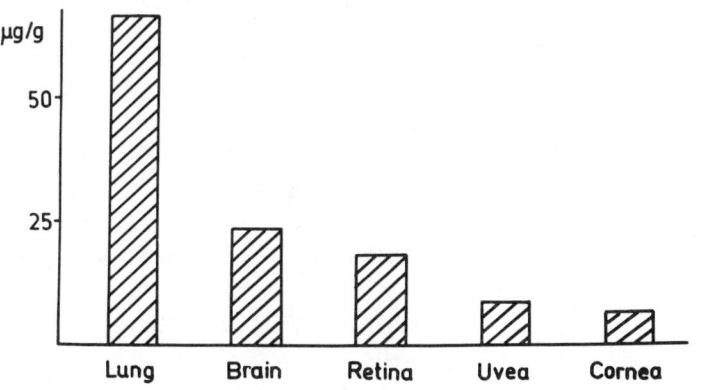

Fig. 6

The properties of Tri-MINO differ in several respects from those of the other Tri-tetracyclines. The main difference is the higher lipid-solubility of Tri-MINO, manifested in a 30-100-fold higher chloroform/water distribution coefficient. As a consequence, several tetracycline-resistant strains, e.g. of Staphylococci, proved to be sensitive to Tri-MINO; serum values are lower and organ values higher. Moreover, whereas the central nervous system is shielded from the penetration of other tetracyclines, it is flooded by Tri-MINO. An excellent site for the investigation of the nervous-tissues affinity of Tri-MINO proved to be the eye: after i.v. administration to rabbits, the highest value was found in the retina /Fig.6/. Following this observation, i.v. administration of 50-100 mg Tri-MINO was tried in 3 cases of heavily-infected eye-injuries with preretinal abscess, and in 2 cases of endogenous uveitis. The highest serum values after 30 minutes were 2 μg/ml, and an average of 12 per cent of the administered antibiotic was found in the collected urine. Only the 3 infected eye injuries were cured, these having previously been treated with Gentamycin without success.

References

Kahán, I.L., Hammer, H. /1974/. In vitro and in vivo study of the biological effects of Tri-tetracyclines /new tetracycline complexes/. Chemotherapy 20, 148.

Kahán, I.L., Hammer, H. /1975/. The parenteral application of a new Methacycline preparation, Tri-metahcycline. Arzneimittelforschung /Drug Research/ 25, 234.

Kahán, I.L., Pápai, I., Hammer, H. /1974/. Intraocular penetration of Tri-tetracyclines after parenteral and subconjunctival administration. Albrecht von Graefes Archiv für klinische und experimentelle Ophthalmologie 190, 257

Kulka, F., Kahán, I.L., Vigh, E. New therapeutic approaches to thoracic empyema:local treatment with Tri-methacycline. To be published.

NIFURPIPONE IN URINARY TRACT ACUTE INFECTIONS

M. Laudi, G. Fontana, U. Ferrando,
C. Benvenuti,* and G. Sesia

*Clinical Research Dept., Recordati SpA
Ospedale Maggiore di San Giovanni Battista e
della Citta di Torino, Italy

Summary

Therapeutic effectiveness and tolerability of nifurpipone, a new nitrofuran derivative, were evaluated in urinary tract acute infections.

Efficacy was assessed by recording body temperature, subjective symptoms and urine culture.

Nifurpipone in capsules proved to be as effective as nitrofurantoin, but in gastro-resistant tablets was better tolerated particularly at gastric level.

Aim of the study

Effectiveness and tolerability of nifurpipone, a new nitrofuran (5nitrofurfurilidene hydrazide of 4-methyl-1-piperazinacetic acid) in acute inflammatory conditions of the urinary tract were stated by three subsequent trials:
- double blind comparison between nifurpipone in capsules and nitrofurantoin;
- evaluation of therapeutic effectiveness and tolerability of gastro-resistant tablets of nifurpipone;
- evaluation of tolerability of gastroresistant tablets of nifurpipone administered in patients intolerant of nitrofurantoin.

* Research Laboratories of Recordati S.p.A. - Milan.

Patients and methods

During our three trials we observed the following parameters every three days: body temperature, urgency, strangury and frequency.

Except for the first sign, a semi-quantitative evaluation was made by arbitrary scoring. For strangury and urgency: from 0 = absent to 4 = very severe; and for frequency (number of micturitions in the 24 hours): from 0 = up to 5 to 3 = more than 12. Students "t" test corrected for continuity was used for statistical analysis.

Before and after the treatment a urinoculture (type and number per ml of bacterial colonies) was carried out.
Tolerability was evaluated by recording gastroenteric disorders (nausea, vomiting, gastric pyrosis etc.) and the most important hematochemicals constants.

1) Nifurpipone versus nitrofurantoin

A double blind comparison between nifurpipone and nitrofurantoin was performed. Both nifurpipone and nitrofurantoin were prepared in indistinguishable capsules, containing respectively 100 mg and 50 mg. Dosage was 4 capsules a day for 9 days.

Patients were 30, 22 male and 8 female, aged from 20 to 79 years, and suffering from an acute inflammatory process of the urinary tract with the following diagnostic distribution: 7 fever after instrumental examination, 3 acute pyelonephritis, 3 acute cystopyelitis, 7 acute cystitis, 6 vesical papilloma with acute cystitic pattern, 1 prostatic carcinoma with acute inflammatory pattern, 1 acute prostatitis, 1 acute urethritis, 1 vesical calculosis with acute cystitic pattern.

2 and 3) Gastroresistant tablets of nifurpipone

In the second and third trial we tested nifurpipone in gastroresistant tablets (cellulose acetophthalate coating) containing 100 mg of drug. Dosage was 4 tablets a day for 7 days. In the second trial 30 patients were treated, all male, aged from 42 to 76 years, with the following diagnoses: 5 cystopyelitis, 3 cystitis, 6 cystitis in vesical ca., 2 cystopyelitis in outcome of adenomectomy, 5 cystopyelitis in prostatic adenoma,

1 cystopyelitis in urethral stenosis, 3 cystitis in vesical papilloma, 1 cystopyelitis in giant hydronephrosis, 1 cystitis in prostatic ca., 2 aspecific urethritis, 1 cystopyelitis in calculosis.

In the third trial 18 men and 2 women, aged from 30 to 79 years, with urinary tract acute inflammatory processes who had manifested, just before, intolerance for nitrofurantoin, were treated with nifurpipone.

Since the per cent incidence of gastric intolerability of nitrofurans is relatively low and a comparison of tolerability between drugs or different preparations would have necessitated a large number of cases, we preferred to treat selected cases.

Results
1) Nifurpipone versus nitrofurantoin

As it regards temperature curve, urgency, strangury and frequency, there was a highly significant difference ($P<0.001$) between baseline values and values of the 3rd, 6th and 9th day of treatment both with nifurpipone and nitrofurantoin. The direct comparison between the two drugs, on the other hand, never evidenced a statistically significant difference as comprehensible by this table:

Drug/Symptom	Urgency	Strangury			Frequency	
Nifurpipone	14 excel.	11 excel.	3 good	1 poor	12 excel.	2 n. resp.
Nitrofurantoin	15	12	2	1	10	5

The number of germs per ml of urine, when initially higher than 100,000, evolved to normal limits after nifurpipone or nitrofurantoin treatment. Neither with nifurpipone nor with nitrofurantoin any significant changes in laboratory examinations were observed. The drugs administered on a full stomach never induced gastric intolerance such as to interrupt treatment.

2) Gastroresistant tablets of nifurpipone

All symptoms were reduced after 3 and 7 days of therapy in all patients.

The final results of strangury were: excellent in 20 patients (complete disappearance of the symptom); good in 5 patients (reduced to level 1); poor in 3 patients (from level 4 to 2).

Overall evaluation of urgency resulted : excellent in 22 patients, good in 2 patients (lowered to level 1), poor in 3 patients (from level 4 to 2), almost nil in 1 patient (from level 4 to 3).

The overall results of frequency (except for 4 patients not considered because permanently catheterized) were: excellent in 13 patients, good in 6 patients (lowered to level 1), poor in 4 patients (from level 3 to 2), almost nil in 1 patient (still remained at level 3).

In all patients the body temperature, if high before treatment, was normalized both after 3 and after 7 days.

Urinoculture was carried out in 26 patients: in all cases the final number of colonies per ml of urine decreased(76.04% average decrease) and, in 13 cases, it fell below 100,000 threshold value of sterility of urine.

The drug showed greatest efficacy on Gram-, Proteus and Escherichia coli germs, and slightly less efficacy on mixed colonies and staphylococci with a very high number of germs per ml.

Only 2 patients in 30 had to interrupt the drug on the 3rd day owing to notable nausea and vomitting, while in 5 patients appeared slight gastric pyrosis, nausea and stypsis. No significant changes were observed in the hematochemical constants.

3) G.R. tablets of nifurpipone in intolerant of nitrofurantoin patients.

Just before nifurpipone treatment, all 20 patients had shown intolerability to nitrofurantoin. In spite of this, during nifurpipone treatment, two patients only complained respectively gastralgia and nausea, but so slight as not to discontinue the therapy.

Diagnoses	Clinical Results		Side effects
	good	fair	
Cystitis	5	1	None
Prostatic adenoma	4	-	None
" ca	1	-	None
Outcome of prostatectomy	2	-	None
Vesical papilloma	1	1	1=Gastr.
" neoplasia	-	1	None
" calculosis	-	1	1=Nausea
Urinary incontinence	1	-	None
Urethral calculosis	1	-	None
Cystopyelitis	-	1	None
Total	15	5	2

Probably the high tolerability of nifurpipone is related to a very low gastric absorption depending on: the gastroresistant coating and the relative maximum of dissociation at acid pH which corresponds to a minimum of gastric absorption since a ion passes biological membranes with difficulty.

Conclusions

We can conclude that nifurpipone can be considered particularly useful in infections of the urinary tract due to germs sensitive to nitrofurans and that gastroresistant nifurpipone can be also used as an alternative to the intolerability to nitrofurantoin.

References

1) Bompani R. et al.: Minerva Urologica, 27, n.1, 12-23, 1975
2) Brodie A.F., Gots J.S.: Arch. Biochem. N.Y. 39, 165 1952.
3) Coscia M.: Minerva Chirurgica, 29, n.3, 146-150, 1974
4) Degen L. et al.: Chemotherapy, 3, 175, 1972.
5) Fontani F., Setnikar I.: Il Farmaco, Ed. Prat. 28, 547, 1973.
6) Laudi M. et al.: Minerva Urologica, 25, n.3, 149-157, 1973.
7) Mintzer S. et al.:Antibiotics, 3, 151, 1953.

8) Nelson W.O.: J. Urol. Balt. 71, 650, 1954.
9) Rottichieri D., Maffeis V.: Urologia, 39, IV,359, 1972.
10) Setnikar I. et al: Abst. VII Int. Congr. of Chemotherapy 1, A-12/15, 1971.

THE USE OF CINOXACIN IN URINARY TRACT INFECTIONS

Alan H. Bennett

Harvard Medical School

Boston, Massachusetts   USA

Cinoxacin, a synthetic organic compound with cinnoline(1-2 benzodiazine) as the basic ring structure has been shown to have a broad antibacterial spectrum, particularly against gram negative bacteria that are most frequently isolated from the urinary tract (1). Administered orally the compound was bactericidal at concentrations close to the minimal inhibitory concentration values. In vivo, doses required for successful therapy were comparable to those for nalidixic acid. Cinoxacin is less bound by human serum proteins than nalidixic acid, has similar antibacterial activity but appears to cause less resistence after treatment.

In this study Cinoxacin was evaluated in the treatment of lower urinary tract infections in twenty ambulatory patients. Ten patients received 250mg po four times a day and ten patients received 250mg po three times a day. Treatment period ranged from seven to ten days. Clean voided specimens were obtained just prior to and three and seven days following initiation of treatment. Cultures were also obtained between 5 and 9 days following cessation of therapy as well as a followup culture at four weeks. Hematological studies including CBC, BUN, serum creatinine, total bilirubin, SGOT, LDH, and alkaline phosphatase were obtained prior to, at the end and 5-9 days following therapy with Cinoxacin.

Nineteen of twenty patients had an excellent clinical and bacteriological response to Cinoxacin therapy. One patient's infection was caused by Pseudomonas which was resistent to Cinoxacin requiring a change in therapy. Another patient whose infection caused by an enterococcus resistent to Cinoxacin sensitivity disc responded both clinically and bacteriologically and was maintained on Cinoxacin therapy.

Table I shows the wide range of pathogenic organisms in this group of patients, the great majority being E.coli. Table II shows the diseases treated with Cinoxacin, the majority being cystitis in females.

None of the twenty patients showed any change in the parameters of liver or renal function studied during administration of Cinoxacin. All patients had normal pre and post therapy values for BUN, creatinine, bilirubin, alkaline phosphatase, SGOT and LDH. Two patients complained of mild nausea while on the drug which was not severe enough to warrant discontinuing therapy. No allergic reactions occurred.

Cinoxacin proved successful in eradicating urinary tract infections caused by susceptible organisms in nineteen of twenty patients studied. Cinoxacin in doses of 250mg po qid and 250mg po tid is well tolerated and demonstrated no untoward effects.

Table I

Pathogens Treated with Cinoxacin

E.coli	13
Streptococcus sp.	2
Enterococcus sp.	1
Proteus mirabilis	1
Klebsiella	1
Enterobacter aerogenes	1
Pseudomonas	1

Table II

Diseases Treated with Cinoxacin

Cystitis	16
Prostatitis	2
Asymptomatic Bacteriuria	1
Pyelonephritis	1

REFERENCES

1. Wick, N.E., Preston, D.A., Wgite, W.A. and Gordee, R.S. Compound 64716, A New Synthetic Antibacterial Agent. Antimicrobial Agents and Chemotherapy, 4:415, 1973.

List of Contributors

Actor, P.
Adam, D.
Adamowicz, P.
Andrews, J.
Arr, M.
Ayliffe, G.A.J.

Ban, Y.
Barrelet, L.
Basker, M.J.
Bedford, K.A.
Bennett, A.H.
Benvenuti, C.
Bergogne, E.
Branefors-Helander, P.
Burgert, A.
Burgio, G.R.

Cavanagh, P.
Ceccarelli, G.
Cioni, L.
Comber, K.R.

Daikos, G.K.
Daroczy, A.
De Carvalho, M.P.
Delagneau, J.F.

Feffeira, A.M.
Ferrando, U.
Ferro, A.
Fontana, G.
Forte, V.
Foster, M.T.

Geddes, A.M.
Gentry, L.O.
Germinale, T.
Giamarellou, T.
Giglio, C.

Godtfredsen, W.O.
Goodwin, C.S.
Graber, H.

Hamilton-Miller, J.M.T.
Harris, A.M.
Hata, T.
Henning, C.
Hernadi, F.
Hill, J.P.
Hossack, G.M.

Ishiyama, S.
Ivic, Z.
Iwai, S.
Iwamoto, H.

Jarosz, J.
Jeppsson, P.H.
Jokinen, K.
Jonsson, S.
Jovin, T.M.

Kaczkowski, W.
Kahan, I.L.
Kaipainen, W.J.
Kamme, C.
Kanellakopoulou, K.
Karjalainen, S.
Kato, H.
Kattan, S.
Kawada, Y.
Kendall, M.J.
Knothe, H.
Krcmery, U.
Kulka, F.

Labia, R.
La Judie, P.de
Lam, C.
Lambert, N.

Laudi, M.
Lim, K.C.C.
Lindroth, M.
Lomar, A.V.
Lucyszyn, G.
Ludwig, E.
Lund, F.

Magni, L.
Marsh, P.D.
Matthew, M.
McGhie, D.
Meyer-Brunot, H.G.
Milani, M.R.
Mitchard, M.
Mizuashi, H.
Moon, C.E.
Moriconi, L.
Murata, I.

Naber, K.G.
Nakasawa, S.
Nakayama, I.
Neu, H.C.
Nishiura, O.
Nylen, O.

Oishi, M.
Oiwa, R.
Olsson, O.
Omura, S.
Orsolini, M.R.

Paddock, G.M.
Paradelis, A.G.
Parry, M.J.
Parsons, R.L.
Paszewski, A.
Patsch, R.
Pedrotti, R.
Pelz, K.
Perenyi, T.
Pesson, M.
Pilone, N.
Piperakis, G.
Pitkin, D.H.
Prince, A.

Raunio, V.
Reeves, D.S.
Regamy, C.
Reitz, I.
Reynier, M.

Rimmer, D.M.D.
Robinson, O.P.W.
Robertson, M.J.
Rouvillois, D.

Sakata, I.
Sandstrom, E.
Sato, H.
Schenk, C.
Schoutens, E.
Selwyn, S.
Sethna, T.N.
Shimada, K.
Shimizu, Y.
Shinohara, M.
Short, H.D.
Singanowitz, E.
Sitka, U.
Sjoberg, B.
Sjouali, J.
Skog, E.
Sommerkamp, H.
Stern, S.R.
Stewart, G.T.
Sutherland, R.
Symonds, J.M.

Tanaka, E.
Tanaka, H.
Thomas, A.L.
Timonen, T.
Tybring, L.

Ursing, B.

Vanderlinden, M.P.
Valler, G.
Vigh, E.
Vischer, W.A.

Waldvogel, F.A.
Wallmark, G.
Weidermann, B.
Weingartner, L.
Weisbach, J.A.
Wessman, J.
Westenfelder, M.
Wilkinson, P.J.
Williams, J.D.
Wise, R.

Yourassowsky, E.

Zak, O.